Care Managers
Working with the Aging Family

Cathy Jo Cress, MSW
Instructor
Emphasis in Geriatric/Home Care Management
Master of Arts Degree Program
San Francisco State University
San Francisco, California

JONES AND BARTLETT PUBLISHERS
Sudbury, Massachusetts
BOSTON   TORONTO   LONDON   SINGAPORE

World Headquarters

Jones and Bartlett Publishers
40 Tall Pine Drive
Sudbury, MA 01776
978-443-5000
info@jbpub.com
www.jbpub.com

Jones and Bartlett Publishers
Canada
6339 Ormindale Way
Mississauga, Ontario L5V 1J2
Canada

Jones and Bartlett Publishers
International
Barb House, Barb Mews
London W6 7PA
United Kingdom

Jones and Bartlett's books and products are available through most bookstores and online booksellers. To contact Jones and Bartlett Publishers directly, call 800-832-0034, fax 978-443-8000, or visit our website, www.jbpub.com.

Substantial discounts on bulk quantities of Jones and Bartlett's publications are available to corporations, professional associations, and other qualified organizations. For details and specific discount information, contact the special sales department at Jones and Bartlett via the above contact information or send an email to specialsales@jbpub.com.

The authors, editor, and publisher have made every effort to provide accurate information. However, they are not responsible for errors, omissions, or for any outcomes related to the use of the contents of this book and take no responsibility for the use of the products and procedures described. Treatments and side effects described in this book may not be applicable to all people; likewise, some people may require a dose or experience a side effect that is not described herein. Drugs and medical devices are discussed that may have limited availability controlled by the Food and Drug Administration (FDA) for use only in a research study or clinical trial. Research, clinical practice, and government regulations often change the accepted standard in this field. When consideration is being given to use of any drug in the clinical setting, the health care provider or reader is responsible for determining FDA status of the drug, reading the package insert, and reviewing prescribing information for the most up-to-date recommendations on dose, precautions, and contraindications, and determining the appropriate usage for the product. This is especially important in the case of drugs that are new or seldom used.

Production Credits

Publisher: Kevin Sullivan
Aquisitions Editor: Emily Ekle
Aquisitions Editor: Amy Sibley
Associate Editor: Patricia Donnelly
Editorial Assistant: Rachel Shuster
Associate Production Editor: Amanda Clerkin
Associate Marketing Manager: Ilana Goddess

Manufacturing and Inventory Control Supervisor: Amy Bacus
Composition: Auburn Associates, Inc.
Cover Design: Kate Ternullo
Cover Image Credit: © Val Thoermer/Shutterstock, Inc.
Printing and Binding: Malloy, Inc.
Cover Printing: Malloy, Inc.

Library of Congress Cataloging-in-Publication Data
Cress, Cathy.
  Care managers : working with the aging family / Cathy Jo Cress.
     p. ; cm.
  Includes bibliographical references and index.
  ISBN-13: 978-0-7637-5585-0 (alk. paper)
  ISBN-10: 0-7637-5585-0 (alk. paper)
  1. Older people—Medical care—Management. 2. Older people—Home care—Management. 3. Continuum of care. 4. Hospitals—Case managment services. I. Title.
  [DNLM: 1. Caregivers. 2. Health Services for the Aged—organization & administration. 3. Aged. 4. Family Relations. 5. Home Nursing—methods. 6. Long-Term Care—methods. 7. Social Support. WT 31 C922c 2009]
  RC954.3.C74 2008
  362.14—dc22
                                                                                    2008027265

6048

Printed in the United States of America
12 11 10 09 08   10 9 8 7 6 5 4 3 2 1

Contents

Contributors

Steven Barlam, MSW, LCSW, CMC
LivHOME, Inc.
Los Angeles, California

Bunni Dybnis, MA, MFT, CMC
LivHOME, Inc.
Los Angeles, California

Claudia Fine, LCSW, MPH, CMC
Senior Bridge
New York, New York

Rita Ghatak, PhD
Director, Geriatric Health
Stanford University Medical Center
Stanford, California

Gwendolyn Lazo Harris, MA, CT
Palliative and End of Life Care Manager
Seniors at Home
San Francisco, California

Diane M. LeVan, MAc
Gerontologist
Notre Dame de Namur University
Belmont, California
Peer Grief Counselor
Palo Alto, California

Frederic Luskin, PhD
Senior Fellow
Stanford Center on Conflict and Negotiation
Stanford University
Palo Alto, California

Julie Menack
Sage Eldercare Solutions
Millbrae, California

Catherine M. Mullahy, RN, BS, CCM
President
Mullahy and Associates, LLC
Huntington, New York

Nick Newcombe, MSW, CMC
A Helping Hand
Seattle, Washington

Leonie Nowitz, MSW, LCSW, BCD
Director
Center for Lifelong Growth
New York, New York

Kali Cress Peterson, MSG, MPA
The VA Greater Los Angeles Healthcare
System Geriatric Research, Education, and
Clinical Center (GRECC)
Sepulveda, California

Anne Rosenthal, PhD, MFT, CMC
Reutlinger Community for Jewish Living
Danville, California

Acknowledgments

For all the assistance she has given me, thanks to Tricia Donnelly of Jones and Bartlett. She has been a joy to work with and her calm organization kept the writing of this book as smooth as a vanilla milkshake.

I would like the think the authors who contributed to this book including Catherine Mullahy, Julie Menack, Steve Barlam, Bunni Dybnis, Anne Rosenthal, Kali Cress Peterson, Gwen Harris, Leonie Nowitz, Claudia Fine, Nick Newcombe, M. Joseph Canarelli, Fred Luskin, and Rita Ghatak. Their knowledge of the peaks and fissures of the aging family have helped to sew this book together. I would like to thank them all for their patience with editing. Their final drafts created a seminal book showing how case managers can solve the problems of the aging family.

I would also like to thank my San Francisco State geriatric care management students Deon Batchhelder, John Doxey, Wendy Ginther, Julie Menack, Pat MacClese, and Dawn Pollack for being my guinea pigs and allowing me to test-drive many of these chapters in class.

Thanks to Maryanne Bee for her reading of the chapter on Hospital to Home.

Finally I would like to thank my own aging family. My 87-year-old dad Harry Cress has such a rich life because of the family members who surround him with love, enrich his life, and blessedly help me care for him. I am grateful to my daughters Jill Gallo and Kali Peterson, my husband Pete Peterson, my grandchildren Julia and Joseph Gallo, my nephew Chris Cress, and my cousins Joy Brad and Gary Cress. Their support helps me balance and tells me more than any research what "it takes village" really means.

Introduction
What Is the Aging Family?

The family is a living, breathing system and the emotional workhorse of our society. In this book we address the needs and challenges of the aging family. To define those needs and challenges, we have to look at the 21st century's redefinition of the family itself. We must reassess this core organism in our culture which magically nurtures us in the present, yet allows us to live in the past, while moving us into the future all at the same time.

The family of today is not always the nuclear family of times past. Divorce, mobility, job pressures that move us away from kin, and other cultural forces have altered the nuclear family in many Western cultures. By dissolving this unit we have ended up with an explosion of family members, expanding our vision of this still-living breathing system.

So the family in its nonnuclear metamorphosis may be spouses and ex-spouses, adult children, distant relatives, friends, gay partners, stepsiblings, and fictive and community siblings.

At the same time the family is not the "vertical top down" model we have depended on for centuries. This new nonnuclear family paints itself out on a broader swath, spreading outward over the horizon, not upward and downward. There is no longer always a father at the top, mother a step below, and children on the lowest rung. We may have a mother, two mothers, two fathers, or a single dad as head of the family. Understanding that family can be this nonnuclear, newly horizontal family is the primary lesson for the care manager. Embracing these broader family members in discussions of care, at the family meeting, in the emergency room, or wherever the care manger serves the aging family is a key step for 21st century care manager

Many of the same forces that pulled the nuclear family apart have morphed the aging family into a new entity. Divorce, mobility, job pressures on adult children, mothers going to work in droves, and longer life spans have repainted the aging family on a larger canvas.

The result of these cultural shifts leaves older people more physically distant from their adult children, who no longer live next door. These cultural shifts remove their traditional caretakers, daughters and daughters-in-law, who now work full time. They still do the caring but must fit it into exhausting overwhelming schedules. In fact these accidental family caregivers are given little training, no money, and negligible support and are made to bear the long-term care system on their breaking backs. It has also given aging family members two or three daughters-in-law, as divorce rates runs over 50% in our society.

Older people now have marginalized stepgrandchildren and traumatized grandchildren who suffered through divorces. Their own children can be at war with each other over "who Mom loved best" or "why did Mom or Dad tear up their childhood nest in divorce?" It leaves their adult children on tenterhooks regarding responsibilities of caring for their parents and also over dividing valuable property and deciding who gets Mom's emotion-laden but monetarily worthless salt and pepper shaker collection.

Medical breakthroughs of the 20th and 21st century have allowed elders to live longer, spawning the more common four-generation family. Yet it has left older people depending more on their tenuous anchors, who now live far away, are divorced, have multiple jobs, and are already balancing the needs of their adult children, grandchildren, and ex-spouses.

In this book we divide the aging family into two broad categories. In these two groupings there are no firm boundaries and aging families can blend into either category. The aging family in this book is seen through two lenses—the nearly normal family and the dysfunctional family. Both types of families are reflected in the evolution of family on American television.

The perfect family reigned in the 1950s and 1960s with popular shows like *Father Knows Best* and *The Donna Reed Show*. As social climates changed, television networks portrayed the working-class family and bigotry in the early 1970s with sitcoms like *All in the Family*. Television began to have people of color in leading roles in *The Cosby Show* of the 1980s. In the late 1980s Rosanne Barr's TV family showed us a blue-collar family facing poverty, both parents working, and old values tangling with feminist ideals. American television moved further away from the perfect family with fathers who leave their jobs and children who are bullies in shows like *Malcolm in the Middle* and *Family Ties*. Now in the 21st century, the family has Hispanic people of color in *Ugly Betty,* and is shown to be dysfunctional through shows like *Big Love, Arrested Development*, and reality TV families such as the Osbornes. The family is still radically evolving in the medium of television and is now light years away from Donna Reed. Our book helps care managers work with the many gradations of the nearly normal and dysfunctional family including facing the difficult and tangled web of the care manager's frequent client: the entitled family.

This book teaches care managers to help the aging family master change. Families are a system and like all systems, are slow to change. Aging families steadfastly resist change and then face massive change when a parent needs extra care. What we explore in many of the chapters in this book is the key development phase: filial maturity. In this relatively unknown new rite of passage, adult children in the aging family have the opportunity to rise above their own needs to accept the mental and physical losses of their elders, and begin to care for their aging family members. The whole aging family must realign and reorganize to change roles and functioning. Adult children must assume the lead in the family in everything from who will hold the Seder to who will cook the turkey, as well as how baby boomers can resist being emotionally and financially dependent on Mom or Dad, and allow her or him to depend on you.

Guiding the whole family through these treacherous waters is a key task of the care manager and this book gives the profession resources and guides to support the aging family through this passage. This book presents navigation tools for the care manager such as forgiveness, acceptance of loss, mirroring behavior, alignment of values, assessing the family caregiver, use of family meetings, working with aging siblings, and many more clinical tools.

Care managers in the 21st century face an aging family with a plethora of problems yet a wheelbarrow full of answers. The contents of this wheelbarrow are deeply explored in this book and meant to allow the care manager to move the aging family to a point where the older family members can be cared for securely, safely, and lovingly in this last phase of their lives, and allow the transmission of care and values to the next generations.

Care Managers Working with the Aging Family in the Medical System

CHAPTER 1

Care Managers–Navigating Families Through the Hospital to Home

Cathy Jo Cress

Hospitalization is one of the most traumatic experiences faced by the elderly and their families. Family members render about three quarters of home care in the United States, yet they are rarely included in discharge planning.[1] Hospitalization can be both a sharp corner in the road and a breaking point for older patients and family caregivers. According to Carol Levine in her executive study, "Making Room for Family Caregivers: Seven Innovative Hospital Programs,"[2] healthcare professionals and family caregivers state that older patients face major difficulties during admission to, stays in, and discharge from hospitals. Family caregivers complain, according to Levine, that they are routinely ignored or made to feel transparent. But at the same time they are asked to play a major part in their family member's care after discharge and receive little training to render what is increasingly highly technical medical care, such as bandaging, caring for wounds, managing pumps, and overall health management. For two decades insurance companies have routinely used medical case managers for both cost containment and for moving patients through the continuum of the hospital. But to make this difficult care transition successful and help avoid the breaking point, all care managers should have a much bigger role with families and elderly patients before, during, and after hospital stays.

The role of the care manager with an elderly client and the family in the hospital mirrors care management tasks in general: educate, assess, advocate, move the client through the continuum of care smoothly, and coordinate for the client/patient and family. All these skills are needed during the entire hospitalization but critically at preadmission and at discharge. The care manager needs to be there for the family at all "care transitions" and especially from the home to the hospital and from the hospital to home. A study from University of California, Berkeley, "From Hospital to Home: Improving Transitional Care for Older Adults," states that hospitalization can be a treacherous switchback for seniors and their families. If the family is not involved, trained, and advocated for in the hospital, then the return to the home can mean derailment and possibly a recipe for disaster, resulting in rehospitalization and increased mortality and morbidity.[3]

The role of the care manager is to coordinate transitional care in the hospital, from preadmission, through admission, hospital stay, and discharge. Case or care management too often only comes when the patient and the family are at home. The skill set of the care manager includes coordination of needed services and moving the older client through the continuum of care. For example, care managers might move an older client to a higher level of care or bring home care out of the continuum to keep an older person at home. In the hospital, the benefits of the care manager of coordinating and helping move a patient through the continuum are incalculable, and the care manager can offer the family and patient critical services by coordinating across care transitions from prehospitalization to home.

Discharge planners, usually nurses and social workers, are overwhelmed by tremendous case loads and no longer have time to give individual service to patients.[4] A case manager's job is always there—24 hours a day—to render highly individualized service. A good case manager can make the discharge planner's job much easier.

BEFORE THE ADMISSION

Risk Assessments

The first task of the care manager is routine risk assessments before the hospitalization. According to the UC Berkeley study "From Hospital to Home," care management risk tools can be of immense help before the hospitalization for both at-risk elderly clients/ patients and their family. Risk tools can include *depression screening, home safety,* and *psychosocial* and *functional* assessment. These risk tools can be of help to alert the hospital staff of risk problems in the hospital and after discharge. For example, an assessment for mental health problems such as depression for both the elderly patient and the family caregiver before the client enters the hospital can be of enormous aid to hospital admissions to ensure that services to treat depression are available during the hospital stay for both the patient and family member. This mental health assessment can also help the discharge planner judge if the family caregiver who will oversee or actually give care may have mental health is-

sues and may need a mental health evaluation at the hospital before the older client comes home. It will help avoid that breaking point if the care manager can determine whether the person who supports, renders, or supervises care for the elderly patient at home can successfully do so or will be impeded by his or her own mental health issues. For depression, the case manager could use a geriatric depression scale that is given routinely before admission to the patient and the family member.

An environmental or home safety assessment done before admission can alert hospital discharge planners to problems in the patient's home environment that must be solved before discharge. For example, if the bedroom for the patient is on the second floor, then care may have to be arranged on the first floor if possible. If there are safety problems, such as loose electric wires or no grab bars in the bathroom, these will impede patient care and safety. Uncovering these environmental problems can assist the discharge planner and family in making a safe discharge to the home. The care manager can arrange for safety changes, if the family agrees to this.

Who Is the Family?

Embracing a family-centered perspective is critical to achieving quality of care for people with chronic or disabling conditions.[5] The case manager must use the lens of the family-centered perspective to view the family so that he or she can successfully help the patient, family caregivers, and friends who encompass the family. The care managers can be a valuable conduit of information to the discharge planner and physician about the family, the family caregiver, or family in general. The first thing needing to be defined is who is the family? The family may be spouses, adult children, distant relatives, friends, or partners. Understanding that family can include people other than the nuclear family and that the care manager should embrace these broader family members in the discussions of care is a key step for the care manager. It is important to distinguish who represents the patient's family, which ones will be caregivers, and who will be the main family spokesperson to the discharge planner and the care managers. Morano and Morano suggest using a genogram to determine who is part of the family system and what their relationship is to the identified client.[6] Because the family may actually render care, the care manager must be gender neutral and be open to male caregivers. The care manager should also help the family identify who will be the family spokesperson. Too many cooks spoil the soup, and the care manager should encourage only one family member to speak for the family, or the client, if the client does not have mental capacity. It may also be that the family will decide that the care manager will serve in this capacity.

JCAHO Requires the Family Be Informed

The Joint Commission on the Accreditation of Healthcare Organizations (JCAHO) has revised its standards of continuity of care to provide new institutional impetus for involving the family in discharge planning (JCAHO standard C6.1.1). The intent of this standard is that patients and families be informed "in a timely manner" of the need for planning and discharge. This means that discussions about discharge between the hospital and the patient and family need to occur from the very point of admission, across the continuity of care in hospital, through patient and family education.[7] Family involvement and education in the process toward discharge is now a JCAHO requirement. The

care manager should remind the family of this requirement if the hospital fails to do so or point it out in the hospital literature.

Assessing the Caregiver

Because informal caregivers face health risks and increased mortality from providing complex care, assessing the family caregiver is critically important.[8] A care manager must not only assess the individuals who compose the family but also the family member who will actually be rendering or overseeing care and, critically, their ability to do this. If the family will be giving direct care, then the care manager should assess their willingness and ability to perform caregiving tasks and make caregiving decisions. The results of these assessments should be passed on to the discharge planner. The assessment of the caregiver should include the family member's ability to help the care recipient carry out activities of daily living (ADLs) and instrumental activities of daily living (IADLs). The assessment should also include caregiver strain and emotional reactions to giving care. According to a 1999 study on caregiver health effects, caregivers who report mental or emotional strain were more likely to die than the noncaregiver controls in the study.[9] Feinberg suggests in her article "State-of-the-Art Caregiver Assessment" there are six pieces of information that should be included in any caregiver assessment:

1. Type and frequency of the current care provision
2. How able the caregiver is to continue with care
3. Whether additional responsibilities or stressors affect care provision
4. The degree of informal support provided
5. What formal services are required
6. The caregiver's overall health status[10]

As Morano and Morano suggest in their article, "Applying the Stress, Appraisal, and Coping Framework to Geriatric Care Management,"[11] this is a valuable time to make suggestions to the family and discharge planner about who will be the care team when the patient goes home, whether the patient needs home care aides or private home care, and which family members have the skill level and emotional stability to render the patient's care at home.

The care manager also needs to assess barriers of care for family members and be able to come up with an alternative plan to suggest to the discharge planner. For instance, long-distance care providers often cannot render care after a hospitalization because they must return home. Some family caregivers may have health problems of their own as a barrier for care. As an example, if a family caregiver, such as a spouse, has mobility problems, he or she may not be able to complete the caregiving tasks needed after the patient is discharged. The care manager needs to assess the family caregivers for their ability to render care and be able to suggest alternatives to care to the family and discharge planner. The care manager should also work with the family to find affordable and acceptable alternatives. For example, the family may have to hire paid caregivers and must be assessed financially as to their ability to pay for this care.

The assessment of the caregiver should also include a plan of care that is developed with the aid of the caregiver. This care plan should define the problems in care that are identified in the assessment and the solutions to those problems. For example, if the care manager is serving a family where the patient is in the hospital for congestive heart failure and the family caregiver has no knowledge of this disease or its care, the care intervention would be education in the hospital via DVDs, reading, and the Internet about care procedures for the family once the patient is discharged, hiring home care to care for the older patient, or suggesting discharge to a skilled nursing facility, if the care cannot be afforded or the family cannot render it themselves.

A caregiver assessment should be done routinely by the care manager (see Chapter 4, "Assessing the Caregiver") to assess the caregiver's ability to take on the caregiving role, which includes physical, emotional, cultural, and educational components, environmental knowledge, and the care recipient's willingness to accept the help and care.[12]

Having the Legal Documents in Place to Enter the Hospital

The care manager needs to make sure the family has the legal documents in place to ensure that the kind of care the older patient wants is delivered. These documents need to be drawn up before a medical crisis occurs. There are several documents that are critical.[13]

The first is the durable power of attorney for health care. This makes sure that there is an individual appointed to make decisions concerning the older patient's medical care if the person is unconscious or can no longer speak for him- or herself. Another form is the advance medical directive. This tells the physician the kind of care the patient wishes in the event that the person can no longer make medical decisions. A healthcare agent should be assigned as part of the advance directive form. A living will is another document the care manager needs to have the client complete before hospital admission. This form of advance directive only takes effect if the patient is diagnosed with a terminal illness. The care manager should also consult with the patient and the family about a do-not-resuscitate order. All these documents should be drawn up with the oversight and consultation of an elder law attorney or the client's family attorney. The care manager should suggest that the family consult with an attorney in all of these legal issues.

It is valuable as a care manager to sit down with the family and the care receiver to discuss these documents before hospitalization. If the client is mentally incompetent, then discuss this with whoever holds the durable power of attorney. Review the documents and what they mean in laypeople's terms with that person. It may also be helpful to use the "Five Wishes" document published by the Aging with Dignity Foundation.[14] It helps to facilitate the discussion. Determine whether the "Five Wishes" document is as a stand-alone document. It can be part of a medical durable power of attorney. Check with the family attorney. At times of medical crisis or matters of life or death, family members can flounder if the doctor asks what they want to do, so a review can help avoid the legally wrong decision.

The care manager must make sure he or she is HIPAA (Heath Insurance Portability and Accountability Act) compliant before the client enters the hospital. At intake the care manager should have had the client or family member (if client lacks capacity) sign a release of information, giving the care manager the right to review both hard copy and database client information. The care manager should also have access to a HIPAA-compliant shared database of the patient's information. In addition the care manager should check with the hospital admissions director to find out what the hospital policy regarding HIPAA and sharing patient information may be. This will ensure that you can obtain information from hospital records while following your client and their family throughout the hospital.

After the documents are in place they should be shared with the discharge planner and the physician before the admission. Copies should go to the physician, the family physician, and the discharge planner to be attached to the hospital chart. They can also be filed in the elderly patient's personal health record, held by the appointed spokesperson for the family.

Insurance Information for Admission

Assessing the client's insurance coverage is critical before the hospital stay. Both the client and the family members need to understand the financial implications of discharge and know whether their older relative's insurance will cover all the expenses of the hospital stay. The family and the patient may expect much more than they will really receive.[15] Care managers need to make sure client insurance information, including Medicare or any private insurance, is given to the discharge planner with the proper name and address of the insurance company, along with the patient's policy number, ID number, and employer if applicable. Medicare will cover any older client who is older than 65, and the case manager will need to provide the actual Medicare card plus date of retirement. The patient's actual Social Security card should be presented to the admission planner. If the insurance is listed under the spouse's name, the same information will be needed from the spouse's insurance. If managed care is covering the hospital stay, the client will need a managed care referral authorization if he or she is covered by an HMO or POS.

Medical Leave for Caregivers

If the family has just flown in from out of town and are involved during the hospitalization sitting at the bedside with the patient, these family members often must take time off from their job. The care manager should make sure family members are aware of the Federal Family Leave Act, which gives them accrued periods of unpaid leave. This is true of ongoing family support systems as well. The law states that covered employers must grant an eligible employee up to 12 work weeks of unpaid leave during a 12-month period if they have to care for an immediate family member, which includes a parent.[16] In states like California, leave for caregiving is paid. The case manager needs to check on her or his state's laws.

Functional Assessment

Assuming the care manager has followed a client for a period of time before the hospitalization, part of the care manager's initial assessment of the client should include a functional assessment. If the care manager is providing ongoing monitoring of the client, this functional information should be updated regularly. Out of this functional assessment the care manager should have critical information to share with the discharge planner upon admission. This should include the client's medical history in writing, a list of the patient's allergies, a list of the client's current medications and dosages and frequency, and a list of all physicians and consultants who are caring for the client along with all contact information. The care manager should have performed a Katz ADL assessment and a Lawton IADL assessment and be able to summarize the scores for the discharge planner. The case manager should also assess the patient for his or her need for a sitter in the hospital, if the hospital does not do this. This can provide respite for the family who may already be sleep deprived and exhausted, and it may also save the discharge planner work. If you as a case manager already know the client is a wanderer or can be obstreperous and unable to control

anger, this can avoid a crisis in care in the hospital before the patient arrives. Patients can fall out of beds, pull out lines, or be overmedicated if they are tied down and have no sitter. Providing this information upon admission can save the discharge planner hours of time, help to improve communication between the care manager and the discharge planner, and avoid the patient's care becoming a crisis.

Psychosocial Assessment

Before hospitalization, upon beginning services for an elderly client, the care manager should complete a psychosocial assessment. In this assessment a genogram should be made to map the family dynamics.[17] The care manager should share the genogram information with the discharge planner. This will give the discharge planner critical information about who is the family, who is to be the family spokesperson, and what family dysfunction may be present that could impede care. For example, if the aging relative was married a second time in their 70s and there are two sets of adult children, the original adult children of the patient and the adult children of the new spouse, there can be incredible friction. Wars over inheritance can erupt, with adult children feeling like they have been replaced by a new unrelated set of siblings. The case manager should identify all these problems by performing the original psychosocial assessment and passing it on to the discharge planner. The case manager should also ensure that he or she is there to work with any family feuds so that the patient is the center of care, not the warring family.

The care manager should also supply the admissions person with a list of informal and formal supports, gathered in the care manager's psychosocial assessment before hospitalization. Informal supports, for example, the family, are documented in a genogram or standard psychosocial assessment. This will be valuable to the discharge planner, telling the planner which family member, if any, will be caring for the older client upon returning home, who will be the family spokesperson, and who will be visiting the hospital. Informal supports include other agencies involved in care or oversight of the older patient. These agencies may be home care agencies providing care, adult protective services, meals on wheels, and so on. These agencies become critical at discharge because they support the older client in his or her return home.

Dementia Patient Admitted to the Hospital

Part of the case manager's psychosocial assessment should be a cognitive assessment. The case manager should have, at intake previous to hospitalization, given the client a cognitive assessment to determine his or her level of cognitive impairment, if any. Results should be verified by the client's physician in an examination. Common instruments that are frequently used to screen dementia are the Folstein Mini Mental Exam, the clock drawing test, the Global Deterioration Scale, the short portable mental status questionnaire, and the Wechsler Memory Scale.[18]

Another cognitive assessment tool that is especially good to help the family is the Functional Assessment Staging Tool. This assessment is specifically for the older person's family and gives information on the order in which various functions are lost.[19]

The result of these cognitive assessments should be shared with the discharge planner at admission so that the discharge planner is aware of both the level of memory loss and resulting behaviors, such as wandering, and the level of services the hospital will have to implement to manage this patient. This will not only help the discharge planner but the

family. Having the hospital have services in place to manage their loved one gives the family peace of mind. Many family members and even perhaps care managers may feel that the hospital staff will be aware of the level of dementia and that this will automatically be passed on to staff. This is not always true.[20] It is especially important to share cognitive deficit information with the discharge planner because communication with the dementia patient will most likely be challenging.

Even acting out behaviors like wandering are a form of communication to the dementia patient. The care manager should share the dementia patient's level of independence and behaviors the care manager and the family are aware of, such as forgetting to use a walker, if needed, or not being able to make decisions because of memory loss. You should share the level of pain and discomfort the patient has with the discharge planner and what appears to make the patient angry or upset. The care manager should tell the discharge planner what might prompt anger or disturbance leading to wandering, incontinence, shouting, or abusive language so that the discharge planner can alert the hospital staff.

Also in preparation for the hospital, the care manager should ask the family or family caregiver to bring items that are soothing to the dementia patient, such as old photos in albums or a favorite item of clothing or a bedspread. This should be checked out first with the discharge planner to find out if such items are permitted in the hospital.[21]

What to Bring and What Not to Bring for the Hospital Stay

The care manager can be of great assistance to the family and client in suggesting to them what they will need for the hospital stay and also what not to bring. What to bring includes sleepwear, electrical equipment, and personal hygiene items. What not to bring includes valuables such as jewelry. The care manager should communicate with the family about their hospital's policy about bringing valuable healthcare items such as dentures, prostheses, and hearing aids.

THE CARE MANAGER'S ROLE DURING THE HOSPITAL STAY

The care manager educates the family to help empower family members to better talk to the doctor, understand patient rights in the hospital, and navigate the healthcare system.

Educating the family members on how to talk to the patient's doctor is a good first step for the care manager when working with families in the hospital. First, the care manager should know how to talk to the physician her- or himself. As Cathy Mullahay states in *The Care Manager's Handbook*, what blocks communication between care managers and physicians is often stereotypical judgments. Physicians are trained to be results oriented and want to "diagnose and treat." Care managers often come from caretaker professions such as nursing and social work and are taught to maintain patient contact to perform their job. In today's American healthcare system, healthcare professionals often are pitted against each other. Often, with issues of cost, access, and insurance, case managers and physicians are wary of each other. Physicians sometimes feel that a care manager is going to take control away from them in order to contain costs. They see care managers as a threat to that control.[22]

The care manager can begin to break through these barriers by improving communications with the doctor. You may have seen the patient/client before the treating physician; if so, you can share valuable information from your functional, psychosocial, and home assessments. This update can

get the physician on your side because you are making his or her job easier.

In your initial phone call to the physician, say you are involved in the case because of your common concern for the patient, your client. Perhaps the client can't return home and needs to go to a nursing home for rehabilitation or to stay for longer. You can communicate that you are there to provide input to the physician, who will make the ultimate decision. Assure the physician that input from your home assessment, functional assessment, and psychosocial assessment can contribute to the doctor's final call. For example, if you've seen and assessed the home and you know there are loose wires all over the place and the house is on a steep hill with steps outside, let the physician know. This is great input if the patient now has limited ambulation, and it may be safer going to rehab instead of getting care at home. Another example is when your psychosocial assessment showed there is no family to care for the client at home and the patient cannot afford home health care.

In your first call to the physician, tell him or her you are the care manager hired by the family of the older client. Tell the doctor the name your company, of the family member who signed your contact, and the reason they hired you, which should be in your original geriatric assessment and in the first call to your agency. For example, this initial family call to the care manager might be because a parent was wandering and the family was at their wit's end. Or family members live far away and asked you to manage the care for the aged client because you are local and know how to navigate the local healthcare system. This will tell the physician what defines your objectives in working with the patient and family.

Stay in touch with the physician once the patient/client is in the hospital. For example, if the family or competent older client wants the older person to return home, if possible, tell the physician you would like to help facilitate that if the physician recommends. Be positive, and show you are focused on the patient. The last encounter the physician may have had with a care manager might have been negative. You need to convey your desire to have a positive working experience with the physician, and that both you and the physician are jointly focused on the patient. Fax him or her your waiver of confidentially or consent from the patient's family or guardian. Assure the doctor that you are not taking over his or her patient and will be a collaborative partner and not try to talk to her or him every day. Assure the physician that you will not be trying to co-op his or her treatment plans. Inform the physician that you will need his or her help to review your treatment and findings, concerns, and care plan.

You should also ask the family member who hired you to call the physician, explain you were hired, and to let the physician's office know that you will be calling. You might also suggest the family members ask the doctor to work with you. This gives a subtle message to the doctor that you can all work together as a team.

When you initially call the physician office, ask the nurse to act as a gatekeeper for her or his schedule. Acknowledge that the physician's time is limited and ask if calling after hours would be best. Once the nurse knows you understand the physician is pressed for time, he or she will usually work with you. Find out when the physician will be in the hospital and making rounds. Fax the physician your credentials or drop by the office and give the staff your business card, brochure, and credentials.

When you call the physician, ask if you could drop by the office and introduce yourself, drop off brochures for the waiting room,

and, if possible, consult about any patients that might benefit by your services. This combines smart marketing with a rapport with the physician that will allow you and the doctor to work as a team for your patient.

If possible, accompany your client to a doctor's appointment with the attending physician before the hospitalization. For example, if the patient is having elective joint replacement, you can introduce yourself, bring your credentials, and try to establish a rapport with the physician at the pre-op appointment.

Be there when the physician makes a hospital visit to your client. It gives you access and can convey that you want to help him or her. Let the doctor know you can be a resource. If dementia is an issue, show the physician a brochure you have from the Alzheimer's Association on the Alzheimer's patient in the hospital and ask if he or she would mind if you passed it on to the family. Write notes on your company stationery complimenting the physician and send copies to the family. Everyone likes praise. Let the physician know you will make referrals to him or her, and add all the physician's contact information to your marketing database. Let the physician know that you will be the person to make sure his or her treatments are carried out. Finally, do not undermine the physician in front of the client or family. Pass on any information in a courteous and ethically and morally responsible way. For instance, if the physician is ordering your client home and you know the family cannot care for this patient at home because the elderly wife is exhausted and there is no money for home care, pass that on as collaborative information. If you find the physician's orders are not being followed, such as physical therapy was started 4 days late, do not be a blamer, but convey the information to the physician with the caveat that you know everyone in the system is pressed and overloaded and you are just trying to make sure that what everyone wants—the best care—is being rendered.

The care manager should help the family spokesperson set up a meeting with the attending physician, because this doctor will be coordinating the care of the patient in the hospital. This doctor will be the primary physician communicating with all the other consulting doctors and will know their recommendations. The care manager should help the family spokesperson find out the best way to be in touch with the attending physician and whether this is by phone or in person. The care manager can find all this information by talking to the physician's office nurse. The care manager should make sure both the family spokesperson and the care manager's name are in the patient's chart along with cell and regular phone numbers.

If a meeting can be set up with the doctor, it may be during his or her rounds, so the care manager needs to discover his or her schedule of rounds. The care manager should also prompt the family spokesperson to list all his or her questions so that when the physician meeting occurs the family spokesperson is prepared and the limited time of the physician is not wasted. At the same time, the care manager needs to encourage the family spokesperson to continue to ask questions until the family spokesperson feels satisfied with the answers. The list of questions should be a running list that is updated each time that family member meets with the attending physician.

The family spokesperson should also be encouraged by the care manager to communicate effectively with the entire healthcare team, which includes the hospital social worker and nurses attending the patient. The RNs can answer day-to-day questions, whereas the physician may only be reached on a more limited basis for significant issues. The RNs can tell the family members about new procedures and the course of treatment. Talking with the RNs will help family members feel less frustrated with having limited access to the attending physician.

Care managers should encourage family members not to communicate with the RNs at change of shift because changes of shifts are extremely busy for the RNs as they receive reports from the previous shift. Family members should be encouraged to ask the RN to review the physician's orders with them, which are usually on the patient's chart. This way family members can not only receive the information but also have it interpreted and have questions answered. The care manager can do this with the family member if the RN staff is busy.

Family Communications in the Hospital

Care managers can refer families to the hospital social worker for additional support and access to services in the hospital. This professional has a psychosocial background. Medical social workers can help with counseling services and be a liaison between the patient family and rehabilitation team, if rehab is ordered, or with other professionals in the hospital setting. For example, if the family members are sleep deprived from emergency travel or care, the social worker can be helpful in setting up a sitter service in the hospital. If the hospital has a palliative care unit and your client is dying, the social worker can provide families and patients with emotional and practical support involving death and dying issues. The social worker can help families and patients talk about their fears and concerns and make additional referrals to hospice. Social workers can sometimes provide family counseling in the hospital and serve as the go-to person for solving hospital problems, such as when services such as rehab are not being delivered as ordered.

The care manager can also suggest that family members communicate with the hospital chaplain, especially if the end of life or terminal issues are at hand. Through your psychosocial assessment, you should have discovered the client and family's religious affiliation, if any. Ask the patient or family if they would like some pastoral care. If they specifically tell you that they would benefit from pastoral care, then contact the hospital pastoral care office, if one exists. The care manager can also call the patient's rabbi, priest, minister, or imam for help if no pastoral care services exist. If religious services are a part of their life, then the stresses of illness, end-of-life issues, and hospitalization may prompt a greater need for spiritual guidance. Older clients and their families may need help in anticipating surgery, feeling anxious about being in the hospital, clarifying options, or understanding their feelings. This can involve visits by hospital chaplains, attending religious services on site (as many hospitals have a chapel), or commemorating major religious holidays. Many pastoral care services are available on a 24-hour basis.

Care management is about knowing the continuum of care, and in this instance it is the continuum of care in the hospital. Social workers and the clergy are your allies and can help you get families additional mental health support in a very trying setting, the hospital.

The case manager should coach family members to communicate with all hospital staff in a respectful way. These staff members are often short staffed, taking on much more than they did in the past. Coach the family spokesperson to introduce themselves, shake the staff member's hand, and to call physicians, RNs, and staff by their names. Encourage family members to ask for what they need in a grateful and polite manner stated in a calm tone. Coach them to not be adversarial, pushy, or rude. Suggest that the family spokesperson carry a small notebook or the patient's personal care record at all times to jot down questions for the hospital staff and the case manager as well. If the family elects not to communicate or cannot because of distance, the case managers can communicate with hospital staff, if the family elects to contract and pay for this.

The Case Manager Dealing with Family Stress During the Hospital Stay

Many family members are incredibly stressed during the hospitalization. They often have been rendering increasing care in the previous weeks before the hospitalization and are exhausted. If they are the spouses, they are often old and suffer some age-related decrements as a result. In times of stress, sleep, when you are able to get it, is not restful. The family, if they are spending much time in the hospital, has poor nutrition, as they are often eating junk food from the hospital vending machines. If they are adult children, they are often neglecting their primary family responsibility to sit a bedside vigil with their older family member. Inability to care for the patient when he or she comes home can result from such stress. Many family members live far away, so have taken emergency flights into the city, have not slept, and if the care manager has not been involved before, are sometimes out of the loop. As a result, when the care recipient is in the hospital, family members are frequently angry, irritable, and feeling guilty.

The care manager can do many things to help the family. Assess the family for sleep deprivation and encourage those suffering from such to go home and arrange for another family member to stay in the hospital or arrange for a sitter service in the hospital. Talk to family members about their stress level. Just having them acknowledge their pain and stress can be a great first step. The care manager can refer the family member to the hospital social worker or pastoral care, who can further talk to them about their stressors. The care manager can ask the nursing team to explain the medical equipment and its purpose and tell the family what the "alarm bells" on the equipment mean. The use of the small notebook mentioned earlier, where the family member can write down questions to ask the attending physician, is again helpful here.

Some hospitals have "patient pathways" outlining the commonly expected daily care plan for different medical conditions. A patient pathway is a general guideline for the care of a common illness and gives suggestions for what will occur in treating that illness during the hospital stay. This can include treatments, consultations, medications, diet, and assessment, teaching, and getting ready for discharge. These are mapped out in a timeline. They are often written in user-friendly language. Pathways help families to be less stressed by being better informed and knowing what will generally happen.

The care manager can ask the RN or attending physician if the care recipient is on a pathway and ask if the family member can have a copy of it. When families have access to pathways they can work together as caregivers or with caregivers to make the hospital stay more comfortable for the patient and less stressful for the family. The family can work together with the doctors, RNs, and hospital staff because the care needs can be anticipated through the patient pathway. Family members can make better decisions about care through the patient pathway be-

cause it gives them additional information to make those decisions. Patient pathways also give the patient and family space to write their own notes so that they can be used for the families own documentation.[23]

Family Meetings in the Hospital

Another service that the care manager can arrange is a family meeting in the hospital. Family communication can break down in the hospital, especially for dysfunctional families. The care manager can ask the hospital staff and attending physician if they would consider scheduling a family conference. This would include, if possible, at least one physician, key nursing personnel, the care recipient if he or she is well enough to participate, and the person who has power of attorney for health care. It is also helpful to include the discharge planner. The care manager can assist by helping the family members list all of their questions, show them how to prioritize the questions, and then encourage family members to ask those questions in the meeting in a polite and noncombative way. The meeting should be headed by the physician, who should review all clinically important information. The care manager can mediate to help family members express themselves and keep the meeting on track, which could involve gently or firmly redirecting family members to the present—not the past—and the focus of the meeting, which are the patient's current conditions and next care transition. Often old family feuds or anger over which child was the favorite boil up in a family meeting and derail the whole agenda. The meeting should result in formulating a plan of care. Ideally, the care manager should be the one who creates the plan of care and then submits it to the family and the attending physician for consideration.

Healthcare Literacy for the Family

Give the family specific information in multimedia formats (print, DVD, etc.) on the patient's individual conditions. Education to increase health literacy is one of the most important supports a case manager can give family members of a hospitalized client. What is health literacy? It is the ability of people to acquire, process, and understand basic health information and to use that data to make healthcare decisions. This literacy allows the family to make healthcare decisions throughout the hospitalization or to help the competent patient to make those decisions. Family members may have to do this with a competent patient who because of hospital procedures, like major surgery, may be unable to make decisions. The average US citizen reads at a seventh- or eighth-grade level, and it is estimated that the average adult over 65 has inadequate or marginal reading skills. Even those with adequate literacy rates have difficulty in understanding health materials.[24]

Family members usually do not know what questions to ask, let alone whom to ask. They need information that covers the specific illness of the care recipient, not general information. When family members have a question they often don't know if they should ask the doctor, social worker, or nurse. Caregivers become very stressed just by trying to unravel their information gap.

The family needs the help of the care manager to interpret the heath information given to them about the procedures done and also to enhance the information about the procedures and the postacute care that will be needed. For example, there are about 900,000 patients admitted to the hospital with congestive heart failure each year. These patients also have the highest rate of readmission of all adult patient groups. If the care manager

is able to gather resources on heart disease, the specific operation, and posthospital care from the community and hospital library in various user-friendly formats such as brochures, videos or DVDs, or Web sites, this would help the caregiver and the older patient. The caregiver can then be better prepared for the care he or she will render or supervise, and the patient, if competent, will better understand his or her hospitalization and recovery. The care manager could call the local American Heart Association and pick up brochures, printed information, and any videos/DVDs, as an example. The care manager can investigate previously mentioned patient pathways, the hospital library, and community agencies like the American Heart Association for educational material about the particular medical problem.

Include the Patient and Family in the Unit of Care

Unit of care is a term that means the focus of a plan of care. In hospice palliative care this is typically the patient and his or her family. Including the family was originally a major goal of hospital discharge planning and hospitalization. However, in the past 30 years, discharges of patients through diagnosis-related groups (DRG) result in quicker discharges, and involving the family became a low priority. Now the Joint Commission on the Accreditation of Healthcare Organizations (JCAHO) has revised its standard on continuity of care.[25] Case managers need a family systems approach where the care recipient is not the client but the "client system," which takes in the family, the family caregiver, and the friends as part of that system, and all become the client. A recent study on family caregivers, "From Hospital to Home: Improving Transitional Care for Older Adults," recommends recognizing caregivers as part of the unit of care and integrating them into the care team.[26] At every opportunity the care manager should work with the hospital staff to have the family involved in the unit of care so that they can more fully participate in decisions, feel more in control of their loved one's care, and be prepared for discharge in a meaningful way.[27]

Follow the Patient Throughout Hospitalization to Keep All Hospital Services Starting in a Timely Way

The care manager's job is to be a "care navigator" and respond to the patient's and family's needs across settings. In the hospital the care manager's role includes helping the care recipient move in a timely way throughout the hospital stay and making sure what was ordered by the physician (such as rehab) is delivered in a timely way. Again, hospital staff are overworked and stressed, and the hospital discharge planner is focused on what will happen after the hospital stay. They are often overloaded with patients, and they can't render this support to everyone. So, the case manager involved with the family and care recipient in the hospital needs to render this service.

Personal Health Record

In following the care recipient and the family throughout the hospital stay, the care manager should encourage the use of a personal health record. This personal health record can help the family feel more in control and allow them to keep track of what is happening to their loved one. As the hospital is a hectic and sometimes very emotional setting, the care manager's encouragement of this record can be a great contribution to family involvement and reducing family stress through knowledge. The personal health record can be managed in collabora-

tion with the care manager's support and will help to formulate the patient's and family caregiver's questions. These questions may include reasons for taking medications, reasons for a worsening condition, or problems in care in the hospital.

A personal health record can be as simple as a piece of paper, held in a file folder. You can encourage the family to transfer the information to a computer disc or USB drive if they wish. There are many personal care record products on the market.[28] The personal health record can include a copy of the case manager's client data sheet including medicines, diagnosis, care plan, and medical history. For families who want the case manager to provide a high level of support, this is an excellent way a case manager can help the family. The family can then add an ongoing list of questions about care, procedures, and problems that they wish to ask staff. Personal health records can include copies of consents for admissions, treatment, surgery, and releases of information that are signed in the hospital. Personal health records can keep notes on meetings with physicians, nurses, social workers, and pastoral care in the hospital. It could include medical records from all the physicians treating the patient previous to the hospitalization. The case manager should have copies of all of this information also. If the family wishes the case manager to compile all this information, then this is another service the case manager can add on to the existing contract. You must have a release of information from the family to get this information. If time is of the essence, as when the family just flew in from out of town, a copy of your client data sheet and questions the family has may have to suffice.

Making the transition from one setting to another, especially into the hospital, can be perilous for older people. The change in surroundings, new providers, and new medicines can be very disorienting. The care recipient many times cannot speak for him- or herself. The family often lacks some degree of health literacy, and many times they are not included in the unit of care. This coupled with the understaffing of hospital staff makes the care manager of great value in ensuring services are rendered in a timely manner.

As an example, if the physician orders physical therapy every day twice a day post hip surgery and the PT is only coming once a day, the care manager can report this to the physician. This report is going to keep the patient moving swiftly through the hospital and onto an earlier discharge. If sitters services were ordered by the hospital and the care manager knows that two shifts were late and one shift did not show, resulting in the patient pulling out lines, the care manager should report this to the physician or charge RN of the unit. If the patient's RN staff was to be educated on a dementia patient's signals to indicate he or she needs to use the bathroom but wasn't, resulting in the patient unnecessarily sitting in urine, this could lead to skin breakdown and create another problem to hold the patient in the hospital longer. The care manager should report this to the physician to keep the patient moving through the hospital in a timely manner.

The Dementia Patient in the Hospital

For the family who has just flown in or driven a long distance to be at the loved one's bedside in the hospital, the care manager's role can include updating the family on the level of mental deterioration the dementia patient has gone through and the typical behaviors the patient had before hospitalization (wandering, forgetting a walker). It is also a good contribution to the newly arriving family to instruct them, if you have not already done so by phone or e-mail, that these behaviors may be a form of communication for their loved one. Nonverbal behaviors such as agitation, restlessness, aggression, and being

combative are often an expression of unmet needs (pain, thirst, and toileting). So, if the family will be sitting at the bedside, they will know what behavior may prompt what need. You can also tell the family whether the loved one can understand yes or no or simple instructions, or if the patient needs physical cues such as gestures indicating eating and making a choice between one thing or another (hospital food). The family can then help communicate the patient's choices or needs to the hospital staff. The care manager can also update the nursing staff as to these behaviors signaling various needs. Although you may have told all this to the hospital discharge planner, the information may not have gotten to the staff. Updating staff yourself provides a safety net for the staff and family in the care and support of the dementia patient.

Provide 24-Hour Advice and Support to the Family While the Patient Is in the Hospital

The nature of geriatric care management is that you are the piano player at Nordstrom's and are on 24-hour call. This may be you or your fellow care managers. This service is especially helpful for the family in the hospital. That you can be reached at any time to answer questions and deal with concerns or a crisis gives the older patient's family great peace of mind. Family members are usually stressed and dealing with an unpredictable medical situation and a hospital setting that is not always supportive of their needs or sometimes even the patient's. Your being available can make this overwhelming experience much easier. It can also be a bridge to the attending physician and the discharge planner. If they understand you are there to support the family 24/7, but not to undermine their authority or take over their patient, this can be a big selling point to both types of very busy hospital professionals.

DISCHARGE

As older patients, like all patients, are now released from the hospital after briefer stays, in weaker conditions, discharge planning from the hospital and postdischarge services at home are even more critical.[29] Improving these "care transitions" should be a primary goal for the care manager. Discharge from the hospital is the realm of the discharge planner and ultimately the attending physician. You as the case manager are invited into the decision making only if the discharge planner and the physician welcome you. It is hoped in pre-admission, admission, and during the hospital stay that you have proven to both the physician and the discharge planner that you are there to support them, handle tasks they are too busy to handle, and use your professional information about the patient and the family to support the unit of care in the hospital. If the hospital discharge planner does not invite you into the process, you still need to work with the family to assess for the return to home. It may be valuable to pass information to the discharge planner through the family or to fax information to the discharge department. Alternatively, you can give information to the attending physician or to the primary physician of the client. You can also have the family themselves advocate for your involvement. Every hospital is different, and some may be resistant to a care manager becoming involved in discharge planning.

Family Members Appealing Discharge

One role the care manager can play is alerting the family to the fact that if they feel discharge is made prematurely, then the family and older patient have a right to appeal the decision.

If the family feels that their relative is not well enough to go home or to subacute care, the family can appeal. Hospitals are required to give every Medicare patient or family caregiver a copy of the statement "An Important Message About Medicare," which discusses appealing decisions about discharge and making sure the family and patient, if competent, understand the process. This document spells out a patient's rights to all needed hospital care and postdischarge follow-up. The hospital must also give a written notice explaining the discharge, a Hospital-Issued Notice of Noncoverage (HINN). The HINN will include the phone number of the local peer review organization (PRO) and other organizations that review contested cases. What the care managers can help the family understand is that the hospital cannot force family caregivers to take patients home or pay for continued care before the PRO makes a decision.[30] The care manager should at this point work supportively, not adversarially, with the discharge planner and physician to mediate the situation, answer the family's or patient's questions about not being ready for discharge, and try to resolve the disagreement so that the patient, family, and discharge planner all get what they need. Physicians and discharge planners are stressed by DRGs and too many patients. So, your extra support as a case manager can provide a way to get the older patient to the point of discharge.

Include Family and Family Caregivers in Discharge Planning

Network with local caregiver information sites to give family caregiver training for postacute tasks (bathing, lifting, injections, and self-care for caregivers).

Health literacy was mentioned earlier in the chapter. At discharge, the family's health literacy becomes critical. While the older family member is in the hospital, the case manager should have already been networking with local, state, and national aging agencies to arrange condition-specific information and training on postacute tasks. For example, if your client has had a stroke, contacting a local or national Web site like the American Heart Association for information about postdischarge care to support the family would be a good idea. If there is a local stroke association or stroke center, the care manager can contact them to find out if they have training for family members to care for family at home and if they might come to the hospital before discharge to do the training.

For discharge training of the family, you should start in the hospital with the physician to find out if occupational therapy (OT) is ordered to train the family and patient in adaptive devices such as needed with stroke-related paralysis. You should also determine if physical therapy (PT) is ordered to train the older person in ambulation and the use of assistive devices. Such training should include family members regarding transfer safety so that they do not injure themselves. The care manager should contact the physical therapy and occupational therapy departments of the hospital to find out what their orders from the physician are.

If the physician or the hospital has not taken a step to involve the family in the unit of care, the care manager must step up to the plate and get the family involved through training at this time. If not, the older patient has a much greater risk of readmission because the family caregiver did not know how to render care. In addition, family members could injure themselves or the patient by rendering care like lifting, giving injections, or managing complex machines that they are not trained to manage. Care managers should ask the physician if the PT and OT can train family members in transfers and use of medical equipment in the hospital before discharge.

Arrange for In-Hospital Assessment to Determine Medicare and Other Insurance Eligibility for Home Care Service

If it has not been done, the care manager should determine if the patient's Medicare or other insurance covers home care service. Care managers should find out what home health agency may follow the patient home after discharge and find out if training of the family member in patient care could be arranged in the hospital before discharge. If the home care agency is a Medicare agency and has PTs and OTs who will follow the aging client, ask if they can train the family members in transferring the patient, safe cooking, and exercises at home.

Home care, except for a very brief coverage after discharge, is not covered by Medicare. Medicare does not cover what it defines as long-term chronic care. The older patient and the family have to pay for home care, unless they have long-term care insurance. Checking for this should have been done as part of the care manager's initial intake in the financial section of the psychosocial assessment. Such information should have been shared with admissions upon the patient entering the hospital. The care manager should use the financial assessment section of the psychosocial assessment to find out if the older patient can afford home care. Home care can be very expensive, ranging around $20.00 an hour. Offering input to the discharge planner and consultations to the family about the older person's finances is an important task for the care manager. With the help of the discharge planner and the hospital staff, the care manager should assess the older patient's present level of care. Level of care is determined by evaluating the client's home environment in combination with the older client's updated abilities to perform

ADLs.[31] For example, if upon discharge from the hospital, the older client cannot transfer by himself and get out of bed to use the bathroom, the client will need a care provider to offer this assistance. If his wife cared for him before hospitalization without transfers and now cannot transfer due to her own physical limitation, you will need to seek a home care agency. If this cannot be afforded, the care manager may use the family continuum of care to see if a family member who can transfer can render that care. If that is not possible, you may suggest placement in a skilled nursing facility.

Provide a Checklist for the Family upon Discharge Outlining What Care Needs They Will Have to Implement

If possible, the care manager should ask the physician if the hospital has a checklist of specific information about the older client's medical conditions and specific needs of the elderly client during the transition to home (discharge).The care manager can also request that the physician, discharge planner, or RN review the checklist with the elderly patient and the family to make sure the family understands the home care needs of the elderly patient. The care manager should make sure that the family and elderly patient have a copy of this checklist upon discharge so that they can refer to both the medical condition guidelines and home care needs when they arise. If the hospital does not provide such a discharge checklist, the care manager can make one by asking the physician for specific information on the older client's medical conditions and home care needs.[32]

According to a brochure from the National Alliance for Care Giving and the United Hospital Fund of New York, "Hospital Discharge Planning: Helping Family Caregivers Through the Process," a checklist should have certain elements. First, the patient's condition and any changes that may have occurred as a result of treatment at the facility should be listed. Second, any likely symptoms, problems, or changes that may occur when the patient is at home should be listed. Third, the patient's care plan, the caregiver's needs, and any adjustments made to meet those needs should be recorded. The care manager should have updated his or her own care plan as a result of the hospitalization, and this could be included in the information. This would also include new skills that the family caregiver or paid caregiver would have to have, such as giving injections, bandaging, operating medical equipment, and so on. Finally, the potential impact on the caregiver including warning signs of stress and techniques in reducing stress should be included on the discharge checklist.[33]

This is a good time to evaluate, with the discharge planner, whether the family member who may be planning to render care can really do that. If the care manager compares the family member's abilities, such as ability to lift, ability or willingness to be trained in giving injections, and ability or willingness to be trained in managing medical equipment such as a Hoyer lift wheel chair, with the change in the older patient's condition since he or she was admitted, the care manager along with the discharge planner can help the family member decide whether care can be rendered safely. For example, if a wife has macular degeneration, and the older husband's care after being discharged now involves injections, can she really render this care?

This is a time when the care manager can help build in a support system for the family that may involve informal support such as private care givers, other family members who can, for instance, give injections, or close neighbors or friends who may be able to be trained to give the injections.

Educate the Family on Community Services They Can Use Such as AAA, Medicare, Medical, and Paratransit

Home- and community-based services from federal, state, and community resources are funded and administered by a patchwork of agencies. Finding the right community services and understanding their eligibility requirements remains a maze after 40 years of trying to make it simple. This is where the care manager can be that central point of entry for the family. The care manager should educate the family about services in the community where they can call for help when the older family members are discharged. This includes national and community agencies mentioned before that can give condition-specific information. The American Cancer Society is one such example, if the older patient has been hospitalized with a diagnosis of cancer. Community support groups for family members dealing with cancer would also be a good resource in such a case. Community assistance can include transportation to chemotherapy through the Area Agency on Aging's (AAA) paratransit program or by American Cancer Society volunteers driving to those appointments. If one of your clients has an elderly caregiver spouse, this can apply to them as well. You can call and arrange the service, or the family can if they choose to take over this task. Your job is to come up with the options.

The case manager should at this point explain and interpret eligibility requirements to the family so that they understand what services are covered by Medicare and their insurance policies and what they must pay for out of pocket for those services. The care manager should review what services are available though their local Area Agency on Aging, if the older client is not presently a user of the service. For instance, senior para-

transit through the Area Agency on Aging can provide low-cost transportation to physician's visits, physical therapy, and chemotherapy. This is especially helpful to families who are very busy with jobs, children, and personal lives and to elderly spouses who do not drive. Meals on wheels is an excellent referral for older people recovering at home and can supply low-salt and some special meals for recovering patients. Again this resource can be accessed through the AAA and help take the burden off the family.

The Health Insurance Counseling and Advocacy (HICAP) program is an excellent place to refer family members if they have questions and concerns about Medicare coverage in the hospital or for services at home. They will review coverage for supplemental (Medigap) insurance, billing and claims procedures, long-term care insurance questions and help the family with understanding medical insurance terminology. The care manager should refer the family to the local Area Agency on Aging, where HICAP services are usually under the agency's umbrella.

Coordinative Information from Risk Assessment with Patient and Family with Discharge Planner

Before hospitalization, as part of the care manager's initial assessment, risk assessments should have been completed, including cognitive, functional, psychosocial, and depression, and any other assessment that is appropriate, such as quality of life or culturally appropriate services. For example, assessing for the cultural needs of a patient who comes from an ethnically diverse population and needs culturally appropriate resources in the community can be exceptionally helpful.[34] A Korean elder may primarily speak Korean and may need a Korean speaker to render home care. The family may need information about caring for the older patient written in Korean. If the older person has no power of attorney for health care it may be important to get a Korean speaker who can arrange that vital task.

The care manager should also have done a risk assessment on the family caregiver if they will be giving direct care to the elderly patient. The information gleaned from this risk assessment is very important at discharge, because it can help the discharge planner and the family choose the right services to support them at home. If the care manager has routinely done a risk assessment for depression, like the Geriatric Depression Scale (GDS), and the client is about to be discharged, the care manager should be sure the treating physician in the hospital is aware of any depression and whether some pharmacological treatment in the hospital might be considered. The care manager could also make sure the patient sees his or her family physician at discharge to see if medication for depression is recommended. If your elderly client was depressed before hospitalization, the care manager can refer the family and client to a mental health service in the community to support the patient. In addition the care manager might improve the quality of life of the patient and allay depression after discharge. The care manager can use a quality-of-life risk assessment to find out what services in the community may allay the depression. For example, in assessing for quality of life, the case manager may find out the patient loves dogs but can't have one. So, the care manager can arrange for a pet visitation program that might help with the depression. If the patient has spiritual connections and wants to pursue them again, arranging for the minister, priest, or imam to visit the patient upon returning home is a good intervention for depression.[35]

The care manager should have completed a risk assessment on the family member who plans to care for the elderly patient when he returns home. For instance, if an elderly spousal caregiver has macular degeneration and must give injections, the care manager can arrange for another family member to give those injections and also arrange for the elderly spouse to be assessed by the local blind center for vision enhancements throughout the home. This might mean the care manager brings in home care services if they can be afforded to give the elderly visually disabled spouse respite and relieve her of some of the tasks that she cannot do because of the increased levels of care (injections) and her own disability.

Assess Patient's Home Before Discharge and Communicate Needs to Family

A critical risk assessment for the care manager is assessing the patient's home before the patient comes home. The care manager should already have done this assessment when he or she did the original intake assessment of the client. What the care manager needs to do before the older patient is released is to reevaluate the home assessment in terms of the older patient's changed condition as a result of the hospitalization. This is important to the older patient and to the family. For instance, if the older client could climb steps before the hospitalization and now cannot, the care manager may have to investigate a ramp, alterative bedrooms, or alternative housing if home modification cannot be made. The family will have to be involved in both the expense of any home modification or ultimately moving to a higher level of care if home modifications cannot be made or afforded.

Summary

From admission through hospitalization to home, the care manager is a key professional to help the older hospitalized client and his or her family move through the continuum of the hospital—from preadmission, admission, hospital stay, to discharge. The care manager does this as a support to the case manager employed by the hospital or the discharge planner, helping these professionals in their already overwhelming job. The care manager can use risk assessments done at intake to inform admissions about client medical conditions, mental health issues, home safety, and family dynamics. The care manager can additionally assess the family caregiver, critically discovering how that caregiver needs to be supported in the hospital and when they return home. During the hospitalization, the care manager can educate the family on issues to empower individual members to talk to the doctor, understand patients' rights in the hospital, and how to navigate the healthcare system.

The care manager can help with family communications in the hospital, both within the family system and between the family and the hospital staff. The case manager can help the family deal with both physical and mental stress during the hospitalization, helping them cope with what is often the most difficult situation in their family caregiving career. Family meetings can be held at the hospital, prompted by the care manager to engender better communication between family members and the hospital staff. Education of the family caregiver on caregiver tasks, the disease process, and skill sets like lifting, can be organized by the care manager in the hospital and through community agencies. The care manager can help make sure that services for the patient start in a timely way throughout the hospitalization and provide 24-hour advice and support to the family during the hospitalization.

Upon discharge the care manager can make sure the family members and caregivers are included in discharge planning, advised on legal rights about discharge, helped to involve a home health agency (if necessary), and educated on community services they can use on discharge; often the care manager can arrange those services. Care managers can coordinate with the discharge planner, sharing risk assessment information and assessing the home for safety issues before the patient comes home. The care manager can be a team member with the hospital staff, a key support to the family caregiver and the family members, and a critical player in making sure the older client gets the right amount of care at the right time from preadmission to discharge in the hospital.

REFERENCES

1. Brown-Williams H. Dangerous transitions: Study shows discharge planning risks. *Aging Today*. 2007;28.
2. Levine C. *Making Room for Family Caregivers*. New York, NY: United Hospital Fund; 2003;111.
3. *From Hospital to Home: Improving Transitional Care for Older Adults*. Berkeley, CA: Health Research for Action; 2006.
4. Brown-Williams H. Dangerous transitions: Study shows discharge planning risks. *Aging Today*. 2007;28.
5. *Caregiver Assessment: Principles, Guidelines and Strategies for Change*. Vol. I. San Francisco, CA: National Center for Caregiving; 2006.
6. Morano C, Morano B. Functional assessment. In: Cress C, ed. *Handbook of Geriatric Care Management*. Sudbury, MA: Jones and Bartlett; 2007:26.
7. *Hospital Discharge Planning: Helping Family Caregivers Through the Process*. New York, NY: National Alliance for Caregiving and the United Hospital Fund of New York; 2006:2.
8. *From Hospital to Home: Improving Transitional Care for Older Adults*. Berkeley, CA: Health Research for Action; 2006:4.
9. *From Hospital to Home: Improving Transitional Care for Older Adults*. Berkeley, CA: Health Research for Action; 2006:6.

10. Feinberg LF. The state of the art caregiver assessment. *Generations*. 2003–2004;Winter:27.

11. Morano C, Morano B. Applying the stress, appraisal and coping framework to geriatric care management. *GCM Journal*. 2007;Spring.

12. *Caregiver Assessment: Principles, Guidelines and Strategies for Change*. Vol. I. San Francisco, CA: National Center for Caregiving; 2006.

13. Tomsko PL, Padwo-Rogers S. Communicating effectively in the hospital setting. *Family Caregiving 101*. Available at: http://www.familycaregiving101 .org.

14. www.agingwithdignity.com

15. *Hospital Discharge Planning: Helping Family Caregivers Through the Process*. New York, NY: National Alliance for Caregiving and the United Hospital Fund of New York; 2006:4.

16. US Department of Labor, Employment Standards Administration, Wage and Hour Division. Available at: http://www.dol.gov/esa. Accessed April 15, 2008.

17. Morano C, Morano B. Functional assessment. In: Cress C, ed. *Handbook of Geriatric Care Management*. Sudbury, MA: Jones and Bartlett; 2007:26.

18. Belson P. Dementia and the older adult: The role of the geriatric care manager. In: Cress C, ed. *Handbook of Geriatric Care Management*. Sudbury, MA: Jones and Bartlett; 2007:407.

19. Reisberg B, Ferris SH, de Leon MJ, Crook T. The Global Deterioration Scale for assessment of primary degenerative dementia. *Am J Psychiatry*. 1982;139:1136–1139.

20. Caring for someone with dementia: Care on the hospital Ward, www.alzheimers.org.uk/caring_for someone.

21. *Dementia: Preparing for Hospital Admission*. http://dementia.youk.com/bm/brain-behaviour/ preparing-for-hospital-admission.shtml. Accessed May, 2008.

22. Mullahay C. *The Care Manager's Handbook*. 3rd ed. Sudbury, MA: Jones and Bartlett; 2004.

23. Making the Right Choice: Should You Be on a Patient Pathway? Yale New Haven Hospital, Yale New Haven Health System. 2004. Available at: http:/www.ynhh.org/choice/pathway.html. Accessed June 20, 2007.

24. *From Hospital to Home: Improving Transitional Care for Older Adults*. Berkeley, CA: Health Research for Action; 2006:9.

25. *Hospital Discharge Planning: Helping Family Caregivers Through the Process*. New York, NY: National Alliance for Caregiving and the United Hospital Fund of New York; 2006:2.

26. Brown-Williams H. Dangerous transitions: Study shows discharge planning risks. *Aging Today*. 2007; 28.

27. *Examination of Family Caregiver Roles Leads to Book Outlining New Policy Recommendation*. Princeton, NJ: Robert Wood Johnson Foundation: http://www.rwjf.org/reports/grr/04715.htm. Accessed June 14, 2008.

28. American Health Information Management Association. Available at: http://www.myphr.com/ your_record/keeping.asp. Accessed June, 2008.

29. UC Berkeley. Dangerous transitions, seniors and the hospital to home experience. *Health Research for Action*. 2006;April.

30. *Hospital Discharge Planning. Helping Family Caregivers Through the Process*. New York, NY: National Alliance for Caregiving and the United Hospital Fund of New York; 2006:10.

31. Cress C. *Handbook of Geriatric Care Management*. Sudbury, MA: Jones and Bartlett; 2007:90.

32. UC Berkeley. From hospital to home: Improving transitional care for older adults. *Health Research for Action*. 2006;19.

33. *Hospital Discharge Planning, Helping Family Caregivers Through the Process*. New York, NY: National Alliance for Caregiving and United Hospital Fund of New York; 2006:12.

34. Hikoyeda N, Miyawaki C. Ethnic and cultural considerations in geriatric care management. In: Cress C, ed. *Handbook of Geriatric Care Management*. Sudbury, MA: Jones and Bartlett; 2007:99.

35. Herdon NP, Thorpe V. Supporting clients' quality of life: Drawing on community informal networks and care manager creativity. In: Cress C, ed. *Handbook of Geriatric Care Management*. Sudbury, MA: Jones and Bartlett; 2006:357.

CHAPTER 2

Care Managers Helping Aging Families Communicate with a Physician

Catherine M. Mullahy

When elderly individuals become patients, their needs vary as they do for any other category of patients entering the healthcare delivery system. The difference, however, is that because of their longevity, older people are much more likely to be experiencing the effects of *several* chronic conditions rather than one acute condition. This factor has introduced formidable challenges in managing the continuum of care for the geriatric patient. Also increasing these challenges is the fact that patients of all ages no longer have the benefit of one treating physician who oversees and coordinates all aspects of his or her patients' care. From knowing what kind of physician should be treating a particular condition and comprehending the effects the various conditions have on the others, to qualifying a provider and monitoring all of the medications and their potential negative interactions, care managers who work with the aging population are indeed in a very challenging area of patient care. This chapter will provide key insights and actionable direction to assist care managers in the management of these complex medical patients.

First, it is important to define and identify this "complex medical patient" and then examine some of the patient's most relevant characteristics. With a better understanding of these traits and the related issues, the care manager can determine the resources, including other care/case management colleagues, who might be needed to ensure a high standard of care.

Although various models of care/case management exist, including within the subspecialty of geriatric care management, the following core functions are common for all care managers:

• Outreach
• Screening and intake
• Comprehensive assessment
• Care planning
• Service arrangement
• Monitoring
• Evaluation and or reassessment

The more complex the patient is, the more important it is to apply all of these components and to provide them across the continuum of care. Additionally, it is imperative that we communicate the findings within these areas with *all* of the individuals involved with this complex medical patient.

So then, who do we define as *complex*? And since we have accepted that *many* individuals are likely to be involved with each patient, with multiple treatment plans formulated by the various treating physicians, how do we communicate effectively with *all* of them? Because communication is the absolute key to successful care/case management, we will focus some much needed attention on our colleagues in the medical profession in order that we are viewed as collaborative professionals, rather than intrusive individuals who they may perceive as bothersome and not very helpful. The Committee on Serious and Complex Medical Conditions at the Institute of Medicine (IOM) attempted to provide guidance to facilitate the implementation of their own definition of serious and complex conditions.

COMPLEX PATIENTS

In a 2000 publication whose purpose was to define and then make recommendations to health plans regarding this special population group, the IOM recommended the following language:

> A *serious and complex* condition is one that is persistent and substantially disabling or life threatening that requires treatments and services across a variety of domains of care to ensure the best possible outcomes for each unique patient or member.[1]

The IOM further compiled a listing, which was not meant to be all-inclusive but rather to suggest criteria for some conditions that might be classified as serious and complex. Several of these include the following:

- Conditions that are life threatening, such as cancer, heart disease, stroke, and HIV/AIDS
- Conditions that cause serious disability without necessarily being life threatening, such as stroke, closed head or spinal cord injuries, mental retardation, and congenital malformations
- Conditions that require major commitments of time and effort from caregivers for a substantial period of time, such as mobility disorders, blindness, Alzheimer's disease and other dementias, emphysema, and depression
- Conditions that may require frequent monitoring, including diabetes, severe asthma, schizophrenia, and other psychotic illnesses[2]

There are others, of course, and it's important to acknowledge that while these conditions *may* be serious and complex for *some* patients at *some* points during the course of their disease, they will not necessarily be serious and complex for *all* patients at *all* times.[3]

Most assuredly, this reality shines a very big spotlight on case managers and the distinct value and contributions they make. It also underscores that this area of case management is *patient* specific, unlike other forms of care management (e.g., disease management or population management). The very elements that are recommended to be included in an overall strategy include those from the Case Management Society of America's Standards of Practice:[4] case finding; screening and selection; problem assessment and identification of strengths; development of treatment or care plans; implementation of care plans with emphasis on proactive interventions; and monitoring of care plan outcomes.

The development of a collaborative care management plan is critical to the provision of care for complex patients. The plan itself serves as a road map and a guide to indicate direction and "touch points" or landmarks toward the achievement of goals; it provides a way to measure progress (or lack thereof) and can serve as an opportunity to delineate the responsibilities of the various providers of care.

Although most care managers would ascribe to the aforementioned strategic approach, unfortunately, many of the elements are applied by some of our colleagues in a less than integrated or goal-directed manner. Many would even acknowledge that much of their day is spent "putting out fires" rather than actually *planning*. It is hoped that the attainment of improved outcomes, heightened satisfaction by patients (and their families) and providers, and a more rewarding and meaningful experience for case managers can be achieved by improving the manner, scope, and process of communication.

Case managers who master the art of communicating with physicians can then use their skills to train and empower their patients to also enhance their discussions with their providers. In effect, case managers should strive to broaden the circle of communications to also include patients and their families. They should share with these individuals helpful tips on how to convey their concerns and feelings, and how to resolve their issues. Equally important, care managers should teach their patients and their family members how to carefully listen to what their doctors are saying. Finally, there are nuances in communicating with each physician, and case managers should share those nuances with their patients and family members. For example, some physicians are somewhat controlling and don't appreciate being challenged, others are very patient and willing to listen to every detail, and still others prefer very short, precise information about the patient's experience.

When thoughtful attention is given to the art of communication, then collaboration becomes a more natural result. Both communication and collaboration are essential components and without incorporating these into their day-to-day interventions, care managers working with an older population may find themselves functioning within a vacuum. Unfortunately, however, there are many obstacles to achieving this objective. Age-old stereotypical judgments between nurses, social workers, and more recently the newer profession of care managers and our physician colleagues hinder the process. The continual changing of our roles and responsibilities, combined with the increased pressures to control costs and manage care more efficiently, further hamper the ability for all

these professionals to work in a collaborative manner. Perhaps by examining each of these factors a little more closely, an understanding of what is necessary to move beyond these issues and toward a more collegial relationship can be realized.

STEREOTYPES BECOME REALITY

Physicians and case managers (regardless of their professional discipline) may share mutual goals of wanting the best outcomes for patients and delivering high-quality care. However, their approaches and philosophies are different and not always compatible. Additionally, while the healthcare delivery system has been changing around us, we often are unwilling to change the way we think or operate, believing that what we did in the past was working, so why change it. Physicians, who, for the most part, have been educated and trained to diagnose and treat, tend to be results oriented and generally have limited or episodic involvement with patients. Our physician colleagues tend to value their autonomy and individuality and see themselves as "lone agents of success or failure."[5] It is relatively safe to say that the subject of communication skills is not something that gets a lot of time in medical school. And while we're on the subject of stereotypes, the majority of physicians in years past were men, and even today, this remains true. Gender disparities do influence people's perceptions, even though it may go against the reality of the situation. Studies continue to bear out what we have instinctively known: that women are more effective communicators than men. Case managers, who, for the most part, represent the nurturing professions of social work, nursing, and so on, have had to maintain ongoing relationships with their patients in order to effectively function in their roles. Because there are more women in these nurturing professions one can readily appreciate how the differences in our styles of communication—or even an ability to communicate at all—would become evident as physicians and nurturing professionals attempt to establish effective relationships. Case managers frequently report that meaningful interaction with providers is one of the most challenging aspects of their job.[6]

BARRIERS: AN OVERVIEW

As previously noted, long-held stereotypical judgments and assumptions are certainly barriers in collaborative communication, and there are other obstacles and challenges as well. The healthcare system itself is now a formidable barrier. Churning with change, it is unwittingly pitting healthcare professionals against each other. Despite a common cause (the welfare of patients), physicians and case managers are becoming adversaries in a system where turf battles and territorial struggles are on the rise. With bureaucracy being what it is, physicians view case managers with a wary eye, wondering if treatment will be challenged or the access to care and services for their patients restricted. In addition to issues of care control, there are issues of cost control. Neither group of professionals, physicians or case managers, is accustomed to considering, much less negotiating, the cost of care. The result of this then is that both groups are placed in uncharted territory with minefields abounding.

Another emerging obstacle to address is the increasing rise of consumerism; patients and their case manager advocates are becoming much more actively involved in care decisions. With real-time access to information regarding a multitude of diagnostic conditions, treatment alternatives, and the rating of providers including physicians by score-cards, the physician is no longer the absolute decision maker regarding treatment for patients. The physician is no longer the deity of health. For many geriatric patients this change is both troubling and frightening. These seniors' experiences with health care are rooted in a system where doctors made decisions, advised patients, and told them not to worry. In an increasingly litigious society, physicians have been cautioned to step back from this role. Today, treatment options may be presented often, unfortunately, in all too brief discussions, leaving patients to make their own decisions. Although this may be good risk management for physician practices, it certainly isn't a level playing field for the patient, especially for seniors who may not have access to credible information or are so inundated with conflicting and confusing information that they become overwhelmed. When patients do question prescribed treatment, or come prepared for a physician consultation with printouts from the Internet or marketing ads for the latest pharmaceutical agent or an innovative technological treatment, physicians are not always appreciative and can become abrasive, condescending, or indifferent. We're also quickly changing from a time of physicians who were rarely questioned to the current day, when baby boomers question everything and want answers yesterday!

ADDRESSING THE BARRIERS

Care managers who work with an older population, like everyone in case management, can address both the stereotypes and the stresses of a shifting healthcare system by opening up positive dialogues with physicians. The initial phone call is an example. It is important to communicate the purpose of that call, which is concern for the patient. Certain cases, by nature of their circumstances, may automatically cause a physician to be on guard regarding the case manager's intent. For example, the care manager may be asked to intervene by a family member on behalf of a patient who has been in an acute care setting for 3 weeks and for whom new healthcare settings are being explored. The care manager may also understand that the patient's insurance benefits for rehabilitation or skilled facility services are *very* limited. The care manager needs to relay these concerns to the physician and request his assistance in working together to make the best use of the available dollars so that funds may be available for a longer period of time. The communication is up front and professional, and the care manager's role is clearly defined.

This kind of direct communication should not be confused with taking a militant or overly aggressive attitude. Too often, and especially in the case of more inexperienced individuals, care managers mistakenly believe that in order to validate their roles, they must become confrontational, or worse, use the "purse strings" or benefit dollars to wield control in situations where private insurance is the primary policy. They soon learn, however, that instead of causing physicians to acquiesce, this approach only serves to alienate them.

Because of the changing working relationship between care managers and physicians, the transition to full collaboration is often awkward. Generally, society places physicians as being at the apex of medicine. Buying into this mythical pyramid, nurses, social workers, and other care managers have failed to recognize their own contributions. Caught in their own and others' misperceptions, care managers may not be confident in dealing with physicians and have difficulty assuming anything more than a secondary or tertiary function. The solution to this obviously is not an easy one. Avoidance

of physician contact only continues and increases the problems, because *without* physician involvement, a successful outcome is unlikely. Attaining confidence and competence as a care manager comes from achieving successful outcomes, one case at a time. So, it's the old chicken and the egg dilemma. Which comes first? Overcoming the anxiety that care managers may experience about speaking with physicians may be resolved by self-exploration of the issues and then addressing each of the issues. For instance, a care manager may have a complex patient whose conditions she has minimal familiarity with and on which her experience is dated. Acknowledging one's lack of experience is the first step in addressing this obstacle to effective communication with the treating physician. Acquiring current information may be accomplished through online research, contact with a professional colleague, or relating this to the physician during the initial conversation. We sometimes believe that we need to be experts in everything and agonize over our lack of expertise. There is absolutely nothing wrong in honestly admitting to a physician that, while you've been referred to his patient, you really have not worked with this particular condition in many years, or ever. Use an opening line, such as, "I am really not familiar with your patient's diagnosis of locked-in syndrome and the elements of your treatment plan. Would you explain them further?" This kind of disclosure is far better and more ethically responsible than allowing others to think that you have expertise or experience that you don't. Most physicians are absolutely willing to share their knowledge, especially if this will result in a better outcome for their patients. Of course, it goes without saying that this kind of conversation and information sharing would be better if the call or a personal visit occurred at a time that is considerate of the physician's schedule and work priorities. The care manager might say, "I understand that Dr. Adams is very busy and may not have time to meet with me during her busy office hours. Would it be possible for me to speak with her after her last appointment?" This approach is especially successful if combined with a statement such as, "I met with Mr. Johnson and his family yesterday, and I believe I have some information that would be very helpful to Dr. Adams."

PATIENTS AND FAMILIES CREATE BARRIERS TOO

Let's face it. Patients (and often their families) can be difficult. Within many families, there are issues of sibling rivalry, unresolved family disputes, disparities relating to inheritances and unequal burdens of responsibility for taking care of an infirmed family member due to logistics, time constraints, or simply certain relatives being more or less caring. Despite the best efforts of doctors and case managers, these and other issues can wreak havoc on the patient's treatment plan. Patients will self-diagnose, second-guess, and self-treat their ailments. Those with several medical conditions are understandably confused and, if dementia is also involved, they do not know what constitutes a reportable symptom or which physician would need to hear about it. Additionally, the treatment of a truly sick, medically complex patient is difficult to track. With the increasing involvement of multiple physicians (due to the need for specific expertise as well as increasing concerns for liability) caring for each complex patient, it is not unusual that no one of them functions in the coordinator role. Therefore, if none of them is the coordinator of care, then who is? Enter the care

manager! Even *if* there is an actively involved physician coordinator, all the talent, caring, and expertise of that individual can't ensure that a patient will adhere to the treatment plan when he or she moves from one care setting to another.

Serving as the physician's eyes and ears, we can often share valuable information and insights that will prevent complications from occurring or prevent the abandonment of what would be an effective treatment plan once the patient returns home. Often, the care manager is the only professional who has actually been to the patient's home and knows what may or may not be suitable. As an example, an electric hospital bed, over-bed table, and oxygen equipment will not fit easily into a studio apartment, or might be refused by a daughter caring for her father in her home because she does not want to convert the family room into a "sick room." Care managers can assist greatly with complex, poorly educated, feeble, or noncompliant patients. Often, families are dealing with critical care for the first time, and they only have one opportunity to get it right.[7] Furthermore, many are uninformed or unprepared for what is involved in their loved one's care. For instance, everyone may want to have their ailing mother cared for at home, but once mom is home, no one realized just how much juggling of schedules and lives would be necessary and that maybe the mother would be better served in another setting. The care manager can help them understand all of the options and the various ramifications of each so that the best decision can be made. Care managers should also advise their patient's physicians that they are assuming the role of "communicator" and impart to their medical colleagues that this intervention will promote greater patient compliance with their treatment plans and, ultimately, help enhance outcomes.

COMMUNICATING WITH PHYSICIANS

As experienced professionals, we assume that we are also experienced in the art of communication, especially when this occurs with those within our field. We share so much—similar jargon, a desire to help, codes of conduct, standard of practice—and yet despite the similarities, there *are* distinct differences. Unfortunately, as with everything else in life, routine tasks, such as communication, can, over time, become less than effective. Fortunately, there are solutions that are easy to implement into a case manager's practice and that greatly enhance relationships with physicians *and* increase the potential for successful patient outcomes. Through personal and professional experience and those of other colleagues in case management, the following practical steps are offered:

- Develop an understanding of the physician's practice setting. If the doctor is a surgeon, calls in the morning may not be best. Determine the best time to call and the best contact person within the physician's office. If there is a nurse available, often the nurse can obtain an answer if a question is properly framed.
- Act like a professional. Have business cards presenting credentials and professional stationery. When leaving a telephone number for a return call, make certain that phones are answered professionally or if an answering machine is used, have a message that conveys a professional image. It amazes me that some professionals who work from home have a one-size-fits-all message like, "Hi, you've reached Sally, Bob, Suzie, and Jimmy too. Leave a message and we'll get back to you." Have a separate business line, and if using a voice message system, assure the caller that this is a confidential line: "Hello, you've reached the office of Sara James, geriatric care manager and my confidential voice mail. Kindly leave a message and I will return the call as soon as possible."
- Attend physician hospital visits or office visits and note that this is being done at the patient's request and with his or her approval. It underscores professional dedication and provides the opportunity to make direct inquiries and ask, "How can I help you?"
- Confirm all your appointments. Emergencies do arise.
- When attending in-person meetings, express appreciation for the time, which is a highly valued commodity for every professional.
- If in-person meetings aren't possible, make it easier for physicians to provide the information needed. Develop a questionnaire requesting information *specific* to the patient, have it typed, and provide a stamped, self-addressed envelope. Don't forget a signed release from the patient. Additionally, in order to enhance a prompt response, avoid asking for comprehensive reports that may need to be dictated and/or prepared by an assistant. Ask open-ended questions to elicit more information beyond a *yes* or *no*, and leave enough space in between questions to encourage a handwritten response (and then hope for legibility).
- Get to know the local physicians in the community, and develop a good relationship with a support person in each office. Remember his or her name, and use it during subsequent calls.
- Don't trust your memory; make notes during your conversation. Working with multiple patients and multiple physicians,

particularly with similar diagnostic conditions or within the same age groups, can result in a certain amount of similarities. Avoid confusing these important details.

- Send a thank-you note following a personal visit or particularly thoughtful response during phone conversations or questionnaire responses. This kind of acknowledgment and expression of appreciation of time and expertise can make a big impact, and it's vital in building relationships.

- Call to share patient information that the physician would want/need to know. It conveys your care and concern for your shared patient and projects you as a collaborative colleague. Asking, "How can I help you with Mr. Johnson?" defines it still further.[7]

- Practice diplomacy, and try to handle problems in an ethically and morally responsible manner. You may discover that one of the medications prescribed by the physician is having an adverse reaction when taken in combination with another medication. Or, you may discover that the patient has forgotten to mention a medication that he or she has been on for 10 years. Present the situation or problems calmly and professionally, without placing blame, and remember your goal (and presumably the physician's as well) is to correct the problem and obtain a better outcome.

CONCLUSION

Communication, although it is something we do every day, is as much a skill as it is an art. When involving the care of complex and often medically fragile geriatric patients, our ability to be successful is exponentially related to the results or outcomes we can achieve on their behalf. The subtle nuances, strategic approaches, and the caring heart of a case manager can greatly increase the potential for success.

REFERENCES

1. Institute of Medicine. *Definition of Serious and Complex Medical Conditions.* Washington, DC: National Academy Press; 1999.

2. Institute of Medicine. *Definition of Serious and Complex Medical Conditions.* Washington, DC: National Academy Press; 1999.

3. Mullahy CM, Jensen D. *The Case Manager's Handbook.* 3rd ed. Sudbury, MA: Jones and Bartlett; 2004.

4. Case Management Society of America. *Standards of Practice for Case Management.* Little Rock, AR: Case Management Society of America; 2002.

5. Berwick DM. Sounding board: Continuous improvement as an ideal in health care. *N Engl J Med.* 1989; 320, 53–56.

6. Pacala JT, et al. *Case Management in Health Maintenance Organizations: A Final Report.* Washington, DC: Group Health Foundation; 1995.

7. Cress, CJ. *Handbook of Geriatric Care Management.* 2nd ed. Sudbury, MA: Jones and Bartlett; 2007.

Care Managers Working with Aging Family Issues

CHAPTER 3

Working with Long-Distance Families: Tools the Care Manager Can Use

Julie Menack

The number of Americans that provide care to an aging family member (typically defined as 50 and older) is estimated to be approximately 34 million.[1] Recent studies indicate that approximately 15% of those caregivers are living an hour or more away from this person,[2,3] with estimates of the number of long-distance caregivers between 5.1 and 7 million.[4,5] Geographic mobility of adult children and retirement-age parents has resulted in this situation. Of the long-distance caregivers, one third live 1 to 2 hours away, and the remaining two thirds live greater than 2 hours away.[6] The National Institute for Nursing Research (NINR) has stated[7] that "one third of informal caregiving occurs at a distance with family members coordinating provision of care, maintenance of independence, and socialization for frail elders living at home."

The challenges of caring for an aging family member are already great; living at a distance can make care provision a complex and difficult challenge, particularly in a crisis situation. According to a recent study of long-distance caregiving by the MetLife Mature Market Institute:[8]

Large geographic distances—and even the time it takes to travel across a big city with congestion and snarled traffic—can add unique and complicated challenges to what is already an often emotion-laden and stressful job: helping a family member whose health and well-being are deteriorating.[9]

Long-distance caregiving poses unique challenges in "assessing the needs of the care receiver and knowing when our help is needed."[10] This is particularly true of the situation where the older adult is experiencing a gradual decline that may not be evident from a distance.

The care manager can help to prepare and empower geographically separated families by providing the following services:

- Can provide assistance on a one-time basis or can provide ongoing assistance depending on the needs of the family and availability of other resources to assist with care planning and monitoring
- Can assess the needs of the care recipient and locate, arrange for, and monitor services as either a one-time service or on an ongoing basis
- Is an expert regarding local resources and knows how to advocate for quality care
- Can provide individual attention to the care recipient
- Can provide regular reports that keep track of all of the caregiving issues
- Can communicate with the family and help them define their concerns and set realistic goals for the future
- Can share any concerns or changes with the long-distance caregiver that might need intervention and can visit as frequently as the long-distance caregiver requests

• Can visit so that the long-distance care-giver does not need to travel for every event, both emergency and nonemergency, reducing the burden of day-to-day care

An important job for the care manager is to identify the long-distance caregivers who live in their own area. Care managers who live in the same location as the long-distance care-giver can share tools and techniques for long-term planning, recommend how to find a care manager in the care recipient's location, and can assist the long-distance caregiver to fa-cilitate moving the care recipient to the long-distance caregiver's location, if needed.

This chapter describes the issues associated with the long-distance caregiver and provides suggestions and tools for the care manager to support the long-distance caregiver.

DEFINITION OF LONG-DISTANCE CAREGIVER

Studies of long-distance caregiving typi-cally define the *long-distance caregiver* as a person who resides at least 1 hour or more away from the care recipient and provides at least some care.[10–13] Parker and others de-fine "distant caregiver" as anyone:

• Who provides informal, unpaid care to a person experiencing some degree of phys-ical, mental, emotional, or economic im-pairment that limits independence and necessitates assistance
• Who experiences caregiving complications because of geographic distance from the care recipient, as determined by distance, travel time, travel costs, personal mobility problems, limited transportation, and other related factors that affect the caregiver's access to the care recipient[14]

This definition does not specify the dis-tance the caregiver is from the care recipi-ent, but focuses on the caregiving experience, and is therefore an excellent working defi-nition for the purposes of this chapter.

LONG-DISTANCE CAREGIVER LITERATURE

The 21st century has brought a virtual ex-plosion of self-help literature geared toward the long-distance caregiver. All of this infor-mation can be useful for the care manager in developing a work practice to support this population. A partial list of this literature is provided in Exhibit 3-1. The first and only book geared specifically toward long-distance caregivers was published in 1993 by Heath.[15] It is still very useful but does not contain information about resources that are Web based or about the vast number of tech-nologies that been developed since the date of publication. There are also several useful stand-alone pamphlet-sized resource informa-tion guides that provide checklists and tips for long-distance caregivers.[16–19] There are also Web-based organizations geared toward care-givers. One in particular, Caring From a Distance (CFAD) is geared toward the long-distance caregiver and provides many case ex-amples, links, an online support community, and recommended activities.[20]

There have been several studies of long-distance caregivers that provide information on demographics and long-distance caregiver needs and experiences.[21–27] A review of the practice literature for work with distant care-givers indicates that there are only a few ar-ticles in professional journals and chapters in books geared toward professionals that provide information on recommended prac-tice guidelines for work with long-distance caregivers.[28–33] One video[34] is available that provides practice guidelines on how to work with long-distance families. This video rec-ommends a number of techniques that the care manager can use including helping the

Exhibit 3-1 Self-Help Literature for Long-Distance Caregivers

---

Books

Heath A. *Long Distance Caregiving: A Survival Guide for Far Away Caregivers.* Lakewood, CO: American Source Books; 1993.

Pamphlets

AARP. *Miles Away and Still Caring: A Guide for Long Distance Caregivers.* Washington, DC: AARP; 1986.

Met Life Mature Market Institute. *Since You Care: Long-Distance Caregiving.* 2005. Available at: http://www.metlife.com/Applications/Corporate/WPS/CDA/PageGenerator/0,4132,P8900,00.html. Accessed June 15, 2007.

National Institute on Aging. *So Far Away: Twenty Questions for Long-Distance Caregivers.* NIH Publication No. 06-5496. Washington, DC: National Institutes of Health; 2006.

Roschbau D, van Steenberg C. *Handbook for Long-Distance Caregivers. An Essential Guide for Families and Friends Caring for Ill or Elderly Loved Ones.* San Francisco, CA: Family Caregiver Alliance National Center on Caregiving; 2003. Available at: http://www.caregiver.org/caregiver/jsp/content_node.jsp?nodeid=1-34. Accessed June 15, 2007.

Web Sites

Caring From a Distance (CFAD): http://www.cfad.org

Children of Aging Parents (CAPS): http://www.caps4caregivers.org

Family Caregiver Alliance: http://www.caregiver.org

National Alliance for Caregiving: http://www.caregiving.org

National Family Caregivers Association: http://www.nfcares.org/

Working Caregiver: http://www.workingcaregiver.com

---

family to get along and the steps that the care manager can take to work with the family and monitor the older adult. This video can be used for training care managers and increasing awareness of the issues of distance.

WHAT MAKES LONG-DISTANCE CAREGIVING DIFFERENT?

It is very common for family members to live in different cities and states. Ours is a mobile society and often both parents and children have moved away from where the family was raised. Sometimes the parent moves to a distant retirement community in a warmer or more appealing climate such as Arizona or Florida. Adult children move frequently with their jobs. Despite the fact that the geographically close family members typically provide the most care, there is still evidence that those who live at a distance provide essential support.[35]

Studies report that long-distance caregivers live an average of between 304 and 450 miles away and spend an average of 4 to 7.23 hours traveling one-way from the care recipient.[36,37] Nearly 50% of long-distance caregivers report that they devote one full work day a week to managing their loved one's needed services, and almost 75% indicated they were spending 22 hours per month providing care.[38] The economic value of all caregiving in the United States has been recently estimated to be approximately $350 billion per year.[39]

Distance is a key or primary factor in determining the role of the family member in a caregiving situation. For long-distance caregivers who are not primary caregivers, the intensity of the caregiver role decreases with distance.[40,41] Geographic distance hinders men more than women from providing care,[42] yet men are more likely than women to be long-distance caregivers because more women live with or near their parent.[43] For all long-distance caregivers, the number of yearly visits decreases significantly with greater distance from the care recipient. In addition, the distance apart determines the nature and type of assistance provided.[44] Military families are a population where typical concerns are made more complex by "relocations, frequent deployments, and other duty commands that may make it difficult for the military member (or family member) to react to an emergency situation or to respond to more chronic problems that require sustained assistance."[45]

Long-distance caregivers manage the care situation with the help of others, primarily relatives.[46] About half report that they provide care as a helper to others, and 23% report that they are the only caregiver. Relatives comprise 83% of the help being provided to long-distance caregivers: nearly one third are helped the most by a sibling who lives near the care recipient, while about 29% report that a relative or other sibling helps with most of the care. Others who help include the caregiver's spouse (20%), the care recipient's spouse (1%), other long-distance caregivers (8%), friends (4%), paid caregivers (4%), or other persons (9%).

The complications experienced by long-distance caregivers[47] make an already difficult job even more difficult. One major challenge is determining whether what is heard long-distance and about the "parent matches the reality of the situation."[48] Older adults often successfully use "geographic privacy" to hide their condition, or alternatively, reports by the older adult or local friends and family may exaggerate the situation. Some unique challenges of long-distance caregiving include[49]:

- Assessing the needs of the care receiver and knowing when help is needed from a distance can be difficult.
- Once the need for assistance has been identified, locating services and monitoring them can be problematic.
- Health professionals sometimes disregard the caregiver's opinions because they are out of town.
- Family relationships may become strained by caregiving responsibilities: often, local siblings resent out-of-town siblings for not doing more, and long-distance caregiving can be difficult when there are no local family members.
- Costs of travel and long-distance calls to assess the needs and arrange for care and time away from work can cause strain.
- The long-distance caregiver experiences emotional burdens of anxiety and guilt for not being as available as they feel they should be.

The care manager should keep in mind that long-distance caregivers may only be able to visit their parents during evenings, weekends, or holidays. Solomon[50] recommends that professionals should make an effort to be available when the long-distance caregiver is available, even if it is during time traditionally considered personal.

WHO ARE THE LONG-DISTANCE CAREGIVERS AND CARE RECIPIENTS?

Long-distance caregivers profiled in published studies are by and large well educated, affluent, and married.[51–54] Table 3-1 summarizes the primary characteristics of long-distance caregivers.

According to many studies, long-distance caregivers are primarily women,[55,56] whereas

Table 3-1 Profile of Typical Long-Distance Caregiver

	Wagner, 1997	*MetLife, 2004*	*NAC and AARP, 2004*	*Watari et al., 2006*	*Koerin and Harrigan, 2002*
Sex	54% female	58% male		78% female	56% female
Mean age (years)	46	51	18% 35–49 15% 50–64	52	42
Marital status	66% married	Almost 75% married		74% married	65% married
Race/ ethnicity	82% white 8% black 4% Hispanic 7% other	95.5% Caucasian		81% Caucasian	32% white 34% Asian 22% Hispanic 12% black
Income	$54,240 average household income	Affluent— 50% income $75,000 or higher	Upper income (19% of those earning $100,000+)		32% >$50,000/ year
Education	58% college or graduate degree 48% high school graduate or some college	70% college or graduate degree	23% college educated	65% college or graduate degree 26% high school graduate or some college	52% college or graduate degree 38% high school graduate or some college
Care recipient relationship to caregiver	55% parent or in-law 11% grand-parent 5% adult child 2% sibling 10% friend 15% other			68% parent 28% other relative 3% friend	66% parent or in-law 18% grand-parent 7% aunt/uncle 5% nonrelative or friend
Employment status	64% full-time 8% part-time 29% not employed	62% full-time 18% part-time	63% full-time		71% employed: 54% full-time 16.5% part-time
Mean household income	$54,240				18% > $75K 14% $50–75K 19% $30–50K 40% < $30K
Distance/ travel time from care recipient	304 miles and 4 hours away	450 miles and 7.23 hours away			

continues

Table 3-1 Profile of Typical Long-Distance Caregiver (continued)

	Wagner, 1997	MetLife, 2004	NAC and AARP, 2004	Watari et al., 2006	Koerin and Harrigan, 2002
How became LD caregiver	48% gradual worsening of chronic condition 30% sudden acute illness/ accident				
Financial contribution	$196/month	$392/month on travel and other out-of-pocket expenses			
Caregiver for how long?	5 years				5.22 years
Primary caregiver, secondary caregiver, share 50/50, only caregiver?	21% primary 49% secondary 31% 50/50 6% only	23% primary	11% primary		10.5% primary 68.4% secondary 21.1% 50/50
Estimated amount of time providing help		Almost 50% spending equivalent of one day per week Nearly 75% helping with IADLs and spending 22 hrs/month			48% 1–3 hours/wk 22% 4–8 hours/wk 30% 10+ hours/wk

From: Wagner, 1997, MetLife, 2004, NAC and AARP, 2004, Watari et al., 2006, and Koerin and Harrigan, 2002.

others[57,58] indicate that there are more men in this role. The average age is between about 46 and 51, they are primarily Caucasian, and between 62% and 70% are employed. Nearly one fourth reported that they were the only or primary caregiver.

Table 3-2 summarizes the primary characteristics of the typical long-distance care recipient who is female, in her late 70s to mid-80s, is married and living with her spouse who may also require assistance. In 1997, 20% of long-distance caregivers reported caring for a person with Alzheimer's or some other form of dementia.[59] This number increased to nearly one third of long-distance caregivers by 2004.[60]

Table 3-2 Profile of Typical Long-Distance Care Recipient

	Wagner, 1997	*Koerin and Harrigan, 2002*	*MetLife, 2004*	*Watari et al., 2006*
Sex	Female (64%)		Female (56%)	Female (67%)
Mean age (years)	78	78	89	79
Marital situation	Married			
Living situation	30% with spouse 30% lives alone 21% nursing home 7% lives w/ sibling 5% group setting (retirement home/assisted living) 2% with friend	56% with another family member/ friend 21% alone in own home 16% apartment or retirement community 5% assisted living 2% nursing home 1% boarding/ group home	35% alone 24% with spouse 13% with another relative 14% nursing home 10% assisted living facility 4% retirement community	40% with spouse 24% alone (more likely to live alone than local care recipients) 19% facility 18% paid caregiver 7% adult child
Income	20% not enough 25% just enough 34% just enough plus a little 20% more than enough			More likely to have a pension than local care recipients
Health condition	1% excellent 12% good 46% fair 41% poor	67% chronic 16% short term 12% both	45% fair 33% poor If living with spouse, ½ spouses also in fair or poor health	Alzheimer's or other dementia
Alzheimer's or dementia	Always: 19% Frequently: 17% Sometimes: 32%	11%	Nearly one third	100%

From: Wagner, 1997, MetLife, 2004, Watari et al., 2006, and Koerin and Harrigan, 2002.

WHAT IS THE EFFECT OF LONG-DISTANCE CAREGIVING?

Providing care at a distance can be stressful in different ways from that for a proximate caregiver: distance can result in a significant drain on emotions, finances, and time. Long-distance caregivers experience uncertainty and guilt due to their inability to provide more care,[61] and financial difficulty and stress can result from taking time off from work to travel long distances. Studies show that long-distance caregivers exhibit more emotional and physical illness, overwhelm, mental health problems, including depression and anxiety, and physical problems such as a weakened immune system.[62] Symptoms of caregiver overload that the care manager should look out for include sleep disorder, marital problems, reduced employment, depression, guilt, anxiety, physical problems, and fatigue.

Contributing to the financial drain of long-distance caregiving are the costs of travel, long-distance telephone, hired help, and missed work. The cost of long-distance caregiving in 2007 was estimated to be higher than for other caregivers—an average of $8728 per year for long-distance caregivers versus an average of $5500 for all caregivers.[63] In addition to financial costs, there is the cost of time. Between 60% and 80% of long-distance caregivers work.[64,65] These employed long-distance caregivers are often required to make significant adjustments to work to accommodate their caregiving responsibilities.[66] Work adjustments are more likely to result in coming in late or leaving early, missing work days, rearranging their work schedule, and the use of unpaid leave in contrast to local caregivers, who are more likely to be able to come in late and leave early from their jobs. According to one study,[67] long-distance caregivers missed an average of 20 hours of work per month. When the long-distance caregiver is the only care provider, they must additionally turn down work-related travel and often lose work-related benefits. Many long-distance caregivers must reduce from full-time to part-time work, give up work entirely, turn down promotions, or choose early retirement.[68] Some long-distance caregivers who are in the military choose to retire or resign.[69]

Long-distance caregivers often feel like they are neglecting their job, spouse, and children when caring for their loved one, and then when they are at home, they feel that they are neglecting their parents. Donna

Schempp,[70] program director of the Family Caregiver Alliance in San Francisco, suggests that the emotions typically associated with family caregivers are taken to a whole new level when distance is a factor. Because the long-distance caregiver is not present on the scene does not mean that he or she does not experience feelings. While emotions including feeling out of control, guilt, ambivalence, and helplessness are an attribute of all caregivers, they are particularly powerful feelings for those at a distance. They experience guilt for not being there with their loved one and for having their own life. Long-distance caregivers may be very demanding of the care manager because they are dealing with their own issues related to "not being perfect." At the same time, they experience ambivalence about a variety of issues, such as getting involved with their parents, not being there, how much to be there, and hiring someone else to do their job. Due to their inability to be present on a daily basis, there are questions about how things are going with the care recipient. Schempp states that it is especially important for the professional to acknowledge these feelings and to build trust so that the long-distance caregiver can be more productive and less stressed.

Schempp also reported that the family dynamics involving long-distance caregivers are unique. When the only caregiver is at a distance, it is important to determine how he or she will communicate and allocate who is supervising the care. When there are both long-distance and local caregivers, the long-distance caregiver needs to learn how to support the parent and participate in the division of labor and decision making. In both cases, it is up to the care manager, if one has been hired, to keep the long-distance caregiver informed. Frequent conference calls to all family members is the best way to do this. That way, everyone hears the same thing at the same time.

WHAT PRECIPITATES NEED FOR A LONG-DISTANCE CAREGIVER AND FOR CARE MANAGEMENT?

A change in conditions can result in a new complex situation requiring the need for the long-distance caregiver to seek out a care manager. The adult child who has not thought about caregiving at all is all of a sudden thrust into the role of caregiver to the parent who lives far away. The precipitating situation might be where the long-distance caregiver made regular monthly visits to their parent(s) and was able to comfortably help them manage their affairs. Then, either suddenly or over time, the primary caregiver either passes away or develops cognitive or physical disabilities and can no longer take care of the other partner who has memory problems. Or, a neighbor reports that the parent is exhibiting signs of not being able to take care of him- or herself. Often, when there is no local family, friends perform some of the roles usually handled by family members. These helpers perform a more limited range of assistance—when there is need for daily household chores or personal care, the family is typically called upon.[71] The exact situation does not matter—the issue is that the situation is now out of control, adding a huge responsibility to the long-distance caregiver's often already overloaded schedule. Various situations that can precipitate long-distance caregiving are described in the publication "So Far Away: Twenty Questions for Long-Distance Caregivers."[72]

Whether the long-distance caregiver is the primary decision maker or helps others, support from family members and friends is key. In recent studies, only 5% to 10% of long-distance caregivers paid for services. Of those who paid for services, women reported spending an average of $751 per month compared to men who spend an average of $490

per month.[73] One significant finding is that paid helpers were most important to the small proportion of long-distance caregivers (5%) who reported that they were the only caregiver.[74] This small group needs access to and information about formal services and might, therefore, be most effectively supported by access to care management.

HOW CAN CARE MANAGERS HELP LONG-DISTANCE CAREGIVERS?

The long-distance caregiver has specific caregiving needs and stressors, so it is essential to design services to provide appropriate support.[75] Care managers can sort through options, help make decisions, and assist with planning and organization.[76,77] Long-distance caregivers need advice regarding decision making, financial assistance, and making arrangements with family members, friends, and neighbors.[78] The special needs of long-distance caregivers include physical assistance with ADLs, companionship, and housekeeping help.[79] There is also a need for information about the care recipient's disease process (e.g., Alzheimer's) and local services or resources.[80]

Long-distance caregivers have also been found to require assistance with family issues. Family disagreement about care is an important factor, as there is "evidence of tensions, rivalries, and communication difficulties between near and distant siblings."[81] Assistance and support may be needed if the long-distance caregiver does not agree with decisions being made by the local primary caregiver.[82] Often, long-distance siblings may hold an idealized view of how care should be provided when the local sibling is dealing with the realities of the parent's situation.[83] As described in other chapters in this book, conflict and perceptions of unfairness in the division of labor between siblings are fairly typical situations even under the best of circumstances. Getting some assistance with an expert family consultant can be beneficial to resolve differences of opinion between the local and long-distance caregivers or to reduce resistance to the long-distance caregiver's help by the primary caregiver or care recipient.[84] The professional also needs to provide the long-distance caregiver with tools for communicating with the care recipient.[85] The long-distance caregiver also needs help managing their own family and work situation; they are often sandwiched between needs of children, spouses, work, and caregiving.

When long-distance caregivers were asked how much formal planning siblings have done to meet parents' needs, how distant siblings view the division of labor, how they view their other siblings' caregiving activities, and how parental caregiving has influenced relationships with other siblings, they reported that they would benefit from the following types of professional assistance[86]:

- "Facilitate family discussion of needs, resources, and division of labor."
- Recommend "proactive preparation and family cooperation in formulating realistic plans" . . . develop a "realistic parent-care plan."
- "Assess strengths and weaknesses of all of the potential caregivers, and help siblings resolve conflicts about care decisions."
- "Help siblings understand one another's strengths and limitations so that they can act together in the best interest of the parent."
- Help put supports "in place to decrease the tension between hometown and long-distance siblings . . . e-mail and regular phone calls (including conference calls), and developing care plans and schedules to improve communication."

- Help "them deal with guilt and frustration that may result from their inability to provide more of the day-to-day care."
- Provide "thoughtful planning in advance of a crisis . . . help families think through alternatives for when parents are no longer able to handle all their needs independently."

For the relatives of individuals with dementia who live in a retirement community care setting, three of the four most commonly identified family caregiving activities can be conducted remotely: coordinating services (78%), emotional support (67%), and managing finances and paperwork (56%).[87] In addition, caregivers reported providing 17 hours per week of assistance before working with a care manager and an average of 6 afterward—a decrease of 65%. After working with a care manager, the caregivers were less stressed overall. They were less afraid their health would suffer, less worried about doing enough, more confident in finding ways to manage the situation, and could better see new problems as opportunities to find creative solutions.[88]

CARE MANAGER PROVIDES ASSESSMENT AND CARE PLANNING

The care manager can help the long-distance caregiver by doing what he or she does best: use the care manager toolbox to evaluate the problem and make recommendations. If a long-distance caregiver has concerns, the care manager will initially conduct psychosocial and functional assessments and assess the needs of the family. The process of geriatric assessment and care planning is described in *Handbook of Geriatric Care Management*.[89] As stated elsewhere in this book, at the time of initial assessment, the care manager should determine how the family, including the long-distance caregiver, defines their responsibilities to the older parent. The caregiver assessment can identify which responsibilities family members see as their own to perform and what they expect and would like to be done for them. If the care manager finds what appears to be a decline in thinking and reasoning on the part of the care recipient or caregiver(s), the initial assessments can be supplemented with a mental status questionnaire and a recommendation for further assessment of cognitive function, if necessary.

The assessment should provide a clear picture of the entire family's situation so that the family can identify and act on all options. If the family wishes, the care manager can prepare a written care plan that incorporates tasks for both local caregivers and long-distance caregivers as well as local resources from the continuum of care. The family along with the care manager can decide who should complete each task, either a family member or the care manager. This will be designated on the care plan, which is shared with all parties, including the care recipient, if appropriate.

According to Solomon,[90] "Even when there is geographic distance between them, elderly parents and their adult children are best equipped through their shared knowledge of family history and dynamics to decide the direction of the treatment plan." She goes on to say that *especially* when there is geographic distance, the worker should present family members the range of viable alternative care plans. The literature suggests that proximity is not as critical in decision making as it is in daily care. The care recipient, long-distance caregiver, and care manager can then select and prioritize care options and develop contingency plans.

HELP THE LONG-DISTANCE CAREGIVER PREPARE BEFORE THERE IS A NEED

Self-help literature geared toward long-distance caregivers commonly recommends that "The best time to establish your support network is before you need it. That way you'll be able to act quickly when a problem arises."[91] In addition, recent research shows that the worry and anxiety of long-distance caregivers who cannot easily visit their elderly parents are significantly reduced when they are satisfied with a realistic "parent-care plan" that is prepared proactively.[92,93] Getting advance support is one of the best things that care managers can do to support the long-distance caregiver to prepare for the unforeseen. In that light, smart care managers develop their business in a way that can support long-distance caregivers both living in their own community and those caring for local parents from far away. The care manager should help families to plan ahead and recognize that they should not wait for an emergency to identify available options. With this in mind, the care manager can support the long-distance caregiver at whatever location is most convenient—either near the long-distance caregiver's home or at a location where it is convenient to monitor the care recipient. The care manager can help the family to do the following:

- Work through the various what-if scenarios so that they can do some contingency planning in the event that funds run out, level of care increases, or availability of family is limited. Also investigate the resources that are available for hospitalization, skilled nursing care, rehabilitation, assisted living, respite, and home care.
- Determine which facilities they would want to consider and which ones they would not want their parents to enter.[94]

- Select a primary caregiver who will typically either be physically closest or the most trusted member of the family.
- Determine how the rest of the caregiving burden will be divided, and identify the caregiving team, both local and distant, who are in regular contact with their loved one.[95]
- Devise a plan for caregiving team communication.

One intervention program that focuses on advance planning, the Parent Care Readiness (PCR) program, was developed and tested in both military settings where the adult children are typically long-distance caregivers as well as by faith-based organizations.[96] The first step of the PCR program is to conduct a detailed assessment that helps to identify and prioritize parent-care tasks. The tasks of

parent care are organized into four domains: medical; legal, financial, and insurance; family and social; and spiritual and emotional, as shown in Figure 3-1. The entire landscape of caregiving tasks is provided in a 50-item PCR assessment summarized in Table 3-3. Each domain in the assessment "reflects a set of real-life challenges (specific parent tasks) that potentially makes up an important aspect of a parent's care plan."[97]

The PCR assessment helps the caregiver prioritize caregiving tasks: the results of the assessment are linked to "prescriptions," which include guidance and resources to help caregivers complete high-priority tasks. The PCR process should be supervised by practitioners who can help the caregivers with the completion of tasks. There can be a gradual approach to the tasks that are more difficult. One benefit of this type of planning is that it

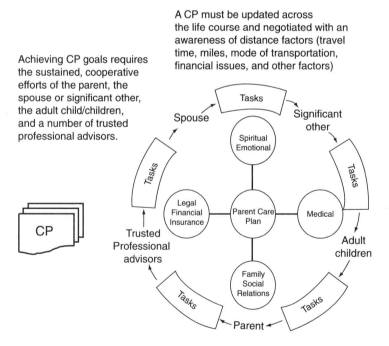

Figure 3–1 Model for Developing and Sustaining a Comprehensive Care Plan

Source: Martin JA, Parker M. Understanding the importance of elder care preparations in the context of 21st century military service. *GCM Journal.* 2003;Winter:3–6.

Table 3-3 Parent-Care Categories and Sample Associate Tasks

Legal-Financial Tasks	Medical Tasks	Social-Familial Tasks	Spiritual-Emotional Tasks
Discuss with parents the need to complete each of the following documents related to estate dispersion and management, advance directives, etc.	Discuss with your parents how involved or knowledgeable s/he would like you to be about their health, medications, and functional status.	Together with your spouse clarify your own values about where parents' care fits with your other life responsibilities.	Make "peace" with your parents.
Estate Dispersion: • Will • Joint Ownership & Tenancy • Trust/Revocable living trust • Durable Power of Attorney • Preferred possession list	Obtain access to results of comprehensive geriatric assessment.	Assess your relationship with your parents, siblings, and other relatives who would be an acceptable and realistic resource for your parents' care.	Secure a video or oral history from your parents.
Advance Directives: • Health care proxy • Do not resuscitate orders • Living will	Log information acquired from medical appointments.	Convene a family conference to formulate plans. Address who can and will do what, when, and how for your parents.	Investigate the nature of religious programs for seniors available for your parents in their home community.
Secure accessible location of legal documents.	Compile a list of parents' healthcare providers and telephone numbers.	Know the name, address, e-mail, and phone number of three people who live near your parents and who you could telephone if required.	Establish an active spiritual life with your parents.
Rule out legal dependency of parents as a way to secure medical and treatment options.	Compile a list of your parents' current medications and obtain a copy of current medical records.	Develop a plan that would allow your parents to remain safely in their home and a plan that includes a move to another location if this becomes necessary.	Identify your parents' wishes for funeral and burial or cremation. If pre-need plans have been made, locate the documentation.
Assist parents in identifying assets, liabilities, income, and expenses.	Verify that primary care doctor or pharmacist is monitoring medications.	Discuss with your parent the possibility of a "panic" button service.	Have a reliable point of contact with at least one member of your parents' church, synagogue, mosque, or religious organization.
Check parents' social security care for accuracy and review parents' credit history (and make sure they have access to joint or separate credit).	Maintain a list of local emergency service providers (addresses, telephone numbers).	Understand long-term care options available in your parents' home community (living options, in and out of home services).	Encourage your parents to complete a codicil to their will that represents what s(he) would like to say to the next generation.
Investigate the costs of long-term care scenarios (e.g., long-term care insurance, savings).	Compile a list of services and programs that encourage successful aging practices and suggest appropriate parental involvement.	Evaluate the safety of your parents' home situation (falls, isolation, scams), and employ appropriate strategies to increase safety.	Understand hospice and palliative care so as to assist your parents in the death and dying process if it becomes necessary.
Determine the full extent of your parents' health/life insurance coverage, as well as Medicare and Medicaid entitlements.	Identify signs that indicate your parents cannot live independently.	Discuss the feasibility of a driving assessment.	Encourage your parents' spirituality.

Source: Used with permission from Dennis Myers, Baylor University.

can help the care recipients get used to the idea that they need to plan and that caregivers are available to help them if needed.

CARE MANAGER PROVIDES ONGOING MONITORING

If there is no local caregiver, the care manager can take on a new role by connecting with the care recipient to provide ongoing services. Care monitoring as described in *Handbook of Geriatric Care Management* includes monitoring the client to measure change.[98] Ongoing services can include:

1. Regular client visits on a weekly or monthly basis to check on the care recipient and reevaluate their changing needs so that the right care is provided.
2. Accompanying clients to important appointments, such as for medical, financial, or legal support.
3. Arrange for or provide transportation for the care recipient.
4. Hire and supervise home care staff or locate housing.
5. Provide regular weekly or monthly status reports to the family of the care recipient's status.
6. Be on call for emergencies.

CARE MANAGER PROVIDES PRINT AND INTERNET RESOURCES

A typical long-distance caregiver experiences "information overload" from the vast amount of information available. Caregivers turn first to the Internet for health information (29%), followed by consultation with doctors (28%), family or friends (15%), and other health professionals (10%).[99] Of the caregivers who use the Internet, 41% are long-distance caregivers who live an hour or more away from the care recipient. Nearly 90% look for health information, more than

half seek information about services available for care recipients, and 40% look for support or advice from other caregivers. More than 33% seek help with information about balancing work and caregiving responsibilities.

Because it is unlikely that caregivers will be able to sort out all of the practical information that is available, one service the care manager can provide is to recommend and supply one or more of these resources. The care manager can recommend practical information designed to support long-distance caregivers such as self-help books, pamphlets, and Web sites (see Exhibit 3-1), many of which are available online. There are also several Web sites and organizations that have recently sprung up devoted solely to supporting this community.

These resources typically provide the long-distance caregiver with "survival" tips on how to take care of an aging friend or family member interspersed with stories of long-distance caregivers. Tips typically include creating a long-distance support system, planning the visit, and developing a care plan. In this way, the long-distance caregiver learns that they are not alone with their concerns and will be better prepared for the care manager's recommendations. These resources often recommend hiring a professional care manager, suggest how to find one, and provide guidelines on questions to ask.[100–103]

One such organization, Caregiving From a Distance (CFAD),[104] was developed by and for long-distance caregivers and has an extensive Web site designed specifically to assist the long-distance caregiver. The site has a library that is rich with information on topics pertinent to long-distance caregiving, and it provides links that have been reviewed and established to be useful to long-distance caregivers, as searching the Web for help can be overwhelming. The CFAD Web site provides an online "family folder" that is a secure place where important information about the care recipient's medical history, community support services, and other pertinent information can be stored.

The care manager can suggest that the long-distance caregiver utilize guidelines and criteria for evaluating health and consumer information on the Internet such as are available from the Setting Priorities for Retirement Years (SPRY) Foundation[105] and CFAD.[106] Some Web pages from reputable organizations provide ratings or can serve as a filter; in this way, the long-distance caregiver can find reliable and current content on important topics. Examples of those include the links page on the CFAD Web site http://www.cfad.org/links/index.cfm and Web pages for services for seniors and family caregivers that have been rated by an organization called "Senior Approved Services" (http://seniors-approve.com/).

CARE MANAGER HELPS LONG-DISTANCE CAREGIVER MAKE THE MOST OF A VISIT

The care manager can help long-distance caregivers plan their "care commute" to make the most of each visit.[107] The purpose of the visit should first be determined. Will this visit be to serve as respite for the primary caregiver, for information collection, or another purpose? How long should the visit be? How frequent? The long-distance caregiver should keep in mind the potential for their own physical exhaustion, conflicts with a job, family responsibilities, and the financial burden of multiple long trips scheduled within a short period of time.[108]

Care Manager Helps Long-Distance Caregiver Avoid "Swooping"

One common pitfall of the long-distance caregiver is "swooping." Swooping is de-

fined on the Caring From a Distance (CFAD) Web site as:

> . . . the way you behave when you fly in from Chicago for the weekend to visit your widowed mom in Boston. If you are a distance caregiver with limited time and a long list, this is what you do. It can be very helpful. It can also be extremely disruptive. You arrive filled with ideas and concerns and a checklist of activities. But your sister, who also lives in Boston, is your Mom's primary caregiver. If you manage your visit well, you can bring your sister some much needed relief, handle a few problems, offer some practical help, and perhaps provide a shoulder to cry on. You can also spend some quality time just visiting Mom and participating in some of the activities of her life. Not doing anything. Just visiting. But beware of the dangers. Your trip can easily turn into a family disaster. Your sister can resent what she thinks is your meddling—and your lack of concern during the months when you were not by Mom's side. Since absence makes the heart grow fonder, your Mom can tend to glorify your presence. Your sister says she is best off staying at home. You think she needs to move to assisted living. You fight. Mom gets upset.[109]

Schempp[110] reports that when the long-distance caregiver visits, they have an agenda and want to get a lot done out of a feeling of loss of control and guilt. The professional can help them just relate to the parent and identify the highest priority issue to focus on. Swooping visits can also be avoided if the care manager supports ongoing communication between the care recipient and other caregivers between visits. That way, all parties can share their concerns and agree on tasks to be divided prior to the visit. When the long-distance caregiver visits, it is important for them to just spend time visiting with the care recipient and local caregivers and not spend all of their time "taking care of business."

When there is a local primary caregiver, the long-distance caregiver should be reminded that there are important tasks that they manage from a distance and not to interfere. The long-distance caregiver can be prompted by the care manager to plan their visit and set priorities by asking the following questions:

- Is this a real medical or care crisis? Ask the physician or call a social worker or nurse for information in their opinion on whether you should travel in—as part of your decision making, not all of it.
- Assess what can be achieved while there and what the consequences are of not going.
- Can someone else locally take care of the issue at hand or eyeball the situation?
- How will this trip affect your own personal situation: children, partner, finances, work, and leave time?
- It's okay for the long-distance caregiver to visit just to put his or her mind at ease, particularly if staying home and worrying is going to be less productive.[111,112]

Another resource to aid long-distance caregivers and care managers alike is a new telecare system called Rest Assured® from ResCare HomeCare. Rest Assured® allows caregivers to make virtual home visits, have two-way audio and visual communication, and be alerted if problems arise such as a fall, a missed medication, or an episode of wandering. Caregivers can check in from any computer with high speed internet access from anywhere in the world, or Rest Assured® staff can assist with monitoring should the need arise.

Care Manager Helps Long-Distance Caregiver to Identify Warning Signs

The care manager can provide the long-distance caregiver with a list of warning signs to look out for during their visit, particularly if the visit is infrequent[113-115] (see Exhibit 3-2). A holiday trip is a good opportunity to see firsthand how well parents are coping.[116] Any one of the behaviors listed may or may not indicate that an action should be taken. If the older adult is currently living independently, warning signs might include unpaid bills, missed appointments, a change in short-term memory, clutter in the home, refusing to go with friends on outings or to religious services, refusing any suggestion or agreeing to everything without consideration, mood swings or getting angry quickly, or refusing to go to medical providers. Other warning signs are when the person cannot perform ADLs such as cooking, bathing, dressing, and housekeeping, or if the person is subject to long-distance undue influence such as contests or sweepstakes.

The care manager should counsel the long-distance caregiver to proceed cautiously if they are troubled by what they see. It is important not to raise the defenses of the parent, because it may stop any future discussions about care.[117] It is also important to look at the whole picture: the way the parent is living may not be the way the long-distance caregiver would prefer, but the long-distance caregiver needs to be respectful and build a partnership with the parent.

Care Manager Helps Long-Distance Caregiver Plan Visit

The care manager can help the long-distance caregiver plan their visit. Planning a visit starts with communication, and the care manager can facilitate communication between the long-distance caregiver and care recipient. First, the care manager should remind the long-distance caregiver that in-person communication is important, particularly for conversations about important eldercare topics such as caregiving and difficult end-of-life issues. The care manager should suggest before placing a telephone call to be aware that

Exhibit 3-2 Warning Signs for Visiting a Long-Distance Relative

- **Curb appeal:** Does the home look maintained, or are there weeds in the yard and general disrepair?
- **Housekeeping:** Are dust and dirty dishes accumulating in this once-fastidious person's home? This could be a sign of depression, dementia, or failing eyesight.
- **Appearance and personal hygiene:** Has this person lost weight? If a male, is he shaving? Does this person shower less frequently, wear dirty clothes, have body odor, bad breath, neglected nails and teeth, or sores on the skin? Have they had physical problems such as burns or injury marks resulting from general weakness, forgetfulness, or possible misuse of alcohol or prescribed medications?
- **Mobility:** Are they having trouble getting around?
- **Odors:** Do you smell urine? Incontinence can be a problem among the elderly, and personal hygiene can diminish.
- **Forgetfulness:** Are there signs of forgetfulness such as piles of unopened mail, stacks of newspapers, unpaid bills, losing or hiding money, unfilled prescriptions, missed appointments, or getting lost?
- **Ordering:** Is there evidence of excessive ordering from catalogs, charity appeals, insurance companies, and television infomercials? Excessive purchases such as buying more than one magazine subscription of the same magazine? Entered an unusual amount of contests or sweepstakes or is their credit card maxed out on shopping channels? Is the mail full of letters from charities, a sign that the care recipient may be giving money to anyone who asks?
- **Medication:** If the person is on medication, can they take it without supervision? What prescription and nonprescription medication is the person taking? Do you have a current list of them?
- **Medical appointments:** Who accompanies the person to the doctor or sees that medical visits are made? How are medical appointments scheduled? Does the care recipient refuse to go to medical providers?
- **Driving/car:** Is this person still able to drive safely? How is their reaction time, confidence, judgment, and general driving skill? Are there signs of fender benders?
- **Answering machine:** Is there an accumulation of unanswered messages?
- **Interaction:** How does the older adult(s) handle extended conversation? Do they increasingly repeat questions? Do they retain what you say? Do they refuse any suggestion or conversely agree to everything without consideration?
- **Refrigerator:** Does the refrigerator contain appropriate and adequate food? Are there several containers of spoiled food? Any fresh vegetables? Fruit? Have eating patterns varied?
- **Trash:** Are bags of trash stashed in basements, garages, closets? How is weekly trash pickup managed?
- **Shopping:** Does this person have difficulty figuring tips, writing checks, or calculating discounts?
- **Eating habits:** Has this person changed eating habits within the last year resulting in weight loss, having no appetite, or missed meals?
- **Behavior:** Does this person exhibit inappropriate behavior by being unusually loud or quiet, paranoid, agitated, angry, exhibiting mood swings, or making phone calls at all hours?
- **Relationship patterns:** Do friends call often? Has this person changed relationship patterns such that friends and neighbors have expressed concerns? Have they decreased or stopped participating in activities that were previously important to them such as bridge or a book club, dining with friends, or attending religious services?

Sources: National Association of Area Agencies on Aging. *Home for the Holidays, Ten Warning Signs Your Family Member May Need Help.* Available at: http://www.n4a.org/locator_holiday_manual_021220. cfm. Accessed October 29, 2007.

Rosenthal A, Cress C. Geriatric care management: Working with nearly normal aging families. In: Cress C, ed. *Handbook of Geriatric Care Management.* Sudbury, MA: Jones and Bartlett; 2006:309–340.

Felt S. Caring from afar—Distance complicates task of looking after your aging parents. *Arizona Republic.* Available at: http://www.foundationforseniorliving.com/cgi-bin/www/displayNews.pl?status=display_news_detail&code=27. Accessed November 11, 2007.

AARP. *Caring for Those You Care About. Providing the Care. Session 2, Long-Distance Caregiving.* Available at: http://www.aarp.org/learntech/family_care/Articles/a2003-05-06-ldcaregiving.html. Accessed June 13, 2007.

AlzNY.org. *Long-Distance Caregiving.* Available at: http://alznyc.org/caregivers/long.asp. Accessed September 29, 2007.

reading facial expressions and body language plays an important part in knowing when to change communication tactics or to back off. It is easier for those who "left home for greener pastures . . . to be in denial a little longer,"[118] so the care manager should be there to support the long-distance caregiver who is not prepared for what they are going to face. Exhibit 3-3 provides suggestions of tasks that the long-distance caregiver can do prior to and during their visit. Prior to the visit, the long-distance caregiver should prioritize things that need to be done during the visit before leaving home so that important tasks are not forgotten.

Life transitions are critical junctures at which time the care manager should recommend that the long-distance caregiver visit if at all possible. For example, when the care recipient is making the transition from living alone at home to having a daily or live-in caregiver, the long-distance caregiver should be involved with selection of the paid caregiver. Or when the older adult is faced with a move to a higher level of care, the long-distance caregiver should plan a trip to help make the ultimate selection of a long-term care facility. The care manager can support the long-distance caregiver along the way by prescreening paid home caregivers

Exhibit 3-3 Tasks That the Long-Distance Caregiver Can Accomplish Before and During the Visit

Before the visit:
- Prioritize things you need to do before you leave.
- Explain to those you are leaving behind the nature of your trip and when you will be returning.
- Make appointments to meet providers—this helps to develop rapport and serve notice that you are an involved caregiver who will be present to monitor services from time to time. Keep a list of people you need to speak with when you visit, and make sure that care providers know where and how to reach you.
- Write out advance questions for providers and be prepared to write down answers.
- Especially if your parent is ill, bring photos of the people he or she loves, or video of family members so that you can spend time together talking about good times.

During the visit:
- Talk to the care recipient so that the two of you can decide together what needs to be done and who can help.
- When working with the care recipient(s) to help them access the services you find, be sensitive to their views of the situation. They may be concerned about having strangers in their home or have trouble facing change. Even though dealing with these issues can be frustrating, it's important to maintain a positive focus. Tips include explaining that the services are designed to help them to remain independent and having someone else your parent respects recommend the service, such as their doctor.
- Use a relaxed approach that doesn't threaten the older adult's independence. One way may be to suggest that they would be doing you a favor by accepting some help.
- Take your elders out while you are visiting to see how they function in the community and with others.
- Take time to reconnect with the person by talking, listening to music, going for a walk, or doing other activities you enjoy together. A visit that is "all business" won't be good for either of you.
- Be with the older person for support when a new service is established, such as a new caregiver, doctor, or living situation.
- Accompany the older family member to a doctor's appointment—speak to his or her physician in person. Establish a relationship with the doctor and office nurse, learn the medications that the older person takes, what pharmacy is used and its telephone number, and understand the conditions. Find out how you might remain in contact with the doctor's office; identify the registered nurse working with the doctor. Be sure that there is a HIPAA Release of Information Form on file at the doctor's office so that you can talk openly with the doctor, and keep one for yourself.

Exhibit 3-3 Tasks That the Long-Distance Caregiver Can Accomplish Before and During the Visit (continued)

- Make sure that doctors and insurance companies are aware of who is the medical or durable power of attorney. The doctor should have a copy in the chart.
- Plan to meet with other care providers and have them bring you up to date with the care recipient's progress.
- Meet with an attorney specializing in elder law to discuss estate planning. Draw up a durable POA and a living will.
- Gather all insurance information and take it to a financial planner to make sure policies are current and appropriate (auto, homeowners, Medicare, Medicaid, Medigap, long-term care, disability).
- Plan periodic visits to give the caregiver a break. You can spend time with the individual, run errands for the caregiver, and participate in planning for care.
- Find all legal documents, take them home, and put them in a binder (if these include original signed documents, make copies and put originals in a safe deposit box or safe place). Key legal and financial documents might include the following:
  - Legal documents
  - Birth certificate
  - Social security card
  - Divorce decree
  - Will
  - Trust
  - Power of attorney
- Set up a filing system at the long-distance caregiver's home for the care recipient and include all pertinent documents involving the care recipient.
- Take home a copy of a fairly up-to-date phone book from the area where the care recipient lives for reference as well as a senior resource guide, if one is available.
- Make a list of the informal local resources: neighbors, religious-activity-related friends, and other relatives, who can be part of the care recipient's support network. Meet with these people so they can share their observations about how the person is doing. Ask if there is any behavioral changes, health problems, or safety issues. Have someone stop by and visit (weekly or daily), and contact you if they observe anything unusual. Also arrange for social visits.
- If the care recipient lives in an apartment or retirement residence, make sure that the staff has your phone number, and let them know that you want to be informed if they notice any problems or changes.
- Assess the home safety each time you visit: locks, telephone access, and test smoke alarms. Look for uneven flooring, loose rugs, and poor lighting. Install grab bars or ramps to make the home safer.
- Monitor neighbors or friends or anyone who might take advantage of the older person, carry out any sweetheart scams, or exert an undue influence.
- Look for sweepstakes mailings, large bank withdrawals, or other evidence of long-distance undue influence.

Sources: Beerman S, Rappaport-Musson J. *Eldercare 911: The Caregiver's Complete Handbook for Making Decisions.* Amherst, NY: Prometheus Books; 2002.

McLeod BW. *And Thou Shalt Honor: The Caregiver's Companion.* Emmaus, PA: Rodale Press; 2002.

Payne B. *Providing Care from Afar.* Available at: http://www.caregiving.com/yourcare/html/weeklytip70.html. Accessed November 13, 2007.

Rosenthal A, Cress C. *Geriatric Care Management: Working with Nearly Normal Aging Families.* In: Cress C, ed. *Handbook of Geriatric Care Management.* Sudbury, MA: Jones and Bartlett; 2006:309–340.

AARP. *Caring for Those You Care About. Providing the Care. Session 2, Long-Distance Caregiving.* Available at: http://www.aarp.org/learntech/family_care/Articles/a2003-05-06-ldcaregiving.html. Accessed June 13, 2007.

AlzNY.org. *Long-Distance Caregiving.* Available at: http://alznyc.org/caregivers/long.asp. Accessed September 29, 2007.

for the long-distance caregiver's final approval or by developing a prescreened list of facilities prior to the visit.[119]

Periodic visits by the long-distance caregiver to a long-term care facility where the care recipient is residing are critical. It is important for the long-distance caregiver to establish good contacts with employees, and let the contact person at the facility know that the long-distance caregiver appreciates what they're doing. It is also important for the long-distance caregiver to establish good contacts with the informal support network of others who see the care recipient regularly (friends, community volunteers, church members). These contacts will be a great source of information when the long-distance caregiver is back home.

It can be very helpful for the long-distance caregiver to accompany the older family member to a doctor's appointment and speak to the physician in person. This is an opportunity to establish ongoing relationships with the care provider and understand the medications the care recipient is taking. Visits are also a good time to gather legal, financial, and insurance paperwork, meet with the appropriate professional in those respective fields, and set up a filing system for all pertinent documents. The long-distance caregiver can take advantage of a visit to meet the care recipient's neighbors and friends and utilize their eyes and ears to informally monitor the care recipient. The long-distance caregiver should closely scrutinize these friends and acquaintances to make sure that there is no potential elder abuse.

Help Long-Distance Caregiver Identify Tasks to Do from Home

The care manager can recommend easily accomplished tasks that will keep the long-distance caregiver involved with the care recipient and local caregivers. Some of these tasks can be done from home, as they do not require proximity to the care recipient, and others are recommended to make the most of a visit. These tasks include information gathering from the Internet, staying in close contact with the care recipient and other caregivers, providing emotional support to others on the caregiving team, arranging for services, taking care of business and financial arrangements, acting as the primary contact for various practitioners, and contributing financially. A list of suggested tasks is provided in Exhibit 3-4.

The National Association of Professional Geriatric Care Managers (NAPGCM) has an excellent binder by Betsy Carey Evatt available in the NAPGCM store called Caregiver Planner: A Notebook to Organize Vital Information. It has most of the tabs mentioned in Rosenthal and Cress,[120] and the family member can add more.

Care Manager Helps Deal with Crisis Situation

The care manager is uniquely qualified to deal with crisis situations as they arise. Exhibit 3-5 lists tips the care manager can share with the long-distance caregiver regarding how to be prepared for the inevitable emergency trip. In a crisis situation, the whole family is affected and time may be at a premium. The care manager can help the family determine whether there is a true emergency. According to Heath,[121] the following are indicative of a true emergency where the long-distance caregiver should visit their relative immediately:

- A health professional requests the long-distance caregiver's presence due to a serious medical condition
- A calamity occurs, such as a fire or natural disaster

Exhibit 3-4 Tasks That the Long-Distance Caregiver Can Accomplish from Home

- Gather information by telephone or on the Internet on medical conditions, medications, local community resources, support groups, and government programs.
- Provide emotional support to others on the caregiving team in a variety of ways including: (1) ask the primary caregiver what they need help with; (2) visit as often as possible, planning trips to give the primary caregiver a respite break; (3) invite the care recipient to their home to provide the primary caregiver respite; (4) write regular notes to the primary caregiver saying how much you appreciate what the primary caregiver is doing and how difficult it is.
- Make regularly scheduled (i.e., weekly or biweekly) phone calls or e-mails to check in with the care recipient and solve problems, as well as provide them with companionship and emotional support. Regular contact by letters, cards, telephone, or by using one of the hi-tech solutions described in this chapter can also include friendly reminders to purchase medication or remember doctor appointments.
- Be on the look-out for changes in the parent's behavior. If changes persist, alert the doctor and call another member of support team and ask to visit the parent and provide a full report.
- Set up an online chat room, manage a round-robin letter, or call other family members with updates on the loved one's situation.
- Provide personal support to the care recipient:
  - Request that other loved ones send photos to the care recipient from faraway special events such as birthday parties, anniversary celebrations, and so on.
  - Send care packages to them—bake cookies with your children or partner and send samples along with pictures of everyone baking in the kitchen.
  - Send flowers, food items, or other assorted gifts periodically. This can easily be done online at a reasonable cost.
  - If the care recipient has access to e-mail, send virtual greetings or virtual flowers or just a note to say hello.
  - Buy postcards of the area where you live and send them with notes.
  - When you travel or if you live overseas, send fun tourist souvenirs.
- Have all business-related mail forwarded to you and take care of banking and bill paying using online services, direct deposit, or traditional mail. Many public utilities now will notify a caregiver, even one at a distance, if the loved one's account becomes past due or if service is in danger of being disconnected.
- Arrange regular visits from religious groups if appropriate.
- Arrange services from the community such as Meals on Wheels.
- Take care of income tax preparation.
- Arrange and monitor hands-on services to help the care recipient. After the initial arrangements, much can be handled through telephone calls and occasional short visits to stay connected with home care providers.
- Maintain the care recipient's informal support network. Let them know how to reach you and that you welcome their calls.
- Act as the primary contact for physicians, care providers, or others. Maintain communication with the registered nurse who works with the care recipient's doctor.
- Contribute financially, as able, if necessary.
- Keep all of the information about the care recipient in a care binder with section dividers to help to organize the information. Keep track of the important information in a care log in a section of this binder.

Sources: Wilson B. *Caregiving Tip Sheet—Practical Tips for Long Distance Caregiving.* Available at: http://www.helpstartshere.org/. Accessed September 29, 2007.

Rosenthal A, Cress C. Geriatric care management: Working with nearly normal aging families. In: Cress C, ed. *Handbook of Geriatric Care Management.* Sudbury, MA: Jones and Bartlett; 2006:309–340.

AlzNY.org. *Long-Distance Caregiving.* Available at: http://alznyc.org/caregivers/long.asp. Accessed September 29, 2007.

McLeod BW. *And Thou Shalt Honor: The Caregiver's Companion.* Emmaus, PA: Rodale Press; 2002.

Rosenblatt B, Van Steenberg C. *Handbook for Long-Distance Caregivers: An Essential Guide for Families and Friends Caring for Ill or Elderly Loved Ones.* San Francisco, CA: Family Caregiver Alliance National Center on Caregiving; 2003.

Beerman S, Rappaport-Musson J. *Eldercare 911: The Caregiver's Complete Handbook for Making Decisions.* Amherst, NY: Prometheus Books; 2002.

Exhibit 3-5 Prepare for an Emergency Trip

- **Travel:** Be ready to travel at a moment's notice. Find out what airlines and/or bus lines travel nonstop or have reduced last-minute fares to the care recipient's location or make sure that your car is in good repair and that you have valid auto insurance and driver's license.
- **Money:** Keep an emergency travel fund in your bank account or have a buffer on your credit card so that you can charge your trip during a caregiving emergency situation.
- **Access:** Have an extra set of the care recipient's house, mailbox, and/or car keys with you and with a reliable neighbor of the care recipient for easy access.
- **Your own household:** Create a plan for your own household: identify several backup and alternate care providers for your own family and pets in case you need to make an unexpected visit and have the numbers for your local newspaper and post office so that you can have deliveries held.
- **Work:** At work, save family leave, personal, vacation, or sick days from work for these visits. Keep track of the amount of Family and Medical Leave Act (FMLA) time that you use on an annual basis; up to 12 weeks per year of unpaid leave are permitted for eligible employees, and some states have laws that extend the duration of the FMLA or provide paid time off for family leave.

- Family or friends report a sharp decline in the older person's physical or mental status, or no one has been able to contact the older person
- Persons assisting the relative tell the long-distance caregiver that the older person has a number of unmet needs that detract from his or her health or safety
- An accident occurs, such as a drug overdose, a car accident, or fall that results in a severe injury

If it is not possible for the long-distance caregiver to be present, the care manager can follow the strategy suggested by Wexler in her book *Mama Can't Remember Any More*:

1. Within a day (and sometimes within hours), I personally visit, or send a trusted associate to visit the patient and make an assessment of the situation. After talking with neighbors, friends, doctors and clergy, in order to get a clear picture of what is going on, I report back to my client.
2. I make sure that the immediate crisis is stabilized.

3. After a crisis is stabilized, I recommend options for the elder family member's best long-term care . . . we also discuss many factors that must go into the family's decision-making process, such as cost, service, availability , and expectations for the patient's future prognosis.
4. I continue to monitor the patient's progress, reporting back to my client on a regular basis.[122]

If it is not possible for the long-distance caregiver to be present throughout a hospitalization, nursing home, or rehab facility stay, additional support in the hospital is a good investment in the care recipient's recovery process. As stated elsewhere in this book, there are so many things that can go wrong in an institutional setting that a few additional sets of eyes and ears are critical. The care manager should act as an advocate and visit often, using his or her healthcare knowledge and the willingness to ask questions to demand good care. The care manager can suggest hiring a private duty nurse's aide to be there a few hours a day to add to the hospital care since hospitals do not provide that type of personal attention.

The care manager should help the long-distance caregiver to develop a plan for communication during a crisis, such as daily updates from the doctor. This plan should include who will collect and convey the information from the doctor to the others who are involved and how the information shall be conveyed, such as by e-mail.

The care manager should coach the long-distance caregiver to speak with their employer in the event of a crisis[123] and:

- If possible, speak frankly with their supervisor or human resources staff about their situation, keeping records of these discussions in case they need to explain their decisions later on.
- Tell the employer that they may need to make calls from the office, or to be absent from work with little or no notice until the crisis is resolved.
- Identify workplace-related benefits such as sick leave, vacation, unpaid leave under the Family and Medical Leave Act (FMLA), the company's Employee Assistance Program (EAP), or eldercare program. Unfortunately, long-distance caregivers who are in the military cannot use the FMLA program since military leave is restricted to 30 days per year.[124]

CARE MANAGER ASSISTS WITH EMERGENCY PREPAREDNESS

One of the essential qualities of care management is crisis intervention and planning. Care managers can and should offer emergency and disaster planning services to all of their clients since disasters can occur anywhere and at any time.[125] Particularly if there is no local family caregiver, care managers should address the needs of the care recipient in the face of a potential disaster. Care managers should ensure that each client has a plan in place to minimize confusion and danger and to maximize health and safety.[126]

In the aftermath of the New Orleans disaster of 2005, it became evident that the elderly and disabled are particularly vulnerable when disaster strikes. Disasters including hurricanes, earthquakes, winter storms, tornadoes, thunderstorms, flooding, toxic spills, fires, and power outages, not to mention terrorism, can wreak havoc on property and interrupt the flow of everyday life. When a person has a mobility impairment or special medical need, it will be even more difficult to deal with an emergency situation.[127]

The care manager cannot promise to be available after a widespread disaster as there may be many clients to service. However, if possible, the care manager should: (1) call or visit the care recipient as soon as possible after the emergency situation to ensure their safety and well-being, and (2) attempt to contact out-of-town family members and take steps to address any needs that have arisen as a result of the disaster.

The care manager should determine the local region's vulnerabilities and help plan accordingly. A list of tips for disaster preparedness for care managers is provided in Exhibit 3-6. Preparation for a disaster includes having a disaster plan, appropriate supplies, and an emergency support network. The care manager should make sure that the care recipient, family, and paid caregivers all participate in the process. The plan should be posted, and all members of the emergency support network should have a copy of the plan.

Care managers should identify a resource and utilize it to develop disaster plans. The Red Cross and FEMA have developed a manual for disaster preparedness entitled *Preparing for Disaster for People with Disabilities and Other Special Needs*.[128] A consumer guide to preparing for an emergency is available for free from the US Department

Exhibit 3-6 Tips for Disaster Preparedness for Older Adults

Overall assessment. The care manager should conduct a comprehensive needs assessment and develop an emergency plan for the care recipient. This plan may involve supplies for remaining at home or help signing up for a special-needs shelter, hotel, hospital care, or travel out of town.

Paid caregivers. The disaster plan should address both the care recipient and paid caregivers who might be with the care recipient during a disaster. If possible, the care recipient should be empowered to do as much preparation as possible on his or her own behalf. When a disaster strikes, it is likely that paid caregivers, even if they are devoted to the care recipient, will be concerned about and wish to attend to their own family and loved ones. It is therefore possible that they may not be able to stay with the care recipient. This possibility should be discussed in advance and incorporated into the disaster plan. To make it easier for the paid caregiver to remain with the care recipient, the care manager should consider including the caregiver's family in the disaster plan.

Emergency supplies. Coordinate and purchase emergency supplies and place in an easily portable container. Review items listed by the American Red Cross and the AOA.

Medications and specialized equipment. The following actions should be taken to prepare an adequate supply of medication and specialized medical equipment:

- The care manager should make sure that there is a labeled supply of any medication that the care recipient takes, adequate for at least 2 weeks. If the care recipient is stranded at home or must go to a public shelter, they may not be able to get more medications easily. An extra pair of glasses and hearing aid batteries should be included.
- If the person requires specialized equipment such as a respiratory system or a medical monitor, the care manager should prearrange for that to be available at the new location, if possible. If there is a way to modify the system without electrical power, the care manager should include those items with other emergency supplies (such as having a manual wheelchair available).
- The care manager should include in the plan how to get prescription refills, oxygen replacements, maintain dialysis regimens, and so on if all services in the area are interrupted.
- The care manager should keep a brief medical history and an updated list of all medical information, including health insurance, Medicare or Medicaid numbers, and the physician, pharmacies, and other healthcare services' names and telephone numbers, a list of medications, and when they are normally taken.
- The care manager should check to see what geographic area the care recipient's health insurance covers.

Emergency support network. There should be at least three people in the care recipient's emergency support network for each location where the care recipient spends time who will know their capabilities and needs and be available within minutes. The plan should be based upon the care recipient's lowest anticipated level of functioning.

Incorporate community disaster plans. The care manager should be aware of community disaster plans such as response plans, evacuation plans, and designated emergency shelters. It is also important to know how local authorities will warn of an impending disaster and how they will provide information during a disaster. There may be special assistance programs available in the event of an emergency for the elderly and those with disabilities. The care manager should register all persons with disabilities with the local fire or police department or the local emergency management office so needed help can be provided quickly. There may also be a neighborhood emergency program where community members who require special help can be registered and identified in advance. If a person is electric-dependent, it may be possible to register with the local utility company.

Exhibit 3-6 Tips for Disaster Preparedness for Older Adults (continued)

Communications plan. The plan should include contact information for family members, members of the support network, caregivers, and the out-of-town contact, meeting locations, emergency services, and the National Poison Control Center (1-800-222-1222). A form for recording this information can be found at www.ready.gov or at www.redcross.org/contactcard. These Web sites also provide blank wallet cards on which contact information can be recorded and carried in a wallet, purse, backpack, and so on, for quick reference. The communication plan should be posted near the telephone for use in an emergency.

Escape routes and safe places. In a fire or other emergency, the care recipient may need to evacuate on a moment's notice, so the care recipient and any caregivers should be trained to be ready to either go to the safest place in the home for that disaster or to get out fast using the best route out of the home. A personal emergency evacuation checklist such as the one available from NFPA should be filled out for each care recipient. A meeting place should be identified: right outside the home in case of a sudden emergency, or a location outside the neighborhood if the care recipient cannot return home.

Choose out-of-town contact. An out-of-town contact should be chosen to call after a disaster because it is often easier to make a long-distance rather than a local call from a disaster area. If the long-distance caregiver lives in a location that will not be affected by the same disaster, he or she is a good person to select as the out-of-town contact.

Review emergency plan. The care manager should review the emergency plan with the care recipient, personal care attendants, and family. The emergency plan should be part of new and refresher caregiver training.

Sources: American Red Cross, FEMA. *Preparing for Disaster for People with Disabilities and Other Special Needs.* 2004. Available at: http://www.redcross.org/images/pdfs/preparedness/A4497.pdf. Accessed November 15, 2007.

National Family Caregiver Support Program. *Just in Case: Emergency Readiness for Older Adults and Caregivers.* Available at: http://www.aoa.gov/PROF/aoaprog/caregiver/overview/Just_in_Case030706_links.pdf. Accessed June 13, 2007.

National Fire Protection Association. *Emergency Evacuation Planning Guide for People with Disabilities.* Available at: http://www.nfpa.org/categoryList.asp?categoryID=824&cookie%5Ftest=1. Accessed November 12, 2007.

Dynamic Living.com. *Planning for a Disaster.* Available at: http://www.dynamic-living.com/news-disaster-preparation .htm.

of Health and Human Services Administration on Aging (AOA) National Family Caregiver Support Program (NFCSP) entitled "Just in Case: Emergency Readiness for Older Adults and Caregivers."[129] This document presents an easy-to-follow approach to emergency preparedness. Some care management software products (for example, Jewel Code's Care Complete) include a disaster planning component. A list of online resources is provided in Karp and Koenig[130] along with a simplified emergency management plan and client emergency management log for a care management's firms existing clients.

One useful tool that can help the care manager to both educate and prepare the care recipient and long-distance caregivers for disaster planning is the video that goes along with the "Just in Case" document. This video can be viewed streaming from the Internet (www.aginginstride.org), or it can be purchased for presentation to groups, along with a presenter's guide to help engage a group of older adults and caregivers. The American Red Cross[131] also has a helpful Web site entitled "Tips for Seniors and People with Disabilities" that lists important items and actions that the care manager should consider including in an emergency care plan.

It is important for the care manager to consider planning for how the care recipient will evacuate their residence in the event of emergency. The National Fire Protection Association (NFPA) has prepared a free downloadable emergency evacuation planning guide[132] that contains chapters on evacuation planning for people with mobility, visual, hearing, speech, and cognitive impairments. It describes the four elements of evacuation information that occupants need: notification, way finding, use of the way, and assistance. The guide includes a handy checklist that can be downloaded that care managers can use to design the evacuation plan.

CARE MANAGER HELPS LONG-DISTANCE CAREGIVER WITH SELF-CARE

Even when caregivers are not physically present and providing support, they are still mentally coping with the personal difficulties associated with the illness. The care manager can assess the distant caregiver over the telephone using one of the caregiver instruments recommended elsewhere in this book.

The adult long-distance caregiver may experience stress due to lingering childhood issues in their relationship with the care recipient or with other family caregivers. The care manager can first discuss these issues on the phone or at an in-person meeting, but should then refer the adult long-distance caregiver to an appropriate treatment person in their own community. In this way, the care manager is a link to distant resources that help to preserve the family unit.[133] The care manager can also offer to mediate sibling or

parent/adult child relationships, or can refer the family to a family therapist.

Donna Schempp[134] recommends that the care manager help long-distance caregivers reframe their guilt into regret for having to make difficult decisions. This is done by helping them realize that they have no control over the situation. In this way, they can try to make peace with not being there to help their parents. This also helps long-distance caregivers to expend less energy on negative emotions and channel their energy into helping the care recipient. She recommends an excellent resource for this task entitled *The Caregiver Helpbook* by Schmall and others.[135]

The care manager can suggest that long-distance caregivers seek emotional support for themselves from others in their local community. It may be helpful to talk to friends, colleagues at work, or find an in-person or online support group where they can talk about caregiving challenges. Discussing their situation, letting their feelings out, and listening to other points of view can be helpful. Participating in support and educational groups is a way to relieve stress because the groups focus on caregiving and provide information on the specifics of the care receiver's disease or chronic condition. Caregiver support groups also provide resources and techniques to alleviate caregiver stress and are a safe haven for caregivers to voice their concerns and frustrations. Some support groups are tailored for long-distance caregivers and others have a combination of long-distance and local caregivers.

The care manager can also suggest that the long-distance caregiver visit a few groups to find the best fit; at a minimum, the group should provide a safe and inviting environment, respect confidentiality, be run by experienced professionals, and occasionally offer guest speakers.[136] There are also on-line virtual support groups for this community of caregivers.

The care manager can help the long-distance caregiver to avoid stress and burnout by coaching them to do the following:

- Develop a list of tasks and priorities while being realistic about how much they can do from a distance.
- Request flexible hours at work (e.g., work 40 hours in 4 days, job sharing, telecommuting, working from home).[137]
- Balance the long-distance caregiving responsibilities against other obligations such as their own health, family, and work.
- Learn to accept and ask for help, especially from family, friends, and community resources (don't be afraid to ask; make tasks sound simple; show appreciation; do not have several people providing the same assistance—if the person feels unneeded, he or she may discontinue helping).
- Use their employer's Employee Assistance Program (EAP) that might include elder care services, or better yet, their company-sponsored elder care program.
- Craft creative ways to use the available benefits, such as the Family and Medical Leave Act (FMLA), and be aware of the following: (1) some states (e.g., California) have a program that is expanded from the national program, (2) the caregiver can use their FMLA benefits incrementally (i.e., hourly, daily, or weekly) so that, for example, a caregiver who must travel can use their benefits in conjunction with a weekend, such as taking 2 days off every other week, resulting in two 4-day weekends per month, a time period where the caregiver can get more accomplished.[138]
- Ask for a family meeting to identify those who can help.
- Set limits and learn when to say no.

CARE MANAGER ASSISTS WITH RELOCATION

As life expectation gets longer, and old-old parents end up requiring more support than they did when they were young-old, long-distance caregivers will be faced with the dilemma of relocation. The many pros and cons of relocation and moving are outlined in detail in Chapter 16 on moving in *Handbook of Geriatric Care Management.*[139] An excellent fact sheet with numerous questions that the long-distance caregiver should ask when considering relocation is available online from the Family Caregiver Alliance and is entitled "Home Away from Home: Relocating Your Parents."[140] There is also an evidence-based guideline entitled "Management of Relocation in Cognitively Intact Older Adults" that can be of help in planning for and evaluating the results of a relocation.[141] Exhibit 3-7 is a checklist that the care manager can provide to the long-distance caregiver to help them evaluate whether it is wise to combine households with the care recipient.

If it is determined that an older adult who is currently disabled requires transportation to a new location that is distant from their home, the care manager can suggest one of several companies that provide transportation support. Although the following companies were recommended as reliable by care managers on the National Association of Professional Geriatric Care Managers (NAPGCM) Listserv in 2007, there may be other reliable companies providing the same or similar service. Note that the NAPGCM Listserv is open to all members of NAPGCM. Some companies provide a medical escort service to support the older adults that cannot travel unattended but need to fly a long distance (e.g., www.medescorts.com/services .html). There are private medical motor

Exhibit 3-7 Considerations for Combining Households

- How do other members of your household feel? Is this a parent who not only finds fault with you, but also doesn't hesitate to find fault with others in your life? If the parent's visits in the past have usually been stressful, then a permanent stay will be even worse.
- Even if the rest of the family agrees this is a good idea, how does your parent feel?
- Does he or she have a circle of friends or is active where he or she lives? If so, will the new community have similar opportunities? Are they easily accessible? Have you checked out these places alone or when your parent has come for a visit?
- Will your parent feel comfortable in a household that may be noisier and messier? Will pets pose a problem?
- Will your parent be able to have a room of his or her own?
- Here are a few things to agree upon before your parent moves in:
  - Is this a temporary stay? If so, for approximately how long?
  - Will your parent contribute financially to the household? (Sometimes even if you don't need the money, your parent will feel better helping out if he or she can afford it.)
  - Will your parent do some chores: cooking a set number of meals, picking up the kids from school, yard work, pet care, and so on? This is a hard one because it involves role reversal. Most parents don't want to feel like guests, yet it's a fine line between helping and interfering. When you ask your parent for help, either explain exactly how you want it done or let your parent do it his or her way and don't complain if you don't like it.
- Ask yourself if your parent moving in is the only choice or are there other options?
  - If you check out community resources for seniors online, you may be surprised at how much is available. A few things to consider are visiting nurses, meals on wheels, low-cost taxi fares, and senior centers or YMCAs with educational and recreational programs.
  - If you and your parent feel it is better to live close by, but not as part of your household full-time:
    - Look into 55-plus communities nearby. Some range from completely independent living to various levels of assisted care all at the same facility.
    - Consider an apartment nearby, possibly shared. Look for someplace near public transportation and, if possible, with a market within walking distance.
    - Create a small apartment unit on your premises with its own kitchen and entrance (an add-on or a remodeled garage) so your parent can live as independently as possible. (Though this may be more challenging if your parent will count on you for all meals and his or her entire social network.)
- And finally, agree up front to revisit these living arrangements every 3 to 6 months. Look at what's working and what's not and make revisions accordingly.

Source: AgeWise Living. Moving in with my daughter. *AgeWise Living Newsletter*. October 2006. Available at: http://www.agewiseliving.com/moving-in.htm. Accessed October 30, 2007.

---

coaches designed specifically for long-distance transfers of the elderly or disabled person who may be nonambulatory, wheelchair-bound, or have a long-term medical condition requiring the assistance of a medical caregiver (e.g., www.medsprinter.com, www.usamedcoach.com). In addition, there are nonemergency air ambulance services throughout the world (e.g., www.airmd.net).

When the move requires that the older adult travels, the care manager should remind the family to make sure that the older adult's medication needs are taken care of. AARP[142] recommends that anyone traveling carry a personal medication record, including over-the-counter drugs and the conditions that they treat; carry medicines in a carry-on bag in case of separation from luggage; bring more than needed (one week's supply is recommended) in the event that travel arrangements change; if medicines need to be kept cool, carry them in a small insulated container; and in the event of overseas travel, make sure that the drugs the person is carrying are acceptable in other countries (e.g., a controlled substance or narcotic, drug requiring a needle). The care manager should also be aware that the need for a personal oxygen supply can be an issue for flights as the airlines either do not provide oxygen, or the level they provide is too low for many clients and typically, personal oxygen tanks are not allowed on flights due to pressurization issues. Cindy Schaefer, a flight nurse and care manager recommends that the care manager speak with the person's physician prior to the flight. She also says that some companies have obtained permission to bring an oxygen concentrator onto a commercial air flight.[143]

CARE MANAGER ENCOURAGES ONGOING COMMUNICATION

The care manager should encourage ongoing communication between the care manager, the long-distance caregivers, the older adult, and local caregivers. It is important to inform the long-distance caregiver that maintaining contact with the care recipient reduces the feeling of isolation that so often happens when a person becomes frail and disabled. Ongoing contact is critical between the caregivers, and if there is a primary caregiver, it is also very important for the other caregivers to provide emotional support to this person.[144] Communication can be in the form of a family meeting, when everyone or nearly all parties are participating. There are several ways that the various parties can communicate, depending upon the comfort level of all involved with available technologies. Table 3-4 lists a few of the communication technologies that may be useful to the long-distance caregiver.

Family Meetings

There is a detailed description of how care managers can facilitate family meetings in another chapter of this book. If the long-distance caregiver cannot be at the meeting location, the meeting can be held long-distance over the telephone, using standard three-way calling (limited to two family members) or using a low cost teleconference or videoconference service. Examples of low cost services include www.conferencecalls unlimited.com and freeteleconference.com. The teleconference can involve anyone from any location with access to a telephone. Just like with any family meeting, the care manager can facilitate and work with the participants in advance to determine what issues to discuss and what decisions to make. The care manager helps everyone to be heard and gets all issues out on the table. One care manager uses a digital voice recorder to record office meetings and conference phone calls via speakerphone.[145] If requested or helpful to the caregivers and client, the care manager can e-mail or save the files to a CD and provide it to any persons who were unable to attend. This guarantees that everyone is privy to the issues addressed in the meeting.

Prior to the meeting, the care manager can work with all of the participants, either by e-mail, fax, or regular mail to develop an agenda. In advance of the meeting, the

Table 3-4 List of Technologies That Can Be of Use to Long-Distance Caregivers

Type of Technology	Technology/Organization	Web link for further information
Home monitoring/health security system	Examples: • Rest Assured® • Xanboo • AT&T Remote Monitor • Quiet Care • Grand Care	http://www.restassuredsystem.com http://www.xanboo.com/ http://www.attrm.com http://www.quietcare.com/ http:///www.grandcare.com/
Electronic pillbox	Example: • Epill.com	http://epill.com
Telehealth monitoring	Example: • iCare Health Hero	https://www.healthhero.com/ partners/partners_icare.html
Secure online personal health record	Example: • LifeLedger	http://www.elderissuespro.com
Virtual Web meeting place for friends and family	Examples: • CarePages • CaringBridge	http://www.carepages.com http://www.caringbridge.org
Video conferencing for caregivers	Examples: • Caregiver Technologies • Virtual Interactive Families	http://www.internetvisitation.org/ http://vifamilies.com/
Affordable teleconference link	Examples: • free teleconference.com • conferencecallsunlimited.com	http://freeteleconference.com/ http://www.conferencecalls unlimited.com/
Vlogging (video blogging)	Example: • Virtual Families and Friends	http://jimbuie.blogs.com/ virtualfamilies1
Computer-based video conferencing software (do it yourself)	Example: • Skype	http://www.skype.com
Web TV	Webtv.com	http://www.webtv.com
Printing mailbox (receives and prints e-mails and attachments)	Presto	http://www.presto.com/
E-mail without computer or Internet access	My Celery	http://www.mycelery.com/

Table 3-4 List of Technologies that Can Be of Use to Long-Distance Caregivers (continued)

Type of Technology	Technology/Organization	Web link for further information
Easy-to-use cell phone	Jitterbug	http://www.jitterbugdirect.com
Digital photo frame and automatic picture updates	CEIVA Digital Photo Frame and Picture Plan	www.ceiva.com
Industry organization	Center for Aging Services Technologies (CAST)	http://www.agingtech.org CAST Product Clearinghouse: http://www.agingtech.org/Browsemain/aspx
Industry organization	Home Care Technology Association of America	http://www.hctaa.org/aging.html
Industry organization	American Telemedicine Association, home telehealth and remote monitoring special interest group	http://www.atmeda.org/ICOT/sighomehealth.htm Buyers guide: http://www.atmeda.org/news/2006buyersguidedefinitions.htm
Corporation conducting research	Intel Research	www.intel.com/research/prohealth/dh_aging_in_place.htm
Nonprofit organization supporting development and implementation of technology for older adults	SmartSilvers Alliance	http://network.smartsilvers.com/ Product list: TechEye for the Older Guy (and Gal!) http://network.smartsilvers.com/index.php?option=com_wrapper&Itemid=10005

participants should be asked to provide the care manager with a list of concerns as well as tasks they are willing to do to support the care recipient. Just like in a family meeting when all members are present, it is the care manager's role to address the caregiving situation from each family member's point of view, create feelings of trust and support, and help the siblings appreciate each other. The main purpose of the family meeting is to find out which members of the family may be able to provide what types of support. The care manager should keep the meeting on current concerns (i.e., care issues) rather than matters between siblings or other family members and make

certain that everyone, including the long-distance caregiver, has an opportunity to express feelings, voice preferences, and offer suggestions. During the family meeting, the care manager can help the family with the following:

- Coach the family members to share tasks and identify tasks that the long-distance caregiver can perform from home.
- Encourage long-distance caregiver to provide respite to local caregivers.
- Determine how the family will communicate so that the long-distance caregivers have equal access to information about what is going on.

• Make a plan for what will happen during an emergency or hospitalization if there is no local family caregiver.

Communication with the Care Recipient

The easiest way for the long-distance caregiver to stay connected with the care recipient is by telephone. The care manager should emphasize that frequent phone calls are a good way to monitor the status of a loved one. The care recipient also feels connected to the long-distance caregiver and it can be a highlight of their day. Hearing the care recipient's voice can help alert the long-distance caregiver to possible problems such as depression or even an illness.[146] You can suggest that the long-distance caregiver may want to set up a schedule so that the care recipient knows when to expect a call. The care manager should encourage other friends and family members to telephone too—perhaps help to set up a calling rotation or a system to alternate daily calls, so someone is always checking in.[147] If the care recipient is disabled or hearing-impaired, the care manager can help acquire special telephone equipment. If the care recipient is mentally and physically able, it may be possible to implement other types of systems as a way of staying in touch with family members such as cell phones, personal tracking devices, non-computer-based communication devices, and virtual visitation devices, all of which are described below. Some systems require the use of computers, and others do not. Use of computers may become more common in the future, as baby boomers age along with their technological know-how.

Cell Phones

Cell phones can be used by the care recipient to improve family communication,

for practical calls when not at home, and for emergencies. Older adults will need a cell phone that is simple to use, with a higher than usual earpiece volume, clear ring, and a larger keypad with a display that is easy to read. Connecting the care recipient to cell service makes it easier for the faraway family member to reach the care recipient when they are not at home or in their room at a long-term care facility. It also gives the care recipient more freedom to go out because they are not sitting by the phone waiting for a call. Cell phones are necessary in this day and age due to the fact that increasing numbers of pay phones are being removed and there is no other way to make a call from a public place. For example, having a cell phone makes it possible for the care recipient to call and find out where their paratransit vehicle or taxicab is located instead of being stranded on the street. A cell phone provides the long-distance caregiver with peace of mind that in the event of an emergency situation, the care recipient will be able to communicate. Some families may choose to all be on the same cell phone plan (sometimes people using the same vendor can speak to each other for free).

Some phones with these characteristics may be available from regular cell phone vendors.[148] There is also one phone and associated service that is specifically tailored for the senior market. The Jitterbug phone offered by Great Call offers two handset styles designed for ease of use by the older adult. One has a normal looking but enlarged keypad and the other has just three buttons: one for the operator, one for 911, and one that is programmed to "my choice"—which brings up a personal phone list. Unlike other cell phones, this phone comes with personalized operator assistance that greets by name, looks up numbers, places calls, and answers questions about how to use the phone.[149] These features might assist an older adult who has memory loss or is used to the functions of a regular home telephone.

Personal tracking devices can be added on to some cell phones or purchased with emergency call capability. Some cell phone services can provide a "friend finder" service that takes advantage of Global Positioning System (GPS) technology. Specific devices that are sold primarily as portable tracking devices with an emergency button and limited cellular telephone capability are also available. Some of these systems allow the care provider to establish a boundary so that the person monitoring the device will be alerted if the person with the device wanders off.

Non-Computer-Based Communication Services

As many care recipients may not be able to utilize a computer, there are several alternatives that make use of widely available technologies and are either easy or require no effort to operate. A receipt-only device that uses a regular telephone line may be used if the care recipient cannot afford or is overwhelmed by a computer.[150] MyCelery (www.mycelery.com) is a two-way communication device that allows the older adult to receive e-mails sent by the long-distance caregiver with text or photos on standard fax hardware. The MyCelery user can then send return notes and they will be received by the distant caregiver's e-mail. The Presto Printing Mailbox and Presto (www.presto.com) service offered by Hewlett Packard is a device that offers one-way delivery of photos and letters. The long-distance caregiver can send an ordinary e-mail to the HP Printing Mailbox, where they are converted into easy-to-read color printouts. Another device, the CEIVA Digital Photo Frame (www.ceiva .com), can be connected to a telephone or DSL line. The long-distance family member can upload photos to the frame at any time if they subscribe to the PicturePlan service. Web TV requires the purchase of a dedicated system that allows the care recipient to send and receive e-mail and surf the Web from an existing television (accessible at www.webtv .com).

Virtual Visitation

Two-way video communication can be conducted between the long-distance caregiver and the care recipient using the virtual visitation or televisiting technique of personal video conferencing. Virtual visitation allows the participants to both see and hear each other in the way that comes most naturally to everyone—traditional face-to-face communication.[151] Several small studies have shown that the frail elderly population is capable of participating in teleconferencing, including those residing in nursing homes.[152–155] It is also an efficient means for elderly family care providers communicating with hospice caregivers.[156] These studies suggest that the face-to-face interaction gives the family members a greater sense of involvement and may be a way to alleviate caregiver anxiety.

This technology can help to maintain the quality of a person's diminishing social network. It is a way to share favorite people (e.g., a new baby, the care recipient's favorite nurses aide), places (e.g., photos or a video of a vacation), and things (e.g., a new home or animal). It is also a way for the long-distance caregiver to monitor the quality of care and it also validates the experience of the older person's demise. It should be noted that limitations, such as physical impairments (e.g., vision, hearing loss), technical difficulties, and impaired cognitive ability may limit the use of this technology by the care recipient. Support from a local care provider can help overcome some of these difficulties. The long-distance care provider may also experience limitations, including resistance either due to feeling too overwhelmed by caregiving responsibilities to take the time to participate, or they may simply not wish to witness their parents' now more obvious decline.

Field videoconferencing is another use of this technology that should be of great interest to the care manager as it has implications for a new way of working. Using portable equipment (laptop, wireless DSL or data card, speaker, and camera), the care manager can show the care recipient and their home to others who are located remotely. The remote person can be the long-distance caregiver or another professional supporting the care manager. The long-distance caregiver might be more easily convinced by visual evidence that their loved one needs assistance (e.g., clutter, poor health, empty refrigerator) than they would by the care manager's report. Other practitioners, such as a physical therapist, occupational therapist, or medical personnel, may be called in remotely by the care manager to do a preliminary assessment of an elder who cannot easily travel or who is situated at a remote location. The care manager can also use it for fun, just to connect the care recipient with a family member or friend who they have not seen for a while. This technique has recently been successfully implemented by the Hawkeye Valley Iowa Area Agency on Aging, using the Web-based technology from Virtual Interactive Families (www.vifamilies.com).[157]

Video calling can be accomplished by using a dedicated videoconferencing phone, computer with speaker and camera, Pocket PC, Palmtop, or other handheld long-distance device, or a cell phone with picture and/or video capability.[158] Having this level of flexibility might enable the long-distance caregiver to contact the care recipient from anywhere in the world where wireless broadband is available.

A guide to videoconferencing entitled *The Virtual Visitation Handbook*[159] prepared for the long-distance parenting community can easily be adapted for the long-distance caregiver community. This guide describes both dedicated video telephone devices as well as how to set up video conferencing using a computer, reviews the various products currently on the market, and describes how to set them up. Several other books also provide detailed information on required equipment and setup.[160,161] For family members such as the elderly who are not comfortable using a computer, a dedicated stand-alone video telephone device may be a good choice.[162,163]

Computer-based video calling requires a basic computer, webcam, headset microphone, free or inexpensive software, high-speed Internet (cable or DSL), and security solutions like a DSL or cable router and firewall software. Videoconferencing can be done using either free software such as Skype or by working with a company that is dedicated to providing videoconferencing to this market, who will provide any equipment that is needed and communication software designed for the caregiver–care recipient dyad.

Several companies have very recently created the market of providing fee-based Internet videoconferencing services tailored for family caregivers and care recipients (e.g., Virtual Interactive Families and Friends at www.vifamilies.com and AttentiveCare at www.caregivertech.com). Features of some of these dedicated systems include all of the controls being at the caregiver's end, dedicated software (or no special software needed), multimedia support including voice and text reminders (the caregiver's voice can say "wake up now," or "take your medications today"), and slide show capability (e.g., old photos) that can be cognitively stimulating to the care recipient. The care manager can help the family to investigate the differences between available options and present them to the family.

For Web-savvy caregivers and care recipients, a new way to share personal information with friends and family is the medium of "vlogging," or digital video blogging,[164] where the family can share digital videos of family events, vacations, and so on with the public on a video blog.

Communication About the Care Recipient

The care manager should be keeping the long-distance caregiver informed of events in the care recipient's life. Much more communication is required from the care manager when the caregiver feels out of control and distant. Because the care manager and long-distance caregiver are typically in different time zones, the care manager should establish that she may not be able to respond to long-distance caregiver concerns or queries immediately, but will respond by the next day at the latest. E-mail is an excellent way to stay in contact with the long-distance caregiver, as it is usually a more efficient form of communication than a telephone call, which can end up taking more time. E-mailing is a way to get the long-distance caregiver's questions answered promptly and prevents the problem of "telephone tag," which often occurs when busy people are trying to connect, particularly care managers who may often be with clients and cannot respond to a telephone inquiry directly.[165]

In order to keep the long-distance caregiver informed and to minimize unscheduled contact, the care manager should provide regular reports. The reporting frequency should

be established up front depending upon how stable the care recipient's condition is, how often the care manager visits, and the wishes of the long-distance caregiver. It is reasonable to provide reports on a weekly or monthly basis. Reporting on a less frequent basis than monthly will make the long-distance caregiver feel out of touch with the situation.

Other forms of communication may be necessary when there is a larger group of caregivers who are interested in staying abreast of the latest information about the care recipient. Communication may be synchronous, where all members communicate simultaneously, or asynchronous, where members can participate as their schedules permit.[166] For example, the care manager can moderate a family meeting teleconference at an established time, and the attendees can be provided with a phone number to call in to. It is also very useful to set up either a private e-mail group, a virtual care meeting place, or a bulletin board, where messages are posted and permanently saved for members of the care team. These technologies enable the members of the care team to share information about important issues whatever time it is convenient, regardless of time zone or location. There are several free Web pages that people can use for this purpose.[167]

Holiday Communication

If the long-distance caregiver cannot visit, particularly around the holidays, Barbara Friesner of AgeWise Living[168] suggests that that the long-distance caregiver might want to send a "holiday in a box." The care manager can suggest that it is a fun way to share the holidays, particularly if the care recipient resides in assisted living or a nursing home. It would be a way that all ages can participate in communicating with the care recipient. She suggests that the long-distance caregiver consider doing the following for the care recipient:

- A Chanukah box might contain an electrical menorah, gifts for each day, a draydel, and Chanukah gelt.
- A Christmas box might contain a small artificial tree with all the trimmings, and special ornaments, cards, and gifts.
- Include special "family tradition" items that will help them recall happy holiday memories.
- Set up a time for a phone call that is good for both of you. If possible, call in the morning and early evening when they may be feeling lonely. And, of course, make sure everything arrives well in advance.

CARE MANAGER ASSISTS WITH TECHNOLOGIES THAT SUPPORT AGING IN PLACE

One major area of development is technology to support the independence, security, and health of an aging population. The care manager can help the long-distance caregiver to identify available and affordable technologies that will enable the care recipient to live in the least restrictive environment for as long as possible. It is the care manager's job to identify the technology that will work for a particular situation since none of these systems are "one size fits all." Table 3-4 lists a few technologies that support aging in place.

Academics use the term *gerontechnology* or *gerotechnology* for technologies that can improve the quality of life for the aging. "Nana technology" is another term that was recently coined for the same phenomenon and has been said to include health products, safety products, cognition products, lifestyle products, and whole-house or whole-facility products.[169]

The Center for Aging Services Technologies (CAST), which is a coalition of more than 400 companies, universities, healthcare providers, and government entities organized to explore ways technology can help seniors, further defines aging-related technologies as the following:

- Enabling technologies (assist persons to age in place)
- Operational technologies (assist aging persons to function in society)
- Connective technologies (assist aging persons to communicate with caregivers, families, and medical resources and vice versa) [described under the section on communication]
- Telemedicine (allows a medical source or caregiver to monitor, diagnose, and/or treat patients from a distance)[170]

The benefit of many technologies is that they can provide a daily outlook on the care recipient and notify caregivers, care managers, and physicians before the symptoms become too serious. These systems have the potential to help keep the care recipient stable in their home, thereby avoiding a stay in the hospital.[171] The discussion in the following sections challenges the care manager with a unique opportunity to get in on the ground floor with early implementation of new technologies that may assist the care recipients of the future to stay at home for longer. Some of the technologies are invisible to the care recipient; others are not. When selecting a technology that the older adult will be involved with, the care manager should keep in mind the applicable considerations listed in Exhibit 3-8. The care manager should also be aware of ethical issues and considerations regarding technologies used to monitor the movements of care recipients.

Exhibit 3-8 Considerations in Selecting Computer-Based Technology for an Older Adult

---

- What is the problem you are trying to solve with the technology?
- Are there reliable sources of information about computer-based technology used to care for older adults with the problem?
- What are the advantages and disadvantages in using the technology?
- Is the older adult a willing partner in the use of the technology?
- How much does the technology cost?
- Is the cost a one-time-only expenditure or will there be further costs for service?
- Will insurance cover all or part of the cost of the technology?
- How does the primary care physician fit into the support system for the technology?
- Is the older adult's home (or other care facility) properly outfitted for the technology? For instance, does it have an Internet connection?
- What agency, if any, has certified that the technology you are considering is effective and safe for use?
- Does the technology protect the privacy of the older adult?
- Is a training program available for the older adult or the caregiver in order to ensure proper use of the technology?
- Is there a reliable "help source" to assist in resolving any operational problems that may occur in using the technology at home?

Source: SPRY. *Computer-Based Technology, and Caregiving of Older Adults: What's New, What's Next.* [Reference manual]. Available at: http://www.spry.org. Accessed November 6, 2007.

Digital Home Technologies

Digital home technologies have the potential to provide increased safety for the care recipient and support long-distance caregivers and the care manager. Systems that are embedded in the home to monitor the care recipient's home environment and respond to perceived problems in the environment can be of use to support the older adult who is at risk of institutionalization due to deficiencies in ADLs and IADLs.[172] Some technologies are already on the market, and there is also extensive research being done to improve and expand what these technologies can do. Once the assessments of the older adult and caregiver(s) are completed, the care manager will be able to recommend a specific technology that will support the care recipient's lifestyle and provide the long-distance caregiver greater peace of mind. Other technologies that may be helpful to long-distance caregivers include those that provide assistance with medications management[173] or health monitoring.[174]

The care manager should be aware of potential impediments to implementation of these systems. According to Susan Ayers Walker of the SmartSilvers Alliance and AARP,[175] the current elder did not grow up with technology and may not be comfortable with it. In addition, the elder may deny the need for care and resent the loss of independence that the technology signifies and sabotage or avoid using it. The care manager's job is to help the family come up with a solution that both helps the caregiver and empowers the care recipient. In addition, many of these systems have recently been released or are in the process of being tested and released. Although the following systems are currently available, those who choose to purchase them should realize that in many cases they are going to be relatively "early adopters." Mahoney[176] suggests that it is not for everyone to be an early adopter and that "it may be wise to defer major purchases of new technologies until their third generation, when they have become debugged, made easier to use, and more compact." The care manager can support participation in feasibility trials to test utility and influence design so that caregiver needs are better met.

Monitoring and Response Systems

Personal Emergency Response Systems

A personal emergency response system (PERS) is a lightweight, waterproof necklace or wristband that is activated by pushing a button, which sends a signal via a telephone line to a response center.[177] The response center staff maintains contact with the long-distance care recipient and can call rescue personnel in the event of an emergency. There are numerous well-established companies that provide this service and the care manager should recommend a service that has 24-hour response by trained operators.

This type of system is in a category of technology called "reactive technology to facilitate communication in case of an emergency."[178] It is excellent in an emergency, but unfortunately, it relies on the older adult's "ability and willingness to press the button and call for help."[179] There are cases when the older adult may not be able (loss of consciousness) or forgets (cognitive impairment) to activate the system during an emergency, rendering it ineffective.

Residential Monitoring Systems

Wireless motion detector and camera-based monitoring systems that track an elder's movement within the home are becoming more widely available.[180,181] These unobtrusive digital systems can be placed in the care recipient's home and can help to ease the long-distance caregiver's mind about safety. They can be "accessed through the Internet, enabling adult children to check in remotely to assess the well-being of an aging parent from far away."[182] Some of these systems allow "participants to monitor the functional health patterns of the care recipient while at work."[183] According to Stevenson,[184] "some systems may watch over elderly people who might not realize they need help, like someone with early stage Alzheimers who might forget to eat or take medications. They can also be used to detect falls or other problems as they happen, or to monitor third parties like home health aides and other home help." A benefit of such a system is that the long-distance caregiver can do a quick check on their computer and avoid lengthy and potentially upsetting telephone calls with the care recipient.[185]

This type of system is in a category of technology called crisis prevention and combines "early detection using the technology with the early intervention by a caregiver to prevent a crisis."[186] According to Gage,[187] the challenge of adoption of this technology by older adults is "helping to overcome denial, the 'I don't need it' syndrome."

Some skilled nursing facilities and retirement communities are using this type of monitoring and permit families remote secure Web-based access to information about the resident. This information includes where the resident is located, the number of assistance calls placed to staff and staff response, in addition to movement, restlessness, sleep habits, weight, participation in social activity, and percentage of time spent with others or alone.[188–190]

The systems utilize a combination of cameras, sensors, and computers. Systems are easily installed because they are wireless and are unobtrusive and inconspicuous because they are relatively small. Sensor systems can monitor when the older person's pattern differs from the routine and send an alarm to a central monitoring location if movement patterns in the home are abnormal.[191,192] The sensors can be strategically placed throughout the home to record activity. For example, when a person enters a bathroom, the sensor records how long the person is there.[193] Repeated trips to the bathroom may be a cause for concern that the patient may not mention to the doctor until the problem requires extensive treatment. Other sensors can be placed at locations to record whether a person took their medicine, how often the refrigerator is opened, whether the bathtub is overflowing, the temperature of the home, when the care recipient gets out of bed (e.g., how many times at night), and other activities.

These systems can be monitored either by the caregiver alone or by a corporate call center. Corporate call centers notify the person monitoring the system (may be a caregiver or care manager) of an abnormal pattern by phone call, e-mail, text message, or personalized Web page. After notification by a call center, verification follow-up is always required. Although these systems generate many false alerts,[194,195] a monitoring service may be less work than and therefore preferable to a stand-alone system monitored solely by family members.

Another way to determine the care recipient's safety is with cameras placed "in the older person's home that allow someone somewhere else to see what the camera sees."[196] Cameras provide "a visual picture of how the older person is doing—to pick up on clues that might not be obvious from a phone call, for instance."[197] Unfortunately, unless monitored constantly, having a camera does not guarantee that whoever is monitoring will see something going wrong as it happens.

Care Manager Involvement in Residential Monitoring Systems

Mahoney,[198] who has conducted studies of a proprietary sensor-based monitoring system, recommends professional involvement in system design, installation, and monitor-

ing.[199] She believes that it is preferable to first conduct a baseline assessment using a "nursing health assessment model"—very similar in fact to the full care management assessment of the care recipient and family caregiver—and put everyone's concerns together. This evaluation can be conducted by the care manager who can then recommend the type and locations for sensors. Table 3-5 illustrates specific care recipient deficits and the related areas that should be monitored by sensors.

Mahoney's model is appealing in that she suggests that each system should be tailored to the particular need and want of the end users, the caregiver and the care recipient. Mahoney[200] envisions "a role for a new type of care manager who can be the overseer and notice particular patterns of alerts and worrisome changes and intervene before a crisis occurs."

Orientation of Care Recipient

Technological support for cognitive aging is sometimes called "cognitive orthotics"[201] or "assistive technology."[202] The care manager can suggest some simple reminder systems to support remembering tasks that need to be performed and carrying out the tasks at the appropriate time. This type of system can be very helpful because it enables an older adult to perform an essential task and reduce the burden on the long-distance caregiver. For example, a computer in the bedroom with a screen that states, "It is nighttime, stay in bed," and a photo of a family member or caregiver was found to reduce the number of telephone calls in the middle of the night by a care recipient with dementia. Orienting messages on the computer about the care recipient's daytime activities can also reduce anxiety and confusion and enrich the life of the person with dementia.[203] Researchers in England have successfully used wireless technology and sensors to reduce caregiving

Table 3-5 Monitoring Recommendations Based upon Care Management Assessment

Care Management Assessment Indicates Deficit or Risk	Monitoring Recommendations
Self-care Bathing, toileting, dressing/grooming, feeding, other self-care skills	Bathroom monitor, Bedroom monitor, Kitchen monitor
At risk for: Deterioration of sensation/perceptive ability Lack of safety precautions Unsupervised bathing Smoking in bed Knives stored uncovered Potential igniting from gas leak, grease on stoves	Fall/activity monitor, Bathroom monitor, Bedroom monitor, Kitchen drawer and room monitor
Health management Adherence problems (noncompliance) Medication management Need for assistive devices Formal caregivers (caregivers and rehab/medical/ social work professionals in the home)	Medication monitor, Assisted device monitor, Room activity monitor, Door monitor
Thought Process Short-term memory deficit Cognitive impairment Impaired recall ability, perception, judgment, decision making	Exit monitors, Activity monitors, Room monitors
Nutrition Dysfunctional eating patterns	Refrigerator monitor, Activity monitor
Urinary/bowel elimination Disturbance in pattern	Bathroom monitor
Sensory: Vision, hearing, touch, smell **Sleep patterns, for example, daytime napping** **Physical mobility**	Activity monitor, specifically tailored monitoring

Based on: Mahoney DF. Linking home care and the workplace through innovative wireless technology: The Worker Interactive Networking (WIN) Project. *Home Health Care Management & Practice.* 2004;16(5):421.

needs by providing gentle prompts or reminders in the form of recorded messages encouraging a person to return to bed at night.[204]

One of the most important examples of a reminder system is medication compliance. For an individual living alone, remembering to take medication at the right time and in the right order can make a difference between remaining independent and not.[205] High-tech pillboxes and medication management systems can do a number of tasks, including alerting people when it's time to take medication, organizing the pills into compartments, dispensing the proper dose, and monitoring when medications are taken. Many of these systems are listed on the Web site www.epill.com. One is a simple wristwatch that vibrates when it is time to take a pill. Others can do a few, but not all, of the tasks listed previously. For a fee, some can be connected to a professional monitoring system that phones, e-mails, or sends text messages to the long-distance caregiver if there is a problem with the care recipient's use of the medication.

Although systems that include professional monitoring exist at the present time, many are in the development phase by technology companies. They may prove useful for cognitively impaired care recipients, although it is difficult to confirm that a person has actually swallowed a pill that they have removed from a dispenser.[206]

Telehomecare or Home Telehealth

The telehomecare or home telehealth industry is growing rapidly. Telehealth is a large field that includes the use of high-tech diagnostic equipment, together with videoconferencing, reminder messaging, and remote sensor technologies that record physiological data.[207] Telehealth and telehomecare are defined as follows by the American Telemedicine Association's Home Telehealth and Remote Monitoring Special Interest Group[208]:

> *Home telehealth* is a service that gives the clinician the ability to monitor and measure patient health data and information over geographical, social, and cultural distances using video and nonvideo technologies. *Telehomecare* is similarly defined as the use of technology to deliver patient care in the home or place of residence, providing patient–provider contact without either having to travel. Importantly, telehomecare tools enable patient data to be transmitted from the home and patient-centered information to be sent into the home. . . . Its objective is enhanced chronic disease management, but it is especially valuable for patients with conditions that make travel physically difficult.[209]

Home telehealth systems have been shown to be of benefit to the long-distance caregiver. Frequent monitoring of these systems results in keeping the care recipient, long-distance caregiver, and care manager connected to the health professional and health condition. It is of particular benefit to those who have chronic conditions requiring intensive management and frequent monitoring and has been shown to cause a decline in the length of hospital stays and the number of emergency room visits.[210] According to a national study on the future of home healthcare technology,[211] "It is clear that the home care field is rapidly moving toward the universal adoption of telehealth systems. Remote monitoring of chronic disease patients can lead to improvements in quality of care." Preliminary results of the study indicate that patients and families like telehealth as it provides a sense of security by consistently updating health status and is an easy way for patients, care providers, and family members to keep track of specific health data with the goal of preventing emergencies. This data can be tracked from a distance, so the long-distance caregiver can be more directly involved in care than they would have been if the information had been written down in the daily notes by the in-home caregiver.

These systems can facilitate disease management for a broad range of chronic conditions including asthma, diabetes, chronic heart failure, chronic obstructive pulmonary disease (COPD), hypertension, wound care, and mental health (anxiety and depression).[212] Home monitoring devices incorporate wireless transmitters into devices that can measure parameters such as temperature, weight, blood pressure, glucose levels, oxygen, and other data. This data is sent to healthcare providers electronically. Along with the healthcare provider, a long-distance caregiver and care manager can access the information.

One very simple system that is readily available is the iCare Health Buddy appliance available at the drugstore.[213] This system is a small electronic device with a text screen and four input buttons that asks a series of daily multiple-choice questions about an older person's vital signs, symptoms, and behaviors and takes only a few minutes to complete. This prompts the older person to respond and provides education, reinforcement, and messages that prompt patient action, which can include taking the required measurements by one of a variety of medical devices that can be connected to the Health Buddy by cable. This information is transmitted to a secure data center, and family members and authorized care providers can view the answers online and look for any telltale changes in health.[214] Nurses monitor the system, although not 24 hours a day, and contact the older person when a question indicates that there may be something wrong. This provides a sense of security for both the older person and the family member. There is a cost for the system purchase and a fee for monthly monitoring. This product was awarded the Best Product by *Business Week* and Best Enabling Tool by the Disease Management Association of America. This system "enables the care manager to target patients most at risk for an impending crisis."[215] This system is also being used by about 10,000 Department of Veterans Affairs patients.[216]

Online Personal Information

Resources are becoming available where the care manager and the long-distance caregiver can share information about the care recipient at a secure location on the Internet. This can be particularly helpful when there is

an emergency situation. All members of the care team can access this information even if they live at a distance, and if they have the care recipient's permission (e.g., legal healthcare proxy), they can grant access to the information to others such as a doctor in an emergency room. One such service, Life Ledger, was developed by certified care manager (CMC) John Boden (www.elder issuespro.com). The Life Ledger is a secure online service where personal documents as well as financial and medical information can be stored (categories include emergency, general, support persons, medical, physicians, health status, insurance, health records, budget planner, and legal and financial plans). Personal documents such as advance directives and wills can be scanned into the personal health record. There is also a place for a family chat room where family members at any location can discuss and solve problems. A progress notes section is available to professional subscribers to the service.

Several major computer companies such as Google and Microsoft have recently or are in the process of developing health platforms to help users access their health information more quickly and easily. These online platforms include information such as personal health records, health care-related search functions, a localized physician and medical finder, a diet and exercise regimen, and other elements. The idea behind these platforms is to make records more accessible and portable for patients and to make the doctor more productive.

Willingness of Older Adult and Caregivers to Use Technology

Deciding Whether to Use the New Technology

The decision to use the technology must be made by both the older adult and the long-distance caregiver. Those adopting new technology must first perceive that the technology is of benefit to carry out the activities he or she wishes to perform. The next step is to determine whether there are any disadvantages to using the system (such as having to learn something or giving up some privacy). A key factor is determining whether the advantages are outweighed by the disadvantages.[217] Each technology and each caregiver–care recipient dyad will have different reasons for choosing or declining to implement a particular type of technology.

Privacy Concerns

Concerns have been raised regarding how to protect privacy and autonomy when monitoring systems that gather information about an individual's daily life and health are utilized.[218–221] Will elders be willing to trade privacy for security and safety? Issues of privacy of the person and of the collected data as well as the security of wireless transmissions and of the health information must be addressed.[222] Cantor[223] suggests that "professionals recommending monitoring devices, device companies, and health care information monitored have the following four safeguards: (1) Informed consent to the initiation of monitoring; (2) continuing assent to monitoring; (3) control over who has access to the monitoring data; and (4) regular access to the monitoring data generated. For those who are cognitively impaired, a surrogate decision maker is required to make decisions on the impaired person's behalf." Mahoney[224] maintains "participants' privacy through the use of login and password codes, encryption, and other security mechanisms designed to ensure only authorized users access the system." Privacy issues drove the choice of motion-sensor technology over video surveillance in Mahoney's study of caregivers monitoring the care recipients from the workplace.[225]

The Care Manager's Responsibility for Technology

Change Organization's Mindset

It is the care manager's responsibility as both a professional in the field and a consumer to challenge him- or herself to think about a new paradigm of caregiving for elders that includes technology-based tools "rather than rely solely on guesswork and manual labor. This is difficult to do, as change is hard, especially when one is busy with the day-to-day crises and duties."[226] The Center for Aging Services Technologies (CAST) developed and distributes a video entitled "Imagine—The Future of Aging" that showcases devices that may be used in the future to support long-distance caregivers. This video can either be viewed online or purchased for a nominal cost.[227] The CAST video guide recommends that the video can be used by groups in the aging services field (such as care managers) to discuss how these technologies can be put in place.[228] The guide also suggests being open to diversifying services in nontraditional ways and being open to partnering opportunities with regard to these emerging technologies. CAST's "Technology Assessment Tool for Providers" can be used to get organizations to "start thinking about how emerging aging services technologies . . . will likely impact your organization's services in the near and distant future."[229] The guide recommends the following activities and provides detailed suggestions on how to navigate each one:

- Start a dialogue between management, staff, and residents or consumers using the Imagine video and capture their reactions, thoughts, and ideas.
- Overcome organizational "technophobia"— find ways to incorporate emerging technologies today.
- Plan today for the technologies of tomorrow.

Evaluate Technologies

It is important for the care manager to have a process based upon specific criteria to "evaluate technology in a way that facilitates implementation in our caregiving routine or workflow."[230] Gage[231] suggests the following criteria:

- Efficacy—Does the technology perform substantially according to expectations?
- Return on investment and cost effectiveness—Does the end result justify the means? This is particularly important given older adults' limited income and the lack of government funding for those not qualifying for Medicaid.
- Ease of use—Do staff, family members, or elders using the technology day to day find it intuitive and user-friendly?
- Low maintenance—Does the solution require significant time and resources to maintain?
- Improved accountability—Does the solution help the professional staff and/or family caregiver to improve accountability and quality of care?

Stay Up to Date with Technology

The care manager can keep abreast of the latest consumer and healthcare technologies as they become more available and affordable to the general public, many of which can help to support the long-distance caregiver. Several organizations have Web sites that summarize current issues and list newly available products that can support the long-distance caregiver (see Table 3-4). Web sites of corporations and universities that do research in this field can also provide information for products that are currently being tested. To find a system that may work for a specific client, it is useful to belong to an Internet community of professionals and have the ability to query an e-mail group such as the one available to members of the National Association of Professional Geriatric Care Managers or other professional organizations.

The Center for Aging Services Technologies (CAST), the Home Care Technology Association of America (HCTAA), the American Telemedicine Association (ATA), and the SmartSilvers Alliance are all organizations in this field. CAST, which is a subsidiary of the American Association of Homes and Services for the Aging (AAHSA), sponsors research and conferences on this subject (for example, the Healthcare Unbound Conferences).[232] The CAST Web site[233] describes the latest products, pilot projects, research and development, and emerging technologies. The HCTAA was established by the National Association for Home Care and Hospice (NAHC), a government and industry lobbying organization for the home-care technology industry that provides education and information to homecare providers about these technologies, including a free online newsletter.[234] The SmartSilvers Alliance is a nonprofit located in the Silicon Valley. The organization works to match up high-tech companies with venture capitalists for product research and development, helps researchers put together trials to test products, and also helps to educate consumers about available products with their online product list and online video presentations of low cost technologies.[235,236] The American Telehealth Association (ATA) also has an online certificate course on home telehealth applications.

Individual corporations, such as Intel's Proactive Health Group, are currently doing a substantial amount of research to "advance the concept of the digital home in which computers and consumer electronic devices throughout the home are linked together in a wireless network"[237] to form a smart environment. Once a model of the person's daily activities is learned by the system, the smart environment can detect changes and anomalies that may pose a health concern. Intel believes that wireless sensor networks that detect activity in the home have great promise in combating the combination of social isolation, inactivity, and failing nutrition. Although as of the date of this publication many of these products are not generally available, they will be available within the next few years.

CONCLUSION

The care manager can help to prepare and empower families who are geographically separated from their care recipients by minimizing the challenges of distance. The care manager should understand how the long-distance caregiver is different from local caregivers; being a long-distance caregiver can be a more significant drain on emotions, finances, and time, and providing care at a distance can be stressful in different ways from those for a proximate caregiver. Feelings of guilt and ambivalence, although an attribute of all caregivers, are particularly powerful feelings for long-distance caregivers. Long-distance caregivers may be very demanding of the care manager because they are dealing with their own issues related to "not being perfect." The long-distance caregiver is ambivalent about a variety of issues: getting involved with their parents, not being there, how much to be there, and hiring someone else to do their job. The care manager can facilitate communication between the long-distance and local caregivers and care recipient and can help the family make important decisions.

This chapter presents a large number of tools that the care manager can use to help the long-distance caregiver. Many tools are taken from the basics of care management—assessment and monitoring, assistance with family communication, advance planning, dealing with crisis situations, and information and referral. Specific topics such as when to make that long-distance trip or "care commute," emergency and disaster planning, self-care, and new technologically based modes of communication and monitoring are also covered. The care manager is empowered to continue to develop expertise in these areas.

REFERENCES

1. National Alliance for Caregiving (NAC), American Association of Retired Persons (AARP). *Caregiving in the U.S.* 2004. Available at: http://www.caregiving .org/data/04finalreport.pdf. Accessed June 15, 2007.

2. NAC, AARP. *Caregiving in the U.S.* 2004. Available at: http://www.caregiving.org/ data/04finalreport.pdf. Accessed June 15, 2007.

3. MetLife Mature Market Institute. *Miles Away: The MetLife Study of Long-Distance Caregiving. Findings from a National Study by the National Alliance for Caregiving with Zogby International.* Available at: http://www.metlife.com/Applications/ Corporate/WPS/CDA/PageGenerator/0,4132,P889, 00.html. Accessed June 15, 2007.

4. NAC, AARP. *Caregiving in the U.S.* 2004. Available at: http://www.caregiving.org/data/04finalreport .pdf. Accessed June 15, 2007.

5. Wagner D. *Caring Across the Miles: Findings of the Survey of Long-Distance Caregivers, Final Report.* Washington, DC: National Council on the Aging (NCOA); 1997.

6. NAC, AARP. *Caregiving in the U.S.* 2004. Available at: http://www.caregiving.org/data/04finalreport .pdf. Accessed June 15, 2007.

7. Benefield LS. Ways to support long-distance family caregivers. *Home Healthcare Nurse.* 2005; 23 (3):196.

8. MetLife Mature Market Institute. *Miles Away: The MetLife Study of Long-Distance Caregiving. Findings from a National Study by the National Alliance for Caregiving with Zogby International.* Available at: http://www.metlife.com/Applications/ Corporate/WPS/CDA/PageGenerator/0,4132,P889, 00.html. Accessed June 15, 2007.

9. Wagner D. *Caring Across the Miles: Findings of the Survey of Long-Distance Caregivers, Final Report.* Washington, DC: National Council on the Aging (NCOA); 1997.

10. Koerin BB, Harrigan MP. P.S. I love you: Long-distance caregiving. *Journal of Gerontological Social Work.* 2002;40:63–81.

11. NAC, AARP. *Caregiving in the U.S.* 2004. Available at: http://www.caregiving.org/data/04final report.pdf. Accessed June 15, 2007.

12. MetLife Mature Market Institute. *Miles Away: The MetLife Study of Long-Distance Caregiving. Findings from a National Study by the National Alliance for Caregiving with Zogby International.* Available at: http://www.metlife.com/Applications/ Corporate/WPS/CDA/PageGenerator/0,4132,P88 95,00.html. Accessed June 15, 2007.

13. Roff LL, Martin SS, Jennings LK, Parker MW, Harmon DK. Long-distance parental caregivers' experiences with siblings: A qualitative study. *Qualitative Social Work.* 2007;6(3):315–334.

14. Parker M, Church W, Toseland R. Caregiving at a distance. In: Berkman B, ed. *Handbook of Social Work in Health and Aging.* Oxford, UK: Oxford University Press; 2006:391–406.

15. Heath A. *Long-Distance Caregiving: A Survival Guide for Far Away Caregivers.* Lakewood, CO: American Source Books; 1993.

16. AARP. *Miles Away and Still Caring: A Guide for Long-Distance Caregivers.* Washington, DC: AARP; 1986.

17. MetLife Mature Market Institute. *Since You Care: Long-Distance Caregiving.* 2005. Available at: http://www.metlife.com/Applications/Corporate/ WPS/CDA/ PageGenerator/0,4132,P8900,00.html. Accessed June 15, 2007.

18. National Instutute on Aging (NIA). *So Far Away: Twenty Questions for Long-Distance Caregivers.* NIH Publication No. 06-5496. Washington, DC: NIH; 2006.

19. Rosenblatt B, Van Steenberg C. *Handbook for Long-Distance Caregivers: An Essential Guide for Families and Friends Caring for Ill or Elderly Loved Ones.* San Francisco, CA: Family Caregiver Alliance National Center on Caregiving; 2003. Available at: http://www.caregiver.org/caregiver/ jsp/content_node.jsp?nodeid=1-34. Accessed June 15, 2007.

20. Caring From a Distance. Caring From a Distance: Dedicated to Serving the Needs of Long-Distance Caregivers. Available at: http://www.cfad.org/. Accessed November 25, 2007.

21. Wagner D. *Caring Across the Miles: Findings of the Survey of Long-Distance Caregivers, Final Report.* Washington, DC: National Council on the Aging (NCOA); 1997.

22. MetLife Mature Market Institute. *Miles Away: The MetLife Study of Long-Distance Caregiving. Findings from a National Study by the National Alliance for Caregiving with Zogby International.* Available at: http://www.metlife.com/Applications/ Corporate/WPS/CDA/PageGenerator/0,4132,P889 5,00.html. Accessed June 15, 2007.

23. NAC, AARP. *Caregiving in the U.S.* 2004. Available at: http://www.caregiving.org/data/04final report.pdf. Accessed June 15, 2007.

24. Evercare. *Evercare Study of Family Caregivers— What They Spend, What They Sacrifice: Finding from a National Survey, November 2007.* Available at: http://www.evercarehealthplans.com/pdf/Care GiversStudy.pdf. Accessed December 9, 2007.

25. Baldock CV. Migrants and their parents: Caregiving from a distance. *Journal of Family Issues.* 2000;21(2):205–224.

26. Chou K, Yeung S, Chi I. Does physical distance make a difference in caregiving? *Journal of Gerontological Social Work.* 2001;35(1):21–37.

27. Koerin BB, Harrigan MP. P.S. I love you: Long-distance caregiving. *Journal of Gerontological Social Work.* 2002;40:63–81.

28. Rosenthal A, Cress C. Geriatric care management: Working with nearly normal aging families. In: Cress C, ed. *Handbook of Geriatric Care Management.* Sudbury, MA: Jones and Bartlett; 2007: 309–340.

29. Roff LL, Martin SS, Jennings LK, Parker MW, Harmon DK. Long-distance parental caregivers' experiences with siblings: A qualitative study. *Qualitative Social Work.* 2007;6(3):315–334.

30. Parker M, Church W, Toseland R. Caregiving at a distance. In: Berkman B, ed. *Handbook of Social Work in Health and Aging.* Oxford, UK: Oxford University Press; 2006:391–406.

31. Solomon R. Who's in Charge? or Issues in Long-Distance Intergenerational Relations. Annual Conference of Jewish Family Services, keynote address. West Palm Beach, Florida, October 20, 1988.

32. Watari K, Wetherell JL, Gatz M, Delaney J, Ladd C, Cherry D. Long-distance caregivers: Characteristics, service needs, and use of a long-distance caregiver program. *Clinical Gerontologist.* 2006; 29(4):61–77.

33. Collins W, Holt T, Moore SE, Bledsoe LK. Long-distance caregiving: A case study of an African-

American family. *American Journal of Alzheimer's Disease and Other Dementias.* 2003;18(5):309–316.

34. Aquarius Healthcare Videos. *Separated by Time and Distance: Long-Distance caregiving* [video]. Medfield, MA: Aquarius Health Care Videos; 2003.

35. Watari K, Wetherell JL, Gatz M, Delaney J, Ladd C, Cherry D. Long-distance caregivers: Characteristics, service needs, and use of a long-distance caregiver program. *Clinical Gerontologist.* 2006; 29(4):61–77.

36. Wagner D. *Caring Across the Miles: Findings of the Survey of Long-Distance Caregivers, Final Report.* Washington, DC: National Council on the Aging (NCOA); 1997.

37. MetLife Mature Market Institute. *Miles Away: The MetLife Study of Long-Distance Caregiving. Findings from a National Study by the National Alliance for Caregiving with Zogby International.* Available at: http://www.metlife.com/Applications/ Corporate/WPS/CDA/PageGenerator/0,4132,P88 95,00.html. Accessed June 15, 2007.

38. MetLife Mature Market Institute. *Miles Away: The MetLife Study of Long-Distance Caregiving. Findings from a National Study by the National Alliance for Caregiving with Zogby International.* Available at: http://www.metlife.com/Applications/ Corporate/WPS/CDA/PageGenerator/0,4132,P88 95,00.html. Accessed June 15, 2007.

39. AARP. *Caring for Those You Care About. Providing the Care. Session 2, Long-Distance Caregiving.* Available at: http://www.aarp.org/learn tech/family_care/Articles/a2003-05-06-ldcare giving.html. Accessed June 13, 2007.

40. MetLife Mature Market Institute. *Miles Away: The MetLife Study of Long-Distance Caregiving. Findings from a National Study by the National Alliance for Caregiving with Zogby International.* Available at: http://www.metlife.com/ Applications/ Corporate/WPS/CDA/PageGenerator/0,4132,P88 95,00.html. Accessed June 15, 2007.

41. Stern S. Measuring child work and residence adjustments to parents' long-term care needs. *Gerontologist.* 1996;36(1):76–87.

42. Franks MM, Pierce LS, Dwyer JW. Expected parent-care involvement of adult children. *Journal of Applied Gerontology.* 2003;22(1):104–117.

43. MetLife Mature Market Institute. *Since You Care: Long-Distance Caregiving.* 2005. Available at: http://www.metlife.com/Applications/Corporate/ WPS/CDA/ PageGenerator/0,4132,P8900,00.html. Accessed June 15, 2007.

44. Chou K, Yeung S, Chi I. Does physical distance make a difference in caregiving? *Journal of Gerontological Social Work.* 2001;35(1):21–37.

45. Martin J, McClure P. Today's active duty military family: The evolving challenges of military family life. In: Martin JA, Rosen LN, Sparancino LR, eds. *The Military Family: A Practice Guide for Human Service Providers.* Westport, CT: Praeger; 2000.

46. MetLife Mature Market Institute. *Miles Away: The MetLife Study of Long-Distance Caregiving. Findings from a National Study by the National Alliance for Caregiving with Zogby International.* Available at: http://www.metlife.com/Applications/ Corporate/WPS/CDA/PageGenerator/0,4132,P88 95,00.html. Accessed June 15, 2007.

47. Parker M, Church W, Toseland R. Caregiving at a distance. In: Berkman B, ed. *Handbook of Social Work in Health and Aging.* Oxford, UK: Oxford University Press; 2006:391–406.

48. Carton E. Long-distance caring. 2000. Caregiver .com. *Today's Caregiver Magazine.* Available at: http://www.caregiver.com. As quoted in Koerin BB, Harrigan MP. P.S. I love you: Long-distance caregiving. *Journal of Gerontological Social Work.* 2002;40:63–81.

49. Koerin BB, Harrigan MP. P.S. I love you: Long-distance caregiving. *Journal of Gerontological Social Work.* 2002;40:63–81.

50. Solomon R. Who's in Charge? or Issues in Long-Distance Intergenerational Relations. Annual Conference of Jewish Family Services, keynote address. West Palm Beach, Florida, October 20, 1988.

51. NAC, AARP. *Caregiving in the U.S.* Available at: http://www.caregiving.org/data/04finalreport.pdf. 2004. Accessed June 15, 2007.

52. Wagner D. *Caring Across the Miles: Findings of the Survey of Long-Distance Caregivers, Final Report.* Washington, DC: National Council on the Aging (NCOA); 1997.

53. Watari K, Wetherell JL, Gatz M, Delaney J, Ladd C, Cherry D. Long-distance caregivers: Characteristics, service needs, and use of a long-distance caregiver program. *Clinical Gerontologist.* 2006; 29(4):61–77.

54. MetLife Mature Market Institute. *Miles Away: The MetLife Study of Long-Distance Caregiving. Findings from a National Study by the National Alliance for Caregiving with Zogby International.* Available at: http://www.metlife.com/Applications/ Corporate/WPS/CDA/PageGenerator/0,4132,P88 95,00.html. Accessed June 15, 2007.

55. Wagner D. *Caring Across the Miles: Findings of the Survey of Long-Distance Caregivers, Final Report.* Washington, DC: National Council on the Aging (NCOA); 1997.

56. Watari K, Wetherell JL, Gatz M, Delaney J, Ladd C, Cherry D. Long-distance caregivers: Characteristics, service needs, and use of a long-distance caregiver program. *Clinical Gerontologist.* 2006; 29(4):61–77.

57. MetLife Mature Market Institute. *Miles Away: The MetLife Study of Long-Distance Caregiving. Findings from a National Study by the National Alliance for Caregiving with Zogby International.* Available at: http://www.metlife.com/Applications/ Corporate/WPS/CDA/PageGenerator/0,4132,P88 95,00.html. Accessed June 15, 2007.

58. MetLife. *The MetLife Study of Sons at Work: Balancing Employment and Eldercare. Findings from a National Study by the Natinal Alliance for Caregiving and the Center for Productive Aging at Towson University, June 2003.* Westport, CT: MetLife Mature Market Institute; 2003. Available at: http://www.metlife.com/Applications/ Corporate/WPS/CDA/PageGenerator/0,4132,P88 95,00.html. Accessed June 15, 2007.

59. Wagner D. *Caring Across the Miles: Findings of the Survey of Long-Distance Caregivers, Final Report.* Washington, DC: National Council on the Aging (NCOA); 1997.

60. MetLife Mature Market Institute. *Miles Away: The MetLife Study of Long-Distance Caregiving. Findings from a National Study by the National Alliance for Caregiving with Zogby International.* Available at: http://www.metlife.com/Applications/ Corporate/WPS/CDA/PageGenerator/0,4132,P88 95,00.html. Accessed June 15, 2007.

61. Watari K, Wetherell JL, Gatz M, Delaney J, Ladd C, Cherry D. Long-distance caregivers: Characteristics, service needs, and use of a long-distance caregiver program. *Clinical Gerontologist.* 2006; 29(4):61–77.

62. NAC, AARP. *Caregiving in the U.S.* 2004. Available at: http://www.caregiving.org/data/04final report.pdf. Accessed June 15, 2007.

63. Evercare. *Evercare Study of Family Caregivers— What They Spend, What They Sacrifice: Finding from a National Survey, November 2007.* Available at: http://www.evercarehealthplans.com/pdf/Care GiversStudy.pdf. Accessed December 9, 2007.

64. MetLife Mature Market Institute. *Miles Away: The MetLife Study of Long-Distance Caregiving. Findings from a National Study by the National Alliance for Caregiving with Zogby International.* Available at: http://www.metlife.com/Applications/ Corporate/WPS/CDA/PageGenerator/0,4132,P88 95,00.html. Accessed June 15, 2007.

65. NAC, AARP. *Caregiving in the U.S.* 2004. Available at: http://www.caregiving.org/data/04final report.pdf. Accessed June 15, 2007.

66. MetLife Mature Market Institute. *Miles Away: The MetLife Study of Long-Distance Caregiving. Findings from a National Study by the National Alliance for Caregiving with Zogby International.* Available at: http://www.metlife.com/Applications/ Corporate/WPS/CDA/PageGenerator/0,4132,P88 95,00.html. Accessed June 15, 2007.

67. MetLife Mature Market Institute. *Miles Away: The MetLife Study of Long-Distance Caregiving. Findings from a National Study by the National Alliance for Caregiving with Zogby International.* Available at: http://www.metlife.com/Applications/ Corporate/WPS/CDA/PageGenerator/0,4132,P88 95,00.html. Accessed June 15, 2007.

68. NAC, AARP. *Caregiving in the U.S.* 2004. Available at: http://www.caregiving.org/data/04final report.pdf. Accessed June 15, 2007.

69. Parker MW, Call VR, Vaitkus M. "Out of sight" but not "out of mind": Parent care contact and worry among military officers who live long distances from parents. *Military Psychology.* 2002;14(4):257–277.

70. Schempp D. (2007). Personal communication, October 5, 2007.

71. Stoller EP, Forster LE, Duniho TS. Systems of parent care within sibling networks. *Research on Aging.* 1992;14(1):28–49.

72. National Instutute on Aging (NIA). *So Far Away: Twenty Questions for Long-Distance Caregivers.* NIH Publication No. 06-5496. Washington, DC: NIH; 2006.

73. MetLife Mature Market Institute. *Miles Away: The MetLife Study of Long-Distance Caregiving. Findings from a National Study by the National Alliance for Caregiving with Zogby International.* Available at: http://www.metlife.com/Applications/ Corporate/WPS/CDA/PageGenerator/0,4132,P88 95,00.html. Accessed June 15, 2007.

74. MetLife Mature Market Institute. *Miles Away: The MetLife Study of Long-Distance Caregiving. Findings from a National Study by the National Alliance for Caregiving with Zogby International.* Available at: http://www.metlife.com/Applications/ Corporate/WPS/CDA/PageGenerator/0,4132,P88 95,00.html. Accessed June 15, 2007.

75. Watari K, Wetherell JL, Gatz M, Delaney J, Ladd C, Cherry D. Long-distance caregivers: Characteristics, service needs, and use of a long-distance caregiver program. *Clinical Gerontologist.* 2006; 29(4):61–77.

76. Benefield LS. Ways to support long-distance family caregivers. *Home Healthcare Nurse.* 2005;23 (3):196.

77. McLeod BW, ed. *Health After 60: Caregiving and Siblings.* 2007. Available at: http://healthresources .caremark.com/topic/siblingstress. Accessed June 27, 2007.

78. Baldock CV. Migrants and their parents: Caregiving from a distance. *Journal of Family Issues.* 2000;21(2):205–224.

79. MetLife Mature Market Institute. *Miles Away: The MetLife Study of Long-Distance Caregiving. Findings from a National Study by the National Alliance for Caregiving with Zogby International.* Available at: http://www.metlife.com/ Applications/ Corporate/WPS/CDA/PageGenerator/0,4132,P88 95,00.html. Accessed June 15, 2007.

80. Watari K, Wetherell JL, Gatz M, Delaney J, Ladd C, Cherry D. Long-distance caregivers: Characteristics, service needs, and use of a long-distance caregiver program. *Clinical Gerontologist.* 2006; 29(4):61–77.

81. Roff LL, Martin SS, Jennings LK, Parker MW, Harmon DK. Long-distance parental caregivers' experiences with siblings: A qualitative study. *Qualitative Social Work.* 2007;6(3):315–334.

82. McLeod BW, ed. *Health After 60: Caregiving and Siblings.* 2007. Available at: http://healthresources .caremark.com/topic/siblingstress. Accessed June 27, 2007.

83. Parker MW, Call VR, Vaitkus M. "Out of sight" but not "out of mind": Parent care contact and worry among military officers who live long distances from parents. *Military Psychology.* 2002; 14(4):257–277.

84. Watari K, Wetherell JL, Gatz M, Delaney J, Ladd C, Cherry D. Long-distance caregivers: Characteristics, service needs, and use of a long-distance caregiver program. *Clinical Gerontologist.* 2006; 29(4):61–77.

85. Schempp D. (2007). Personal communication, October 5, 2007.

86. Roff LL, Martin SS, Jennings LK, Parker MW, Harmon DK. Long-distance parental caregivers' experiences with siblings: A qualitative study. *Qualitative Social Work.* 2007;6(3):315–334.

87. Knutson K. Care management eases the emotional burden of caregivers with dementia relatives in a retirement community setting. *GCM Journal.* 2007;17(1):8–11.

88. Knutson K. Care management eases the emotional burden of caregivers with dementia relatives in a retirement community setting. *GCM Journal.* 2007;17(1):8–11.

89. Cress CJ, Barber C. Care planning and geriatric assessment. In: Cress C, ed. *Handbook of Geriatric Care Management.* 2nd ed. Sudbury, MA: Jones and Bartlett; 2007:73–97.

90. Solomon R. Who's in Charge? or Issues in Long-Distance Intergenerational Relations. Annual Conference of Jewish Family Services, keynote address. West Palm Beach, Florida, October 20, 1988.

91. Beerman S, Rappaport-Musson J. *Eldercare 911: The Caregiver's Complete Handbook for Making Decisions.* Amherst, NY: Prometheus Books; 2002:111.

92. Parker M, Church W, Toseland R. Caregiving at a distance. In: Berkman B, ed. *Handbook of Social Work in Health and Aging.* Oxford, UK: Oxford University Press; 2006:391–406.

93. Parker MW, Call VR, Vaitkus M. "Out of sight" but not "out of mind": Parent care contact and worry among military officers who live long distances from parents. *Military Psychology.* 2002;14(4):257–277.

94. Payne B. *Providing Care from Afar.* 2001. Available at: http://www.caregiving.com/yourcare/ html/weeklytip70.htm. Accessed November 13, 2007.

95. Rosenblatt B, Van Steenberg C. *Handbook for Long-Distance Caregivers: An Essential Guide for Families and Friends Caring for Ill or Elderly Loved Ones.* San Francisco, CA: Family Caregiver Alliance National Center on Caregiving; 2003. Available at: http://www.caregiver.org/caregiver/ jsp/content_node.jsp?nodeid=1-34. Accessed June 15, 2007.

96. Parker M, Church W, Toseland R. Caregiving at a distance. In: Berkman B, ed. *Handbook of Social Work in Health and Aging.* Oxford, UK: Oxford University Press; 2006:391–406.

97. Parker M, Church W, Toseland R. Caregiving at a distance. In: Berkman B, ed. *Handbook of Social Work in Health and Aging.* Oxford, UK: Oxford University Press; 2006:391–406.

98. Cress CJ, Barber C. Care planning and geriatric assessment. In: Cress C, ed. *Handbook of Geriatric Care Management.* 2nd ed. Sudbury, MA: Jones and Bartlett; 2007:73–97.

99. NAC, AARP. *Caregiving in the U.S.* 2004. Available at: http://www.caregiving.org/data/04finalreport.pdf. Accessed June 15, 2007.

100. Heath A. *Long-Distance Caregiving: A Survival Guide for Far Away Caregivers.* Lakewood, CO: American Source Books; 1993.

101. Beerman S, Rappaport-Musson J. *Eldercare 911: The Caregiver's Complete Handbook for Making Decisions.* Amherst, NY: Prometheus Books; 2002:111.

102. Berman C. *Caring for Yourself While Caring for Your Aging Parents.* 3rd ed. New York, NY: Henry Holt and Company; 2005.

103. National Instutute on Aging (NIA). *So Far Away: Twenty Questions for Long-Distance Caregivers.* NIH Publication No. 06-5496. Washington, DC: NIH; 2006.

104. Caring From a Distance. Available at: http://www.cfad.org/. Accessed November 2, 2007.

105. Setting Priorities for Retirement Years Foundation. *Evaluating Health Information on the World Wide Web: A Hands-on Guide for Older Adults and Caregivers* [reference manual]. Available at: http://www.spry.org. Accessed November 6, 2007.

106. Caring From a Distance. *Links.* Available at: http://www.cfad.org/links/index.cfm. Accessed November 2, 2007.

107. Heath A. *Long-Distance Caregiving: A Survival Guide for Far Away Caregivers.* Lakewood, CO: American Source Books; 1993.

108. AARP. *Miles Away and Still Caring: A Guide for Long-Distance Caregivers.* Washington, DC: AARP; 1986.

109. Caring From a Distance. *Swooping.* Available at: http://www.cfad.org/choices/swooping.cfm. Accessed November 2, 2007.

110. Schempp D. Personal communication, October 5, 2007.

111. Caring From a Distance. *Swooping.* Available at: http://www.cfad.org/choices/swooping.cfm. Accessed November 2, 2007.

112. Wilson B. *Caregiving Tip Sheet—Practical Tips for Long Distance Caregiving.* Available at: http://www.helpstartshere.org/. Accessed September 28, 2007.

113. Felt S. Caring From Afar—Distance Complicates Task of Looking After Your Aging Parents. *Arizona Republic.* 2006;Nov. Available at: http://www.foundationforseniorliving.com/cgi-bin/www/displayNews.pl?status=display_news_detail&code=27.

114. National Association of Area Agencies on Aging. *Home for the Holidays, Ten Warning Signs Your Family Member May Need Help.* Available at: http://www.n4a.org/locator_holiday_manual_021220.cfm. Accessed October 29, 2007.

115. Sorenson D. *Going Home Again: Holiday Homecoming.* Available at: http://www.professionalcareforyou.com/holidayhomecoming.htm. Accessed October 12, 2007.

116. National Association of Area Agencies on Aging. *Home for the Holidays, Ten Warning Signs Your Family Member May Need Help.* Available at: http://www.n4a.org/locator_holiday_manual_021220.cfm. Accessed October 29, 2007.

117. Felt S. Caring From Afar—Distance Complicates Task of Looking After Your Aging Parents. *Arizona Republic.* 2006;Nov. Available at: http://www.foundationforseniorliving.com/cgi-bin/www/displayNews.pl?status=display_news_detail&code=27.

118. Sorenson D. *Going Home Again: Waxing Nostalgic.* Available at: http://www.professionalcareforyou.com/waxingnostalgic.htm. Accessed October 12, 2007.

119. Ramey C, Cress C. Integrating late life relocation: The role of the GCM. In: Cress C, ed. *Handbook of Geriatric Care Management.* Sudbury, MA: Jones and Bartlett; 2007:283–307.

120. Rosenthal A, Cress C. Geriatric care management: Working with nearly normal aging families. In: Cress C, ed. *Handbook of Geriatric Care Management.* Sudbury, MA: Jones and Bartlett; 2007:309–340.

121. Heath A. *Long-Distance Caregiving: A Survival Guide for Far Away Caregivers.* Lakewood, CO: American Source Books; 1993.

122. Wexler N. *Mama Can't Remember Any More: Care Management of Aging Parents and Loved Ones.* Holt, MI: Partners Publishers Group; 1997:100–101.

123. Fleck C. *Long-Term Care: Crisis Control.* AARP Bulletin Online, May 2006. Available at: http://www.aarp.org/bulletin/longterm/cost_elder_care_sb.html. Accessed April 5, 2008.

124. Martin JA, Parker M. Understanding the importance of elder care preparations in the context of 21st century military service. *GCM Journal.* 2003;Winter:3–6.

125. Karp E, Koenig A. Preparing for emergencies. In: Cress C, ed. *Handbook of Geriatric Care Management.* Sudbury, MA: Jones and Bartlett; 2007:239–250.

126. Sorenson D. New Orleans disaster brings out the best in care management and services. *GCM Midwest Chapter Newsletter*. 2005;14:1.

127. Dynamic Living.com. *Planning for a Disaster*. Available at: http://www.dynamic-living.com/news-disaster-preparation.htm. Accessed October 15, 2007.

128. American Red Cross, FEMA. *Preparing for Disaster for People with Disabilities and Other Special Needs*. 2004. Available at: http://www.redcross.org/images/pdfs/preparedness/A4497.pdf. Accessed November 15, 2007.

129. National Family Caregiver Support Program. *Just in Case: Emergency Readiness for Older Adults and Caregivers*. Available at: http://www.aoa.gov/PROF/aoaprog/caregiver/overview/Just_in_Case030706_links.pdf. Accessed June 13, 2007.

130. Karp E, Koenig A. Preparing for emergencies. In: Cress C, ed. *Handbook of Geriatric Care Management*. Sudbury, MA: Jones and Bartlett; 2007:239–250.

131. American Red Cross. *Tips for Seniors and People with Disabilities*. Available at: http://www.redcross.org/services/disaster/beprepared/seniors.html. Accessed October 28, 2007.

132. National Fire Protection Association. *Emergency Evacuation Planning Guide for People with Disabilities*. 2007. Available at: http://www.nfpa.org/categoryList.asp?categoryID=824&cookie%5Ftest=1. Accessed November 12, 2007.

133. Solomon R. Who's in Charge? or Issues in Long-Distance Intergenerational Relations. Annual Conference of Jewish Family Services, keynote address. West Palm Beach, Florida, October 20, 1988.

134. Schempp D. Personal communication, October 5, 2007.

135. Schmall VL, Cleland M, Sturdevant M. *The Caregiver Helpbook: Powerful Tools for Caregiving*. Portland, OR: Legacy Health System; 2000.

136. AGIS. *Tips for Finding a Support Group*. Available at: http://www.agis.com/Document/24/tips-for-finding-a-support-group.aspx. Accessed November 6, 2007.

137. MetLife Mature Market Institute. *Since You Care: Long-Distance Caregiving*. 2005. Available at: http://www.metlife.com/Applications/Corporate/WPS/CDA/PageGenerator/0,4132,P8900,00.html. Accessed June 15, 2007.

138. Yost W. Making the paid family leave program work for you. *Family Caregiver Alliance Update*. 2007;24(3):1,4.

139. Ramey C, Cress C. Integrating late life relocation: The role of the GCM. In: Cress C, ed. *Handbook of Geriatric Care Management*. Sudbury, MA: Jones and Bartlett; 2007:283–307.

140. Family Caregiver Alliance. *Fact Sheet: Home Away from Home: Relocating Your Parents*. Available at: http://www.caregiver.org/caregiver/jsp/content_node.jsp?nodeid=849. Accessed October 30, 2007.

141. Hertz JE, Rosetti J, Koren ME, Robertson JF. Evidence-based guideline: Management of relocation in cognitively intact older adults. *Journal of Gerontological Nursing*. 2007;33(11).

142. AARP. *Using Medications Wisely: Traveling with Your Medicines*. Available at: http://www.aarp.org/health/rx_drugs/usingmeds/ traveling_with_your_medicines.html. Accessed December 4, 2007.

143. NAPGCM Listserv. Posting to NAPGCM Listserv. October 31, 2007, by Cindy Schaefer, A.P.N. Travel Care & Logistics, Inc.

144. McLeod BW. *And Thou Shalt Honor: The Caregiver's Companion*. Emmaus, PA: Rodale Press; 2002.

145. Leverette L. Personal communication, September 27, 2007.

146. Levison N. *Long-Distance Caregiving*. Available at: http://www.strengthforcaring.com/daily-care/practical-care-long-distance-care/long-distance-caregiving/. Accessed November 15, 2007.

147. McLeod BW. *And Thou Shalt Honor: The Caregiver's Companion*. Emmaus, PA: Rodale Press; 2002.

148. Bernatchez E. *The Best Cell Phones for Elderly/Senior Citizens*. Available at: http://cellphones.about.com/od/topcellphones/tp/cell_senior.htm. Accessed November 11, 2007.

149. Walker SA. *Gadget Reviews: This Simple Cell Phone Makes Calling Easy*. 2007. Available at: http://www.aarp.org/learntech/computers/gadgets/simple_cell_phone_makes_calling_easy.html. Accessed November 15, 2007.

150. Walker SA. *Life Online: Demystifying the Communications Gap*. 2007. Available at: http://www.aarp.org/learntech/computers/life_online/demystifying_the_communications_gap.html. Accessed November 15, 2007.

151. Gough M, Rosenfeld J. *Video Conferencing over IP: Configure, Secure, and Troubleshoot*. Rockland, MA: Syngress Publishing; 2006.

152. Mickus MA, Luz CC. Televisits: Sustaining long-distance family relationships among institution-

alized elders through technology. *Aging & Mental Health*. 2002;6(4):387–396.

153. Oliver DP, Demiris G, Hensel B. A promising technology to reduce social isolation of nursing home residents. *Journal of Nursing Care Quality*. 2006;21(4):302–305.

154. Hensel BK, Parker-Oliver D, Demiris G. Videophone communication between residents and family: A case study. *Journal of American Medical Directors Association*. 2007;8:123–127.

155. Savenstedt S, Brulin C, Sandman PO. Family members' narrated experiences of communicating via video-phone with patients with dementia staying at a nursing home. *Journal of Telemedicine and Telecare*. 2003;9(4):216–220.

156. Oliver DP, Demiris G, Day M, Courtney KL, Porock D. Telehospice support for elder caregivers of hospice patients: Two case studies. *Journal of Palliative Medicine*. 2006;9(2):264–267.

157. Dorhout J. Personal communication, November 27, 2007.

158. Gough M, Rosenfeld J. *Video Conferencing over IP: Configure, Secure, and Troubleshoot*. Rockland, MA: Syngress Publishing; 2006.

159. Gough M. *The Virtual Visitation Handbook: A Guide to Personal Video Conferencing*. Available at: http://www.internetvisitation.org/.

160. Abdulezer L, Abdulezer S, Dammond H. *Skype For Dummies*. Indianapolis, IN: Wiley Publishing; 2007.

161. Gough M, Rosenfeld J. *Video Conferencing over IP: Configure, Secure, and Troubleshoot*. Rockland, MA: Syngress Publishing; 2006.

162. Gough M. *The Virtual Visitation Handbook: A Guide to Personal Video Conferencing*. Available at: http://www.internetvisitation.org/.

163. Gough M, Rosenfeld J. *Video Conferencing over IP: Configure, Secure, and Troubleshoot*. Rockland, MA: Syngress Publishing; 2006.

164. Virtual Familes and Friends.com. Available at: http://jimbuie.blogs.com/virtualfamilies1/audio_video_podcasts_vcasts/index.html. Accessed September 20, 2007.

165. Greenman C. Keeping up with mom and dad and their elder-care provider. *New York Times*. August 3, 2000.

166. Hart AY. Connecting caregivers through technology. In: Levine C, ed. *Always on Call: When Illness Turns Families into Caregivers*. Nashville, TN: Vanderbilt University Press; 2004:235–250.

167. Alter J. *During Illness, a Bridge to Family and Friends: Free Web Site Allows Loved Ones to Keep Track of Condition, Treatments*. Available at: http://www.msnbc.msn.com/id/17986179/. Accessed October 21, 2007.

168. Freisner BE. 6 tips to make the holidays less stressful & more enjoyable. *CAPSule: Children of Aging Parents*. 2005;Fall:25–27. Available at: http://www.caps4caregivers.org/newsletter.htm. Accessed October 31, 2007.

169. Professor says much of new technology should be known as nana technology: Creates term to define technology to improve life for senior citizens. *Senior Journal*. Available at: http://seniorjournal.com/NEWS/Features/6-08-16-Professor Says.htm. Accessed November 27, 2007.

170. US Department of Commerce, Technology Administration, Office of Technology Policy. *Technology and Innovation in an Emerging Senior/Boomer Marketplace*. 2005 White House Conference on Aging. December 11, 2005.

171. Ray S. *Telehealth Moves from the Doctor's Office to the Home*. Available at: http://www.caregiver.com/channels/tech/articles/telehealth.htm. Accessed September 29, 2007.

172. Stevenson K. *Elder Web: To Watch or Not to Watch?, Cameras, Ethical Considerations, Sensors, Systems in Operation, What About the Targets?* Available at: http://www.elderweb.com/home/book/export/html/3001. Accessed August 5, 2007.

173. Kawamoto D. Managing the Meds from Miles Away. *CNETNEWS.com*. Available at: http://news.com.com/Managing+the+meds+from+miles+away/2100-11393_3-6188642.html?tag=item. Accessed July 22, 2007.

174. Larson C. In elder care, signing on becomes a way to drop by. *New York Times*. February 7, 2007. Available at: http://www.nytimes.com/2007/02/04/business/yourmoney/04elder.html?ex=1328245200&en=ec63007ce80dfadc&ei=5088&partner=rssnyt&emc=rss. Accessed July 1, 2007.

175. Walker SA. Personal communication, November 29, 2007.

176. Mahoney DF. The future of technology in mental health nursing—A nurse geropsychtechnologist? In: Melillo KD, Houde SC, eds. *Geropsychiatric and Mental Health Nursing*. Sudbury, MA: Jones and Bartlett; 2007:392.

177. Blanchard J. Ethical considerations of home monitoring technology. *Home Health Care Technology Report*. 2004;1(53):63–64.

178. Gage A. Advanced technology helping to meet the challenges of aging and caregiving. *Journal*

of the Minnesota Association for Guardianship and Conservatorship. 2007;18(2). Available at: http://www.quietcare.com/uploads/resources/MAGiC%20article_rev%20FAP.pdf. Accessed December 5, 2007.

179. Gage A. Advanced technology helping to meet the challenges of aging and caregiving. *Journal of the Minnesota Association for Guardianship and Conservatorship.* 2007;18(2). Available at: http://www.quietcare.com/uploads/resources/MAGiC%20article_rev%20FAP.pdf. Accessed December 5, 2007.

180. Blanchard J. Ethical considerations of home monitoring technology. *Home Health Care Technology Report.* 2004;1(53):63–64.

181. Shellenbarger S. Remote control: Frail seniors embrace home monitoring. *Wall Street Journal*, November 29, 2007.

182. Intel. *Digital Home Technologies for Aging in Place.* Available at: http://www.intel.com/research/prohealth/dh_aging_in_place.htm. Accessed July 22, 2007.

183. Mahoney D, Tarlow B. Workplace response to virtual caregiver support and remote home monitoring: The Worker Interactive Networking (WIN) project. Consumer-Centered Computer-Supported Care for Healthy People. Proceedings of the Ninth International Congress on Nursing Informatics. Seoul, Korea, June 9–14. *Studies in Health Technology and Informatics.* 122:676–680.

184. Stevenson K. *Elder Web: To Watch or Not to Watch?, Cameras, Ethical Considerations, Sensors, Systems in Operation, What About the Targets?* Available at: http://www.elderweb.com/home/book/export/html/3001. Accessed August 5, 2007.

185. Mahoney DF. Linking home care and the workplace through innovative wireless technology: The Worker Interactive Networking (WIN) Project. *Home Health Care Management & Practice.* 2004;16(5):417–428.

186. Gage A. Advanced technology helping to meet the challenges of aging and caregiving. *Journal of the Minnesota Association for Guardianship and Conservatorship.* 2007;18(2). Available at: http://www.quietcare.com/uploads/resources/MAGiC%20article_rev%20FAP.pdf. Accessed December 5, 2007.

187. Gage A. Advanced technology helping to meet the challenges of aging and caregiving. *Journal of the Minnesota Association for Guardianship and Conservatorship.* 2007;18(2). Available at:

http://www.quietcare.com/uploads/resources/MAGiC%20article_rev%20FAP.pdf. Accessed December 5, 2007.

188. Larson C. In elder care, signing on becomes a way to drop by. *New York Times*, February 7, 2007. Available at: http://www.nytimes.com/2007/02/04/ business/yourmoney/04elder.html?ex=1328245200&en=ec63007ce80dfadc&ei=5088&partner=rssnyt&emc=rss. Accessed July 1, 2007.

189. Lundberg S. Elite care brings elder-friendly technology to Oregon. *Aging Today.* 2007;September–October:9.

190. Elite Care. *Elite Care Home Technology.* Available at: http://www.elitecare.com/technology. Accessed October 21, 2007.

191. Ray S. *Telehealth Moves from the Doctor's Office to the Home.* Available at: http://www.caregiver.com/channels/tech/articles/telehealth.htm. Accessed September 29, 2007.

192. Stevenson K. *Elder Web: To Watch or Not to Watch?, Cameras, Ethical Considerations, Sensors, Systems in Operation, What About the Targets?* Available at: http://www.elderweb.com/home/book/export/html/3001. Accessed August 5, 2007.

193. Larson C. In elder care, signing on becomes a way to drop by. *New York Times*, February 7, 2007. Available at: http://www.nytimes.com/2007/02/04/ business/yourmoney/04elder.html?ex=1328245200&en=ec63007ce80dfadc&ei=5088&partner=rssnyt&emc=rss. Accessed July 1, 2007.

194. Mahoney DF. Personal communication, November 8, 2007.

195. Kinney JM, Kart CS. Not quite a panacea: Technology to facilitate family caregiving for elders with dementia. *Dimensions.* 2006;30(2):64–66.

196. Stevenson K. *Elder Web: To Watch or Not to Watch?, Cameras, Ethical Considerations, Sensors, Systems in Operation, What About the Targets?* Available at: http://www.elderweb.com/home/book/export/html/3001. Accessed August 5, 2007.

197. Marsa L. Aging under a high-tech eye. *Los Angeles Times,* October 11, 2007. Available at: http://www.latimes.com/features/printedition/home/la-hm-connect11oct11,1,1434083.story?ctrack=1&cset=true. Accessed November 28, 2007.

198. Mahoney DF. Linking home care and the workplace through innovative wireless technology:

The Worker Interactive Networking (WIN) Project. *Home Health Care Management & Practice*. 2004;16(5):417–428.

199. Mahoney DF. Personal communication, November 8, 2007.

200. Mahoney DF. Personal communication, November 8, 2007.

201. Horgas A, Abowd G. The impact of technology on living environments for older adults. In: Pew RW, Van Hemel SB, eds. *Technology for Adaptive Aging*. Washington, DC: National Academies Press; 2004:230–252.

202. Gage A. Advanced technology helping to meet the challenges of aging and caregiving. *Journal of the Minnesota Association for Guardianship and Conservatorship*. 2007;18(2). Available at: http://www.quietcare.com/uploads/resources/MAGiC%20article_rev%20FAP.pdf. Accessed December 5, 2007.

203. Baruch, J, Downs M, Baldwin C, Bruce E. A case study in the use of technology to reassure and support a person with dementia. *Dementia*. 2004;3(3):372–377.

204. Dementia Caregiver's Toolbox. *Dementia Caregivers Have Technology Assistance*. Available at: http://nurturingnuggets.typepad.com/the_nurturing_nuggets_blo/2007/03/two_new_technol.html. Accessed March 21, 2007.

205. Horgas A, Abowd G. The impact of technology on living environments for older adults. In: Pew RW, Van Hemel SB, eds. *Technology for Adaptive Aging*. Washington, DC: National Academies Press; 2004:230–252.

206. Kawamoto D. Managing the meds from miles away. *CNETNEWS.com*. Available at: http://news.com.com/Managing+the+meds+from+miles+away/ 2100-11393_3-6188642.html?tag=item. Accessed July 22, 2007.

207. Stachura ME, Khasanshina EV. *Telehomecare and Remote Monitoring: An Outcomes Overview*. Available at: http://www.advamed.org/NR/rdonlyres/2250724C-5005-45CD-A3C9-0EC0CD3132A1/0/TelehomecarereportFNL103107.pdf. Accessed November 10, 2007.

208. ATA Home Telehealth & Remote Monitoring SIG. Available at: http://www.atmeda.org/ICOT/sighomehealth.htm. Accessed November 10, 2007.

209. Stachura ME, Khasanshina EV. *Telehomecare and Remote Monitoring: An Outcomes Overview*. Available at: http://www.advamed.org/NR/rdonlyres/2250724C-5005-45CD-A3C9-0EC0CD3132

A1/0/TelehomecarereportFNL103107.pdf. Accessed November 10, 2007.

210. Stachura ME, Khasanshina EV. *Telehomecare and Remote Monitoring: An Outcomes Overview*. Available at: http://www.advamed.org/NR/rdonlyres/2250724C-5005-45CD-A3C9-0EC0CD3132A1/0/TelehomecarereportFNL103107.pdf. Accessed November 10, 2007.

211. HealthTechWire. *Philips Announces Results of National Study on the Future of Home Healthcare Technology*. Available at: http://www.healthtechwire.com/Pressrelease.146+M585d6525c62.0.html. Accessed October 21, 2007.

212. Stachura ME, Khasanshina EV. *Telehomecare and Remote Monitoring: An Outcomes Overview*. Available at: http://www.advamed.org/NR/rdonlyres/2250724C-5005-45CD-A3C9-0EC0CD3132A1/0/TelehomecarereportFNL103107.pdf. Accessed November 10, 2007.

213. Datta SSR. *Health Care Moves Home*. Available at: http://money.cnn.com/2006/10/03/magazines/business2/healthcare_home.biz2/index.htm. Accessed October 26, 2007.

214. Larson C. In elder care, signing on becomes a way to drop by. *New York Times*, February 7, 2007. Available at: http://www.nytimes.com/2007/02/04/ business/yourmoney/04elder.html?ex=1328245200&en=ec63007ce80dfadc&ei=5088&partner=rssnyt&emc=rss. Accessed July 1, 2007.

215. Versweyveld L. Could home telehealth make nursing homes obsolete for baby boomers? *Virtual Medical Worlds Monthly*. Available at: http://www.hoise.com/vmw/07/articles/vmw/LV-VM-02-07-28.html. Accessed November 11, 2007.

216. Datta SSR. *Health Care Moves Home*. Available at: http://money.cnn.com/2006/10/03/magazines/business2/healthcare_home.biz2/index.htm. Accessed October 26, 2007.

217. Rogers WA, Fisk AD. Cognitive support for elders through technology. *Generations*. 2006;30(2):38–43.

218. Cantor MD. No information about me without me: Technology, privacy, and home monitoring. *Generations*. 2006;30(2):49–53.

219. Larson C. In elder care, signing on becomes a way to drop by. *New York Times*, February 7, 2007. Available at: http://www.nytimes.com/2007/02/04/business/yourmoney/04elder.html?ex=1328245200&en=ec63007ce80dfadc&ei=5088&partner=rssnyt&emc=rss. Accessed July 1, 2007.

220. Mahoney DF. Linking home care and the work-place through innovative wireless technology: The Worker Interactive Networking (WIN) Project. *Home Health Care Management & Practice.* 2004;16(5):417–428.

221. Stevenson K. *Elder Web: To Watch or Not to Watch?, Cameras, Ethical Considerations, Sensors, Systems in Operation, What About the Targets?* Available at: http://www.elderweb.com/home/book/export/html/3001. Accessed August 5, 2007.

222. Blanchard J. Ethical considerations of home monitoring technology. *Home Health Care Technology Report.* 2004;1(53):63–64.

223. Cantor MD. No information about me without me: Technology, privacy, and home monitoring. *Generations.* 2006;30(2):49–53.

224. Mahoney DF. Linking home care and the work-place through innovative wireless technology: The Worker Interactive Networking (WIN) Project. *Home Health Care Management & Practice.* 2004;16(5):417–428.

225. Mahoney DF. Linking home care and the work-place through innovative wireless technology: The Worker Interactive Networking (WIN) Project. *Home Health Care Management & Practice.* 2004;16(5):417–428.

226. Gage A. Advanced technology helping to meet the challenges of aging and caregiving. *Journal of the Minnesota Association for Guardianship and Conservatorship.* 2007;18(2). Available at: http://www.quietcare.com/uploads/resources/MAGiC%20article_rev%20FAP.pdf. Accessed December 5, 2007.

227. CAST. *Imagine—The Future of Aging.* Available at: http://www.agingtech.org/imagine_video.aspx. Accessed August 2, 2007.

228. CAST. *Imagine—the Future of Aging: Vision Video Introductory Guide.* Washington, DC: American Association of Homes and Services for the Aging; 2007.

229. CAST. *Technology Assessment Tool for Providers.* Available at: http://www.agingtech.org/ArticleDetail.aspx?id=48. Accessed November 30, 2007.

230. Gage A. Advanced technology helping to meet the challenges of aging and caregiving. *Journal of the Minnesota Association for Guardianship and Conservatorship.* 2007;18(2). Available at: http://www.quietcare.com/uploads/ resources/MAGiC%20article_rev%20FAP.pdf. Accessed December 5, 2007.

231. Gage A. Advanced technology helping to meet the challenges of aging and caregiving. *Journal of the Minnesota Association for Guardianship and Conservatorship.* 2007;18(2). Available at: http://www.quietcare.com/uploads/resources/MAGiC%20article_rev%20FAP.pdf. Accessed December 5, 2007.

232. TCBI. *Fourth Annual Healthcare Unbound: A Conference & Exhibition on the Convergence of Consumer & Healthcare Technologies, Special Focus on Remote Monitoring & Home Telehealth for Managing Diseases & Promoting Wellness.* Available at: http://www.tcbi.org/hu2007/folder/TBCI_HU2007_Brochure.pdf. Accessed August 3, 2007.

233. CAST. *CAST Clearinghouse.* Available at: http://www.agingtech.org/Browsemain.aspx. Accessed August 2, 2007.

234. HCTAA. *Home Care Technology Association of America: Aging in Place.* Available at: http://www.hctaa.org/aging.html. Accessed August 5, 2007.

235. SmartSilvers Alliance. *The SmartSilvers Alliance: Using Technology to Foster Active Aging.* Available at: http://network.smartsilvers.com/. Accessed November 15, 2007.

236. SmartSilvers Alliance. *The SmartSilvers Common Sense Guide to Aging in Place Using Low Cost Technology.* Available at: http://network.smartsilvers.com/index.php?option=com_content&task=view&id=37&Itemid=1. Accessed November 28, 2007.

237. Intel. *Digital Home Technologies for Aging in Place.* Available at: http://www.intel.com/research/prohealth/dh_aging_in_place.htm. Accessed July 27, 2007.

CHAPTER 4

Assessing the Caregiver

Cathy Jo Cress

Assessing the family caregiver is a new but crucial concept for care managers. As care managers, we are health and social services oriented. For almost three decades we have assessed the care receiver for problems with function, social connection, and psychological issues. If we suspect depression we have completed that screening. If our client plans to move, has cultural needs and preferences, exhibits signs of dementia, needs ways to improve quality of life or a spiritual connection, we have assessed the care receiver for those problems. All our assessments have left out a major fact—care is an exchange. To receive care, the patient/client usually needs a family caregiver to give or supervise it. That family caregiver is the glue that holds it all together, and his or her inner bond begins to weaken and can break under the strain of caring.

Other countries have seen what the United States has yet to grasp. In 1995, the United Kingdom passed the Recognition and Services Act, which provided British caregivers a statutory right to request an assessment at the same time that a frail elder or adult with disabilities is assessed.[1]

When the viselike pressure of caregiving reaches a crisis (burning pots, wandering, incontinence), the family may bring in a care manager. That care manager assesses the care receiver and brings in a range of resources to ensure that the frail elder can stay at the appropriate level of care, usually at home. The success of that frail elder staying at the right level of care many times relies on the outside resources (meals on wheels, friendly visitors, paid caregivers), but more likely the key is the informal caregiver system of the aging family. These family or informal caregivers represent 78% of the long-term care system and are the backbone of long-term care.[2] Professional care managers have paid little attention to this backbone of long-term care: the aging family. This blind spot leaves the care receiver and the aging family ready to crumble and break unless the family caregiver is urgently assessed for their own needs. The care manager and the rest of the long-term care system must now meet the caregiver's needs.

From a critical policy perspective, the federal government and the long-term care system in the United States cannot afford to neglect the burnout and strain of millions of Americans caregivers. Despite the rewards caregivers get from giving care, we know from years of research that being a family caregiver results in significant losses. These degradations and deficits include role conflict and overload from the never-ending tasks demanded of a caregiver. Left in a permanent state of worry and anxiety, caregivers often work in a deteriorating and unpredictable situation. Caregivers can feel entrapped by the restrictions on their own life.

They are often beset by fiscal worries because they are not paid except in some states, like California under Medicaid. Yet the caregiving situation explodes in cost through medical bills, medical equipment, and informal care that must be brought in, if the family can afford it. Family caregivers face a quagmire of legal problems including untangling wills, trusts, and inheritance issues, which generally complicate care both emotionally and physically. Many times these family caregivers compound their fiscal woes by having to quit their job, running the risk of being hired again, if they can eventually return to work. The caregivers' own physical and mental health is often ravaged. They are asked to do medical tasks that caregivers 10 years ago were never assigned, thus increasing their risk of personal injury through turning, lifting, and transferring the older patient.[3]

In fact, as Nancy Guberman points out, if these family caregivers were working for any other health agency, home care agency, or any other profession, worker compensation boards would be waging major prevention campaigns, and there would be workers' compensation claims galore from the caregiver tasks, strain, and burnout these family caregivers endure.[4]

The needs of the family caregiver are different from the needs of the care receiver, and the care manager must differentiate those needs to make sure the care receiver's functional and psychosocial needs are met. The care receiver and the family caregiver are part of one homeostatic system encompassing the whole aging family. To keep that family healthy and whole, in the middle of swirling care crises, the care manager must first recognize that there are multiple clients, including the person who gives or supervises care. Egregiously, family members who give care are often referred to by the inanimate wooden term *resources*. They have also been referred to as *informants*. This stripping of personhood denudes them of their status as individuals We must not be blind to caregivers' humanity and thus their own needs.[5]

HOW DID WE GET HERE?

Care managers have lived through the major healthcare changes of the last 40 years. So has the aging family. We now die of chronic diseases such as cancer, dementia, and the degradations of old age. We used to succumb to acute care diseases such as measles, diphtheria, and pneumonia. We died in childhood. The parent's heartbreak of losing a baby was transformed when medical science created inoculations for polio and measles and antibiotics for such infections as pneumonia. We now fall victim to long-term chronic illnesses and disabilities that often take several years or decades to develop. With so many people living so long using very expensive treatments for chronic healthcare problems, the federal government turned to cost containment during the last 40 years and radically shortened hospital stays. The average hospital stay for someone 65 or older in 1970 was 12.6 days. This was sliced by more than half through cost-cutting efforts. Today's older patients are often pushed out of fiscally bleeding hospitals "sicker and quicker" into the arms of their very unprepared family members. Patients' homes are turned into hospitals, and the wives, daughters, and daughter-in-laws become the nurse/caregivers, all completely untrained for the job.[6]

After a huge surge in the 1990s, Medicare-funded home care was placed under restrictive prospective payment reimbursement system rules. Families, in spite of their uninvited burden, turned their homes into hospitals, themselves into untrained medical personnel, and contributed up to $257 billion in free care in 2000. They had no lobby to gain relief from the tidal wave of caregiving that washed over them.[7]

WHO IS THE FAMILY CAREGIVER?

Who are these family members who become accidental caregivers? According to the National Center for Caregiving at the Family Caregiver Alliance, a family caregiver can be defined as any relative, partner, friend, or neighbor who has a significant personal relationship with, and provides a broad range of assistance for, an older person or an adult with a chronic or disabling condition. These individuals can be primary or secondary caregivers and live with or live separately from the person receiving care.[8] The family caregiver does not have to give direct care but can supervise, arrange, or give a broad range of assistance.

Family caregivers number approximately 44 million, are 18 or older, provide unpaid assistance, and support older people and adults with disabilities in the community. Family members or relatives represent 83% of caregivers. Most are middle aged and their ages range from 35 to 64 years old. Ethnicity varies, with 21% for both white and African-American, 18% Asian, and 18% Hispanic. About 1 out of 2 caregivers are women. Slightly half of caregivers (48%) are employed outside the home with full-time jobs.

The amount of care these family caregivers render varies widely from 8 hours to more than 40 hours a week. These caregivers give care for an exhaustingly long time—an average of 4.3 years.[9]

Spouses who care for their wife or husband at home are, according to Dr. Steven Zarit of the Zarit–Burden scale, between 69 and 73 years old. So they are already somewhat frail themselves to be taking on sometimes complicated major medical tasks.

Carol Levine, a pioneer in the caregiver assessment movement and a female caregiver herself, points out that the broader view we must take as professionals is that family caregivers are mostly wives, daughters, and daughters-in-law.[10] The majority felt they had no choice but to assume this role. It was not their calling, they felt, but their fate.

SOCIAL TRENDS IN FAMILY CAREGIVING

According to Zarit, there is a hierarchy in the family as to who the family caregiver is. It begins with the spouse when both parents are alive. The daughter will be the main support of the spouse and the disabled elder when both parents are living. When one parent dies or both are incapacitated, the daughter usually steps up to the plate as the main caregiver. Brothers will help sisters but are usually not the lead caregiver, unless there is no sister. Daughter-in-laws come forward then. The daughters who care are balancing 100 plates, with their own children, husband, and their own work. They often have to rearrange their work schedule or leave work altogether to offer this caregiver support to their parent or parents. With the birth rate dropping and a continuing 100-year trend toward smaller families, the caregiving of a parent or parents is resting on fewer and fewer adult children. In fact the midlife couple is apt to have more parents than children.[11] Growing rates in divorce in the United States and worldwide create questions as to which child or set of children becomes the family caregiver—his or hers. Divorce brings a new dynamic to the situation. Will children who did not grow up with a parent be willing to care for them? If a father never paid child support, will his son or daughter be there to offer the caregiving he never gave?

Finally, as Zarit points out, caregiving is not a one-way street but an exchange. Their aging parents may care for adult children who care for a parent financially at the same time. So caregiving in the family is dynamic and has a history of interchange between generations.[12]

WHAT IS A CAREGIVER ASSESSMENT?

A new caregiver assessment tool needs to be added to the care manager's arsenal to assess these beleaguered and tottering struts holding up the older care receivers' world. A caregiver assessment is defined by the National Center on Caregiving at the Family Caregiver Alliance as follows:

> A systematic process of gathering information that describes a caregiving situation and identifies the particular problems, needs, resources, and strengths of a family caregiver. This new measure approaches issues from a caregiver's perspective and culture, focuses on what assistance the caregiver may need, examines outcomes the family member wants for support, and seeks to maintain the caregiver's own health and well-being.[13]

We have crafted an assessment tool for care managers (see Exhibit 4-1). In general, research into caregiver assessment tells us that assessments should be tailored to the caregiving context, service setting, and program. There is no single protocol for all caregiver assessments. The National Center on Caregiving at the Family Caregiver Alliance has suggested that no one approach is optimal in all care settings and situations.[14] We have devised a caregiver assessment tool that you can alter as you see fit.

We also offer the Stress and Appraisal Coping Framework, developed by Pearlin and suggested by Barbara and Carmen Morano in their excellent article on caregiver assessment in the *GCM Journal*,[15] as another excellent caregiver assessment tool that care managers can use for family caregivers. Both are good choices for care managers to begin assessing beleaguered and long-neglected family caregivers. There are many other excellent assessment tools that are listed in this chapter for a care manager to choose from.

Who Is My Client?

The caregiver assessment concept brings care managers back to an age-old question: Just who is my client? Is the care receiver your client or is the caregiver your client? For care managers to see the caregiver as a client is a major challenge. Our focus as care managers has always been on the care recipient as the client. The National Center for Caregiving suggests professionals in any agency see both the caregiver and care receiver as clients, but for this to happen a shift must take place in the entire agency. Both administration and frontline care managers need to build a consensus that the caregiver is a client as well. If your care management practice is a solo practice, you have no problem, but if you have partners or work in a large agency you must create a consensus that you will include the caregiver as a client so that frontline care managers get the necessary support. Questions such as whether caregivers have their own records and what the budgetary impacts and pressure on staff will be will have to be answered.

Concerns may come up with other staff such as increased paperwork, taking time away from the care receiver, lack of resources in the community to meet the caregiver's needs, and the caregiver's reluctance to share information.[16]

Whose Problem Is It?

After climbing through the barbed wire of "who is my client" the care manager faces the next question: whose problem is it?

Exhibit 4-1 Caregiver Assessment Tool for Care Manager

What triggered the caregiver assessment? _____

1. Basic caregiver information

GCM assessors name _____   Date of interview _____

Caregiver's name _____   Care Receiver's name _____

Caregiver's telephone _____   Caregiver's sex   F   M

Caregiver's address _____   same as care receiver   N   Y

Caregiver relationship to care receiver_____

2. Hour's caregiver cares for care receiver.

All the Time   N   Y

Days circle   M   T   W   T   F   S   SU

Hours per day M_____, T_____, W_____, T_____, F_____, S_____, S_____

How long has caregiver been caring for care receiver __years__mo

3. Informal Supports for caregiver (friends, neighbor family who help with ADL's IADL's)

Informal Supports for caregiver

Help provided _____

Name_____ Location _____Phone_____

Relationship to care receiver

Help provided _____

Informal Supports for caregiver

Name_____ Location _____Phone_____

Relationship to care receiver

Help provided _____

Use back of page for more listings

Is there anyone else that might help you with care receiver?

4. Formal Supports (homecare agencies, Adult day care, senior transportation, elder law attorney)

Present Formal Supports to help caregivers-

Name _____

Help provided _____

Name _____

Help provided _____

Name _____

Help provided _____

Name _____

Help provided _____

Use back if more

continues

Exhibit 4-1 Caregiver Assessment Tool for Care Manager (continued)

5. Cultural Needs

Language spoken by Caregiver _____ Language spoken by care receiver _____

Informal or formal Supports needed by Caregiver if languages are different N   Y   what _____

Translator needed if Caregiver does not speak care manager's language N   Y _____

6. Limitations of care giver

Poor Health   N   Y   diagnosis _____

Disabled   N   Y   disability _____

Doing tasks that are repulsive N   Y what _____

Frail N   Y describe_____

Employed elsewhere   N   Y   days___hours

Providing care to others   N   Y   who_____ hours _____

Lack knowledge/skills   N   Y   what _____

Poor relationship with care receiver   N   Y   describe _____

Long distance care provider   N   Y   lives where _____

Alcohol, drug abuse   N   Y   describe _____

Unable to do ADL's   N   Y   what _____

Unable to do IADL   N   Y   what _____

Financials strain   N   Y   describe _____

Dependent on Care Receiver for housing   N   Y   describe

_____

7. Additional assessments for caregiver

Score on Zarit Burden _____

Score on GDS given to caregiver _____

8. Intervenyions needed for Care Giver

Formal Supports needed by Caregiver   N   Y   describe

_____

Training needed by Caregiver   N   Y   describe

_____

Education Resources needed for caregiver _____

Organizing Tools needed for caregiver (calendar) _____

Referral to Physician needed for caregiver   N   Y   describe

_____

Stress relief needed for caregiver   N   Y   describe

_____

Respite needed for caregiver   N   Y   ___ describe

_____

Exhibit 4-1 GCM Field Evaluation/Care Management Service (continued)

Advocacy needed for caregiver   N   Y   describe?

_____

Family dysfunction impairing care   N   Y   describe

_____

Emotional or mental health resources   N   Y   describe

_____

Support group needed   N   Y   describe

_____

9. Caregiver care plan

Problems = list

Fill in what is needed if Y circled in section 8

Formal Supports needed _____

Respite _____

Education _____

Training needed _____

Impaired Health _____

Hours need reducing _____

Depression_____

High Stress level _____

Lives Long Distance _____

Alcohol, Drug abuse _____

Family Dysfunction _____

Other _____

Use problems checked off in problems list above to create care management care plan for caregiver

Caregiver Care Plan

Problems   Interventions

Many times caregivers seek help from a care manager or other professional, asking them to fix the care receiver's problems. Though the caregiver asked the care manager to find a solution to the problem, the care receiver or patient may deny anything is wrong. So when the care receiver or patient won't work with the care manager, the care manager may have to "fix" the person who asked for help in the first place—the caregiver. Steven Zarit points out that this is often the case with patients with Alzheimer's disease. Rarely do dementia victims seek help for themselves. Instead, often the family member approaches the aging professional on behalf of the "patient." Usually this is because problems have begun to erupt in the caregiver's life related to the care receiver. The problems that come up for the family caregiver depend on how the family member appraises the situation and then takes responsibility for the older person. In the meantime the older family member with the problem usually does not acknowledge that there is any problem at all.[17]

Thus one reason the care manager may want to assess the caregiver is based on systems theory. The solution a care manager brings to the situation in the form of a care plan—defining the problems and offering solutions—almost always involves working with the caregiver to make changes in the situation. If the problem is that the care receiver can't remember to take his or her medications, it is usually the family caregiver who either sets up the meds or actually gives them to the patient. If those meds involve medications for anxiety on the care receiver's part, this may stop her from calling the family member over and over. So when the family member tells the care manager that she is being driven crazy by her mother calling her over and over, the daughter as caregiver is part of the problem. The care manager must design a solution that takes this into account. In this case the care manager wants to fix the problem of the mother calling over and over by using the daughter to fix the mother's problem that then fixes the daughter's problem. So using a caregiver assessment usually has a dual result of defining a problem and finding a solution to an interaction between the caregiver and the care receiver.

WHY ASSESS THE CAREGIVER?

A caregiver assessment gives the care manager the ability to understand the caregiver's needs and then define the caregiver's problems. A caregiver assessment arms the care manager with the ability to pinpoint the resources of the caregiver and the family so that the family can muster those resources.

The care manager will gain invaluable information from assessing the family caregiver. First of all, a systematic assessment of the caregiver allows the care manager to clearly identify the caregiver's problems. Since, as mentioned earlier, solving the caregiver's problems is often a way of solving the care receiver's problems, this is the great enhancement to creating the care manager's care plan.

Let's take Ms. Handy, who lives in Petaluma, California. She is the family caregiver for her father, Mr. Wilson, who has vascular dementia and lives with her. She also has two school-age children and one 3-year-old in day care. She works as a social worker for a children's agency during the day. Mr. Wilson attends an adult day program 5 days a week and goes to the Catholic Church on Sunday, where the church picks him up and brings him home. So Ms. Handy already has a good care plan involving outside resources as support for her and her father.

But Ms. Handy says she is exhausted because Mr. Wilson won't go to bed until midnight and she has to get up and slowly convince him to take off his clothes, put on a new adult diaper, and get into bed. If she does not do this, he will sit up in his recliner all night watching TV and be too tired to attend the respite programs during the day. His physician does not want to prescribe sleeping medications for fear he will fall at night if he gets up. Once the daughter's up, she can't go back to sleep, so then she is awake for a few hours and wakes up exhausted. She has also missed several days of work from being too tired to go to her job, and it has become an issue at her agency. She has run out of vacation and sick days and will now lose pay for every day not worked because of her exhaustion.

Ms. Handy does not have the financial resources to afford a care provider. Her husband is also very frustrated because the emotional and sexual relationship with his wife has deteriorated. The teacher of her oldest child also reports problems in school because Ms. Handy does not have all the time she needs to nurture her children and help with homework.

The care manager Ms. Helpmate is called by Ms. Handy, who is thinking of placing her father in a facility. Ms. Helpmate does a caregiver assessment. She also does a geriatric depression assessment, and Ms. Handy has a score of 17, indicating depression. The care manager then suggests that Ms. Handy begin getting her father ready for bed at 10:00 PM. The daughter is reluctant because she is still locked in her old role of "I'm the kid, and he's the dad." She fearful to change her father's routine, even though she is so tired after months of this that she is at the breaking point.

After much coaching by the care manager, the daughter starts to stay up until 10:00, go through all the prompting to get her father changed, then turns off the TV. The father is angry and resistant at first, but gradually goes to bed at 10:00. The care manager coaches the daughter over the next few weeks, and the father slowly adjusts to this new routine, giving Ms. Handy encouragement to continue. Ms. Handy then is able to sleep all night, pulling her off the edge of the cliff where her next step was nursing home placement for her father.

What the care manager has done, through the caregiver assessment, is to identify the caregiver's problem and then identify the resources the family has to change the situation. The daughter made the change with the care manager's encouragement and coaching, allowing her to see new choices in her care and relationship with her father. Sometimes

the obvious is hard to see in families because of their extreme state of overwhelm. The daughter had the ability to change her dad's routine, and the care manager's coaching gave her both the insight and the courage to alter her father's schedule, even if he at first was angry and balked. So the care manager then identified the caregiver's role, changing the time of bed, turning the TV off, and gently helping the daughter deal with the father's angry reaction to going to bed earlier. The care manager has identified the inner resources the daughter already had to make this change.

The third thing the care manager has identified is the family caregiver's pressing need, which was a night of uninterrupted sleep. Babies usually start to sleep all night at 6 months. With older clients the sleeplessness goes on, sometimes till they die. This daughter had been sleepless for 8 months and was at the point of placing her father in a facility. So Ms. Helpmate's caregiver assessment was an indispensable part of creating a new care plan for the care receiver. She has identified the caregiver's problem and then successfully intervened with the caregiver, not with the patient. But both the care receiver and caregiver have changed, plus the ultimate goal of keeping Mr. Wilson at home has been achieved, all through a caregiver assessment.

The care manager then created a new intervention in her care plan for the daughter's exhaustion. That was to have the daughter attend a caregiver support group in her local community. The care manager knew that the daughter could only afford to have the care manager monitor the situation once a month. In a free support group setting, Ms. Handy would get positive enforcement of her need to care for herself. The daughter would learn from other caregivers the importance of taking care of themselves. The care manager also used technology as another intervention. She identified several sites on the Internet where the daughter could learn about caregiver stress and the effect of sleeplessness on her own body. So the daughter could then use the World Wide Web, very cost-effectively, to educate herself about her problems.

The caregiver assessment gives the care manager the ability to identify the primary caregiver and the informal caregivers.[18] While asking questions, the care manager found that the daughter was the oldest of five siblings. The care manager suggested a family meeting, between all the siblings, to discuss some support for the exhausted daughter. The care manager agreed to facilitate that meeting.

At this gathering of the family, Ms. Helpmate used respite care as a new intervention to the daughter's problem. At the meeting, the two siblings who lived nearby agreed to spend one night a week each at the daughter's home and get the father to bed, so Ms. Handy had two nights respite a week. A third sibling who lived a distance away agreed to come to visit for 1 week every 5 months and take over the care of the father. In addition, a fourth sibling, who lived some distance away but never had a good relationship with the father, wanted to support his sister the caregiver. He agreed to pay for a private home care service that his siblings can call if they cannot relieve Ms. Handy. Ms. Handy could also use this service, if she is ill. This is budgeted at 3 days per month but can be increased.

Ms. Helpmate was able to use a family-centered approach to this family as a result of her caregiver assessment. Mr. Wilson may have been identified as the client, but his problem of a looming inappropriate placement was a problem for his entire family. This involved his primary caregiver daughter, Ms. Handy, but also all of his adult children. Ms. Helpmate made changes in his care, involving the entire family system to meet his needs plus his daughter's. The care manager needs to see the family from a homeostatic point of view. Ms. Handy may have been the primary caregiver, but in essence all his children were potential caregivers. Tapping into their unmined resources made the entire caregiving situation change. The care manager also realigned this family around the care of the father, in the interest of supporting their oldest sibling.

Finally the care manager, while doing the caregiver assessment, discovered home safety problems. The drivers who picked Ms. Handy's father up for day care and church often complained of the uneven pathway they had to negotiate to get Mr. Wilson to the van. The care manager identified this as an environmental problem and referred Ms. Handy to two licensed contractors who would repave walkways for fall safety.

Through the caregiver assessment the care manager has identified the caregiver, Ms. Handy's, problems. The care manager identified the resources that Ms. Handy and her family had to change the situation. The care manager also provided direct services herself in the form of counseling and coaching. The care manager also gave Ms. Handy community resources in the form of information about private formal caregiving services. The care manager offered the daughter technological solutions to research the effects of her sleeplessness. The care manager offered training of the caregiver by showing her an alternative to getting up in the middle of the night to get her father to bed. The care manager, finally also used the tool of a family meeting to identify family resources, respite care, and financial support for paying the private home care agency.

So a caregiver assessment will give the care manager the ability to understand the caregiver's needs, and then define the caregiver's problems. It will give the care manager the ability to define the care manager's resources and make referrals to those resources.

Another benefit of a caregiver assessment is to give the caregiver a voice. The research from California's Caregiver Resources Center (CRCS), a program that has been doing caregiver assessment since 1988, tells us that caregivers who care for family members with cognition impairment really appreciate a caregiver assessment and see it as an opportunity to express their own needs and have their care taken seriously.[19] Ms. Handy was able to speak of her own pain in the situation and be heard by the care manager and her family.

You can see from the example of this caregiver that the caregiver assessment gives the care manager an opportunity to define the caregiver's problems, which will also help define the care receiver's problems. Mr. Wilson would benefit best by staying home with his family's care, but this warm nest was endangered by the daughter's problem of recurrent sleeplessness. The care manager also can define the caregiver's resources and make referrals from a caregiver assessment. Ms. Handy had resources within herself to stop seeing her father as he was at 40, when she was 12. She was coached by the care manager to be filially mature and see herself as 47 and her father as 75, in the here and now. She just needed encouragement and clinical direction from the care manager to be a mature adult and do what was needed for her impaired older father. She also had resources in her family, who after a family meeting, agreed to offer respite and financial support to their sister to help with their father's care. Through her knowledge of the continuum of care in the community, the care manager has referred Ms. Handy to a caregiver support group and the Internet, where she can access many sites on caregiver burnout and the effects of sleeplessness.

Another benefit to the care manager is that he or she can determine eligibility for support services through a caregiver assessment. As Mr. Wilson is not on Medical (Medicaid in other states), he is not eligible for in-home support services, which could pay Ms. Handy in the state of California, if her father was on Medical. The federal Medicaid laws give states the option to pay family members, excluding those who are legally responsible for the care of individuals such as parents and spouses. In addition Medicaid can pay family members, friends, and neighbors.[20]

Another financial support available to some family caregivers comes from the Cash and Counseling Demonstration programs implemented in New Jersey, Arkansas, and Florida, which provides a cash allowance to recipients of Medicaid personal care services and community-based services.[21]

Financial support can strengthen the girders that hold up family caregiving. One way to do this is through a stipend or allowance for caregivers that allows them to defray the cost of caregiving. A second approach is to give them vouchers or direct payments to provide respite care. By assessing the family caregiver, the care manager can also find environmental problems that impede care. Ms. Handy's sidewalk leading to the street was cracked and uneven. To prevent her father from falling, she needed to have it repaired. In her state of overwhelm from sleeplessness she had neglected to see this as a priority. The care manager was able to refer her to licensed and bonded contractors that she had in her resources database.

ELDER ABUSE AND CAREGIVER ASSESSMENT

The care manager giving a caregiver assessment can prevent elder abuse. Depression is highly predictive of caregiver stress and can be an indicator of elder abuse if the caregiver's stress level reaches a clinical level.

So the care manager completing a caregiver assessment in tandem with a geriatric depression scale or other depression scale may detect the roots of some elder abuse and find solutions for this. The main focus of elder abuse appears now to be in past relationships between the caregivers and the care receivers. So a caregiver assessment in tandem with a psychosocial assessment is a good way for a care manager to tap into these past relationships and see if there are any red flags for elder abuse. Caregivers who have quality past relationships with their care receivers are less likely to experience stress in caregiving and less likely to be violent. Care receivers and caregivers who had a violent relationship in the past are more likely to have a present violent relationship in caregiving. If caregivers are not receiving adequate help from family, this can to be another alarm bell for elder abuse. If a caregiver feels isolated and actually is not, this is another sign of potential abuse. Abusive caregivers state that certain behaviors create a great deal of stress for them. These include verbal aggression, refusal to eat or take medications, calling the police, invading the caregiver's privacy, vulgar habits, disruptive behavior, embarrassing displays, or physical aggression. Finally, cohabitation is another indicator of elder abuse. This appears to apply to only adult children, friends, or relatives, not spouses. Many of these behaviors can be discovered in a caregiver assessment.[22]

The caregiver assessment can also give the care manager a way to stop the loss of a primary caregiver before they succumb to their job.[23] The caregiver is the linchpin to the care plan for the care receiver, and without this crucial family member the care plan may fall apart. The well-being of the family caregiver is the key to the care plan and the care recipients getting the help they need at home rather than placing them inappropriately in a skilled nursing facility.[24] Without the caregiver assessment, Ms. Handy would have placed Mr. Wilson in a nursing home. A caregiver assessment additionally gives the care manager an opportunity to see the everyday working of the caregiver's and care receiver's experience. By filling out the caregiver's assessment, the care manager saw the virtual morning in the Handy home. She viewed, through the daughter's answers, a tired Ms. Handy getting her father dressed and seeing him off while he walked down the uneven driveway. She figuratively saw the afternoon, with Ms. Handy working and then worn out, coming home to three kids and her aging father. Then the care manager viewed the virtual evening and night through the daughter's answers: Ms. Handy getting up at midnight and taking an hour to get her dad undressed, diapered, and ready for bed, followed by a few hours of lying sleepless in her bed.

WHAT DOES THE CAREGIVER GAIN FROM A CAREGIVER ASSESSMENT?

A caregiver assessment legitimizes the needs of family caregivers themselves as a distinct entity from the care receiver. It also legitimizes the caregiver's right to be heard.[25] It is a first step in helping the family caregiver maintain his or her own health. Ms. Handy was physically running out of steam as a result of lack of sleep and caregiver overload. The caregiver assessment can also be the first step in defining caregiver depression and anxiety. Caregivers report higher levels of depression and mental health problems than their noncaregiving peers; 20–50% report depressive disorders and symptoms.[26] It can also be a way that family caregivers can understand their own mortality. Additionally, the assessment is also the first step caregivers can take toward balancing work

What Does the Caregiver Gain from a Caregiver Assessment? 103

and family. Two thirds of caregivers report that they need help balancing work and family responsibilities and managing their emotional and physical stress.[27] Ms. Handy had three children, a job, a husband, and her father to take care of. Who she was not taking care of was herself, the linchpin of the whole family and producer of half the income of the family. Family caregivers face workplace issues, financial burdens, and financial insecurity.[28] Ms. Handy had been absent from work several days because she was so tired in the morning, and this was becoming an issue at her job.

The caregiver assessment also gives the caregiver the ability to understand their own role and what abilities are needed to carry out required tasks. Ms. Handy was shown that a change in her father's bedtime routine plus calling on the resources of her family gave her the ability to carry the responsibilities of her father, her job, her family, and her own health. The daughter had a better grasp of her role and her abilities to carry out the tasks of caregiving and take care of her own family through the caregiver assessment. The caregiver assessment can also help the caregiver understand the effect of lost wages on the family. Ms. Handy ran out of sick days and vacation time at her job and will not be paid for any more absences from work. This could mean a financial burden for her family in the short term and perhaps the loss of her job in the long term. About 14% of caregivers report financial burdens. In a 1996 national survey of caregivers for a relative 50 years or older, about two thirds of the caregivers were working, and about half reported changes in their work schedule because of caregiving. In one study women who reduced work hours to care for their parent gave up an average of $7800 in pretax wages in 1994, which was 20% of the median family income for these women.[29]

An assessment can also help the family caregiver to realize how much caregiving takes away from spending time with his or her family. Mr. Handy was increasingly frustrated by his wife's diminished emotional and sexual relationship in their marriage. In addition, one child was having problems in school, and all three children were living with a more distant mother-and-child relationship, just when they needed it most. Assessing the caregiver can give the caregiver a wake-up call about a need for help. Ms. Handy was on the brink of imperiling her marriage and family, her health, and her father's need to stay at home. A caregiver assessment can also give the caregiver insight into community services and the caregiver's eligibility for services. Ms. Handy had formal respite home care available through her brother and joined a caregiver support group as a result of Ms. Helpmate's caregiver assessment. The caregiver assessment can also be therapeutic for family members and help them understand each other. The members of Ms. Handy's family, by participating in a family meeting arranged and mediated by Ms. Helpmate, were able to comprehend their sister's state of overwhelm. They were able to take the next step and glean what each of the siblings could offer to assist their sister in caring for their father. This was based on their relationship with their father and sister. It also gave the family a role in the treatment process and validated their knowledge and experiences. Through the family meeting both Ms. Handy and her siblings all willingly assumed a role in both the treatment of Ms. Handy and their father, Mr. Wilson, based on their financial status and how far they lived from their sister.[30] This family understood each other better as a result of the care manager's intervention and the caregiver assessment.

Finally the caregiver assessment can give the caregiver an ability to have a voice and express his or her own needs. The assessment helps to identify the caregiver as an individual, not as an anonymous adjunct to an elderly client. Ms. Handy's unmet needs were impeding her elderly confused father's ability to remain at home, his best option for care. Through the caregiver assessment, the father could stay at home, his family could recognize what large problems their sister was having, and the family could coalesce to meet their sister's individual needs, their father's, and ultimately their own.

WHO SHOULD ASSESS THE CAREGIVER?

The National Consensus Development Conference for Caregiver Assessment held in San Francisco in 2006 agreed that the professional who does a caregiver assessment should have education and training that not only equips them to understand the caregiving process and its impacts but also to be knowledgeable of the benefits and elements of an effective caregiver assessment.[31] A care manager who has either an educational certificate or degree in care management, or a practitioner with at least a bachelor's degree in the human services field and at least 2 years of supervised care management experience should be qualified to give a caregiver assessment. Practitioners should also be credentialed in care management either as a Certified Case Manager (CCM) through the Commission for Case Management Certification or through the National Academy of Certified Case Managers (CMC). Care managers can also be certified as a National Association of Social Workers Advanced Social Work Case Manager (C-ASWCM) or as a certified Social Work Case Manager (C-SWCM). All care managers with such credentials should have the background to assess a caregiver.[32] In essence the profes-

sional who should perform a caregiver assessment should be a care manager, social worker, nurse, physician, or rehabilitation specialist such as a physical therapist, occupational therapist, or speech therapist.[33] Even though differences will be present in the approach these professionals bring to an assessment, the variances can be strengths that benefit the family. So if you are a physical therapist (PT) that also does care management with aging families, you will bring those strengths from your PT background. The care manager should keep a consumer focus; this will help bridge professional differences.

Also working as a team across disciplines can be of help. If you are a care manager RN serving an aging population and you team up with a care manager social worker focusing on aging clients, there is a sharing—a communication and collaboration—that occurs across these disciplines. The caregiver benefits from the combined perspectives of both care managers. As a team you can see the caregiver's problems and solutions all the more clearly because of your combined backgrounds.[34]

The care manager who gives a caregiver assessment should have a specific knowledge base, abilities, and skills. Care managers are excellent candidates for assessing a family caregiver because they are experts in the continuum of care and the resources needed for building an aging community support network for the caregiver. A care manager with a background in aging is pivotal in doing an aging family member's caregiver assessment. A knowledge base of mental health issues in aging is also a requirement. The case manager who gives caregiver assessments must have the ability to listen and to be open to emotional responses from the interviewee. The care manager must also have interviewing skills and be able to engage people who at times are not really asking for help but really need it.[35]

WHAT TO ASSESS

Most caregiver assessment tools focus on the dimensions of caregiving and the caregiver. They assess the caregiver's specific burdens and the caregiver's health status. What is seen through a good caregiver assessment is not only the type and frequency of care provision, such as help with ADLs and IADLs, but other parts of the caregiver's life as well, such as employment and informal support. The caregiver assessment will also determine formal services needed; personal health issues that function as barriers to providing care at times; caregiving skills, ability to continue care, and standard demographic and contextual information such as living arrangements and cultural needs. Areas that should be added and are often neglected are actual tasks performed beyond personal care. Caregiving often goes beyond ADLs.[36] Carol Levine, in "Notes from the Abyss," reports her anger that a caregiver's tasks are only measured in ADLs. Levine has been a caregiver for her husband along with being the director of the United Hospital Fund of New York and the author of a book called *Family Caregivers on the Job: Moving beyond ADLs and IADLs*. She recounts a time when her husband, who had a serious car accident and for whom she had cared for 16 years, had a deep wound from surgery on his back. The home care RN who came to monitor her husband's condition probed the wound with a long implement and said to Levine, "This is how you clean the site." Levine who is not an RN countered, "No, this is how *you* clean the site. I'm not a nurse, and I am not trained to do this." The moral of the story is a caregiver assessment needs to ask not just what the caregiver does but what the caregiver's reactions are to certain tasks instead of whether they do it or how long it takes. In other words, Levine sagely tells us

that we as care managers should look at what the caregiver finds onerous or just cannot do. Determining which tasks are viewed negatively by the caregiver can go a long way in preventing burdens for the caregiver.

CULTURALLY COMPETENT CAREGIVER ASSESSMENT

Caregiver assessment should also reflect a culturally competent care management practice and approach.[37] A care manager cannot assume that the wording of items or the construction of the caregiver assessment being used translates well for groups whose primary language is not English. Cultural groups speak many languages that the care manager may not understand. But the care manager, by communicating with an instrument like a caregiver assessment, may be communicating poorly just by the way the questions in the assessment tool are worded. Even in one language such as Chinese, there are two distinct dialects. The care manager's best bet may be to get a translator to ask the questions.[38]

ASSESSING CAREGIVER STRESS

A study done by Schultz and Beach in 1999, called the Caregiver Effects Study, revealed the maudlin and all too sad finding that caregivers who experienced the greatest levels of stress were 64% more likely to die within 4 years than noncaregivers.[39]

Morano and Morano have adapted Pearlin's stress, appraisal, and coping framework to both geriatric care management and assessing caregiver burden.[40] They state that there is a preponderance of research that tells care managers that this framework can be used to understand stress in the caregiver, predict how caregivers react to that stress while giving care, and design interventions to that stress.

Understanding the origins of caregiver stress and how to relieve it is one of the most important reasons for a care manager to do a caregiver assessment. Caregiver burden many times equals caregiver stress, and when too much stress builds up the caregiver can become overloaded and begin to break down physically and emotionally, leaving them unable care for the older person or themselves any longer. Ms. Handy's example in this chapter shows that she was so stressed by a lack of sleep that she was thinking of placing her father in a home. The main objective of the caregiver assessment was to determine the primary stressor—her lack of sleep caused by caring for her father—and the secondary stressor—how she coped with the lack of sleep. She coped by letting other items in her life go, which were her family and her work.

One primary stressor for the caregiver is the caregiver's perception of the health and functional status of the care recipient. Part of Mr. Wilson's ADLs were his inability to take off his clothes, change his adult diaper, and get to bed. All of his undressing and diapering and getting into bedclothes had to be prompted by his daughter, Ms. Handy. He could not carry out these ADLs without help because he had vascular dementia and memory loss. But he also had a behavioral problem. His routine, which was still intact despite his dementia, was to go to bed at midnight after watching TV, perhaps a habit from watching Johnny Carson for many years. A primary stressor is one that the care manager needs to first see objectively, like a detective—just the facts. Mr. Wilson would not go to bed until late and his daughter needed to go to bed early as she had a job, three kids, and a husband. She was tired. However, Ms. Handy was going to bed at 9:00 PM and getting up again at midnight, her father's routine bedtime, then prompting him to take off his clothes and get ready

for bed. She then could not go back to sleep for a few hours and woke up exhausted.

The subjective part of the primary stressor, Mr. Wilson going to bed at midnight, is the impact this midnight bedtime had on Ms. Handy. Some caregivers who had less to do or were night owls themselves would not have been stressed by Mr. Wilson's routine. But Ms. Handy was neither a night owl nor without many other responsibilities.

Ms. Handy's perception of her father's midnight bedtime was that it was very stressful to her. There are several ways a care manager can assess this caregiver's reaction to the primary stressor. First, the care manager can see how the caregiver perceives the event, in this case Mr. Wilson going to bed at midnight. Ms. Handy perceived this as upsetting. She was torn between her desperate need for sleep and her need to respond to her father as she had been when he was 40 and she was 12. "I won't overtly cross my Dad" was her subconscious family rule from her original family. Ms. Handy was not filially mature enough to switch out of feeling 12 years old, when she was in real time 47 years old.

Another way the care manager can look at the subjective component of the primary stressor is to assess role overload, role captivity, and loss of relationship. Role overload assesses the impact caring has on the caregiver's time and energy. In our theoretical case, role overload was sapping all of Ms. Handy's time and energy. Role captivity traces how much the caregiver feels trapped by the situation. Ms. Handy felt so desperately trapped in her routine of giving in to her father's going to bed at midnight that she was ready to place him in a skilled nursing facility. The third measure for the care manager to use is their perception of the extent they have lost intimacy with the care receiver. Ms. Handy had distanced herself enough from her father to place him in a facility. The warm feeling and filial obligation she felt to take him in to her home originally diminished as her role overload built.

Secondary stressors can spill over or proliferate in other areas of the caregiver's life. They are not secondary in terms of importance, but are secondary because they do not arise directly from the patient's illness. Pearlin and his colleagues offered two types of secondary strains. The first is role strains or secondary tensions and conflicts that arise in maintaining other roles in the caregiver's life, such as employment and family relationships. In Ms. Handy's case she was in trouble at work for missing so many days. She ran out of sick and vacation days. She had used up all her sick time and was being docked for every day she took off, which was going to affect her and her family financially. The other conflict that arose in Ms. Handy maintaining her role in life was the conflict with her mother role and wife role. The school was reporting her oldest child was falling behind because Ms. Handy could not help with homework. Her kids were feeling neglected. In addition, her husband was frustrated because her lack of sleep and odd sleeping hours was affecting their intimacy as a couple.

Ms. Helpmate tracked the roles that Ms. Handy the caregiver had, which were wife, mother, and employee, in addition to caregiver. Roles are also good to track through demographic questions in a caregiver assessment when assessing strain and burden. So the secondary stressors of Ms. Handy's role of mother, wife, and employee spilled over into other areas of her life. She was overwhelmed by these role stressors by the time she called the care manager Ms. Helpmate to do an assessment because by then she was thinking of placing her father in a nursing home.

The second type of secondary stressor identified by Pearlin and his associates is intropsychic strains. These strains erode a person's self-concept in four identified areas.

These domains are self-esteem, competence in caregiving, feelings of gain in caregiving, and one's sense of self. We could say that Ms. Handy's self-esteem was being worn down because she knew the human resources department at her work was keeping an eye on her for her many absences at work. She was also being accused of being a poor wife by her husband by avoiding sexuality and intimacy, and she was being judged by her oldest child's teacher as a poor parent for not helping with homework and letting her child's academic goals fall short. Ms. Handy may have suspected she should change her father's routine for bed but was stuck in what so many adult children are stuck in, which is a lack of filial maturity. They are not able to approach their parent in the here and now and respond to their here-and-now needs. Instead they continue in their original parent–child role of their childhood. Ms. Handy was allowing herself to be 12 years old in her mind and not change her father's bedtime for her own and her parent's ultimate good. This affected her own sense of well-being and sense of self.[41]

Care managers using a stress and appraisal model, according to Morano and Morano, can predict how caregivers will react to stress when providing care to a person with dementia. The Moranos suggest using a model based on Pearlin that allows care managers to see how personal characteristics, age, gender, and appraisal (primary and secondary) have a direct or mediating effect on depression and life satisfaction and coping. Ms. Handy's situation was predictive of her being depressed, and indeed Ms. Handy was depressed as evidenced by the Geriatric Depression Scale score of 17.

Ms. Handy also appraised her caregiving situation as a burden. This is part of the secondary appraisal, the subjective part of the primary stressor. She was still getting her father to be bed at midnight even though she had to awaken to do that. Ms. Handy felt stuck in this very stressful routine, not able to call on relatives or change the bedtime to 10 PM. She felt she did not have the skills to cope with the care of her father or to change the way she was handling the situation. The stress and appraisal framework introduced in the Morano article and based on research by Pearlin tells us if all this is true, then the caregiver is likely to place a loved one in an institutional setting, which Ms. Helpmate the care manager found Ms. Handy poised to do.

The care manager helped Ms. Handy understand that her stress was originating from her father's noncompliance with a better bedtime for her (10:00), not his care needs, which were prompting to get undressed and ready for bed. Ms. Handy then could see that she could cope with his primary care needs. Her appraisal of the primary stressor was that she was giving in to her father's mandates. The care manager helped her reframe her appraisal and see that she could handle her father's care needs if she just changed the time she got him to bed. The care manager helped her to understand that she could, again, handle his care needs if she asked her siblings for help in the form of respite. Her original appraisal of the primary stressor was that she could not ask her siblings to help. The care manager helped her understand that she could ask for help, and if she did she would be able to keep her father at home.[42]

The care manager also used a neurolinguistic programming model developed by Grinder and Bandler called generalization. This model is based on using language with words that stop us from changing. In a generalization the person, or in this case the caregiver, uses universal quantifier's such as *never, nowhere, none, no one, nobody, never, always*, and *can't*. Ms. Handy had created an impoverished model of coping that blocked her coping with her father. The care manager

Ms. Helpmate reconnected Ms. Handy's model with her experience, which was that her father, her family, and Ms. Handy herself had changed many time in their lives, which meant change was possible. The care manager helped Ms. Handy reduce the perceived insurmountable obstacles that she had built for herself: "My Dad will never go to bed earlier," "My family will never help me with my Dad's care," and "I always have to take care of my Dad because I am the oldest daughter."

The care manager, by identifying Ms. Handy's impoverished model of her experiences, was able to create a rich new model of reality for Ms. Handy by creating choices based on distinctions that were previously not there. Ms. Handy's sisters and brother would help her by offering respite, Mr. Wilson could change his bedtime, and Ms. Handy could endure her father's anger at changing his routine, with the caregiver's support.[43]

ASSESSING THE WELL-BEING OF THE CAREGIVER

The caregiver assessment should include assessing the well-being of the caregiver. Well-being is defined in the recommended domains and constructs of a caregiver assessment, according to a national Family Caregiver Alliance conference.[44] Well-being is broken down into self-rated health, health conditions and symptoms, depression and emotional stress, and life satisfaction and quality of life.

Caregiver's mental health is critical to assess. Caregivers suffer from high rates of depression, anxiety, and feelings of anger. It's estimated that 40–70% of caregivers of older adults with these various disorders have clinically significant symptoms of depression.[45] Performing a geriatric depression scale or another depression scale is always a good idea for a care manager in tandem with a caregiver assessment.

Among the costs of caregiving is the caregiver's health. About one in five caregivers report that their physical health has suffered by being a caregiver.[46] The care manager should ask the caregiver for a simple rating of his or her health. This includes asking whether their health is changing, if they currently have health problems, including diagnosed symptoms and illnesses. The care manager also should ask if they are getting treatment for these symptoms. Some caregiver's put off going to the doctor if they have heavy caregiving demands.

A care manager should also do a functional assessment of the care receiver.[47] This will measure the caregiver's burden. This should be done to find out whether the caregiver should carry out the tasks that must be done to functionally care for the care recipient. These tasks are usually ADLs, IADLs, and medication management. First, the care manager identifies the care receiver's health status and problem, and then by performing a functional assessment determines the care receiver's ADLs, IADLs, and medication management and transfer needs. The care manager can then compare this list of requirements with the caregiver's own abilities to ensure they match. For example, if a caregiver reports during a caregiver assessment that she has a bad back and is seeing the physician for this and the care receiver needs to be lifted, then the tasks and the caregiver's health abilities do not match, and the care manager may suggest additional paid caregivers or placement.

As part of the a basic psychosocial assessment of the care receiver the care manager should find out if the care recipient has memory loss or cognitive impairment, behavior problems, or a mental health diagnosis.[48] This will also tell the care manager what psychosocial needs the care receiver has compared to the ability of the caregiver to render that care. For example, if a caregiver is given a GDS score as very depressed herself, this may be a barrier to caring for a dementia patient. The care manager might consider the care receiver seeing her own physician to evaluate for medication and bringing in other family supports, as in the case of Ms. Handy.

In the caregiver assessment and the care receiver's psychosocial assessment the care manager should identify all the demographic information about the caregiver and the family including names, where they live, the care receiver's and caregiver's relationship with the family, and history and potential stressors in that relationship. In Ms. Handy's family there was a brother who had a bad history with his father Mr. Wilson. Ms. Handy was the oldest sibling and a female, so assumed all the burden. The other sisters lived nearby and were open to respite after a family meeting held by the care manager. This was all gathered in the caregiver assessment and psychosocial assessment of Mr. Wilson by care manager Ms. Helpmate.

Finally, the care manager should assess the caregiver's willingness to provide care and what tasks the caregiver may find onerous and uncomfortable. The caregiver's willingness to assume individual tasks and care in general is often neglected and really central to assessing the caregiver. The story of Carol Levine, mentioned earlier, where cleaning her husband's wound was something she did not want to do and was untrained to do is a good example of what must be discovered by the care manager. Questions about what the caregiver finds uncomfortable and what they have no training for are important. For example, if a caregiver must check blood pressure but was never shown how, then it is important for the care manager to pick up on this.

WHAT TRIGGERS A CAREGIVER ASSESSMENT?

Care managers should routinely assess caregivers after they have completely assessed the care receiver. The National Center for Caregiving suggests the professional assess the caregiver after all services are in place, because the caregiver is too focused on the care receiver to put the microscope on themselves. If a second visit is planned by the care manager, perhaps to monitor services that she or he has put in place, then this might be a good time to assess the caregiver.

However, events can trigger performing an immediate assessment. Examples include when a family caregiver burns out and is ready to place their aging family member in a facility, or when a family argument ignites over care issues and the care manager is called in by a family member. Another trigger can be a care manager being contacted to help move an older person, when the underlying reason may be caregiver burnout. A care manager should consider assessing the family caregiver ideally after a client assessment, if there is a family caregiver. This is of course if the family agrees to the assessment. Some families will not pay for a family caregiver assessment, and you may have to respect their wishes.

SPECIFIC OUTCOMES TO A CAREGIVER ASSESSMENT

Caregiver assessment is not an end in itself but should help caregivers to make informed decisions themselves. It should also prompt the care managers to help the family caregiver connect to the continuum of care in his or her community so that the care receiver can stay at the right level of care. The outcome of the caregiver assessment should be the care manager's care plan. A care plan is a list of all the caregiver problems the care manager has discovered and a list of the interventions the care manager has generated. Care planning is a developed skill in a care manager.[49]

The care manager's care plan should address the health of the caregiver and any interventions to medical problems of the caregiver. It should address the caregiver's emotional well-being including depression and any interventions for depression, such as seeing their physician for medication, evaluation, or bringing in respite care. The care plan should address stress in the caregiver's life and any solutions to reduce that stress, such as placement of the client in community programs, like adult day health care, to relieve the stress of caring.

Another outcome of a caregiver assessment is placement of a care receiver in a nursing home. Although only 8% of elders end their days in nursing home and the overall objective of care managers is to keep older people at home, at times the care manager must suggest placement of a care receiver in a skilled nursing facility. Home care is not a guaranteed constructive outcome. Ongoing home care can burn out caregivers if they do not have the help they need or do not have the sufficient financial or family resources to get that help. Sustained home care can also lead to elder abuse if the caregiver and care provider have a prior contentious background. Family caregivers often put off getting outside help until fairly late in the disease process. The result is caregivers turn to needed assistance, such as formal home care too late, when they have already burned out. As a result, skilled nursing facility placement, assisted living placement, and placement in some type of residential care is another outcome that results from a care manager's caregiver assessment.[50]

A caregiver assessment outcome can be reduction of a crisis and the establishment of more preventative maintenance for the caregiver family and care manager. Rather than lurch from crisis to crisis, like repeat emergency room visits, falls, or family arguments over care, the care plan can provide relative stability.

An excellent outcome can be that the relationship between the caregiver and the care receiver is transformed because of the caregiver assessment. The caregiver, after finding ways to improve his or her own self-esteem, stress level, health problems, family support, or depression, can many times see a way to reunite him- or herself with the reason that he or she decided to be a caregiver in the first place. This initial decision to be a caregiver is frequently a genuine wish to help a family member. After a caregiver assessment identifies ways to help negative health problems in the older mother, father, or relative, such as getting them to a physician to prescribe medication to mediate violent outbursts, the relationship can be transformed as well.

Another outcome is to improve the emotional well-being of the caregiver. The caregiver may find that the interventions in the caregiver assessment gave them more freedom to have a life of their own, maintain their own health, prevent social isolation, have more peace of mind, and get appropriate support from formal and informal sources.

An outcome of a caregiver assessment can be the improvement of environmental problems. When the care manager visits the home to do a caregiver assessment he or she may notice home safety issues in the caregiver assessment. It is a good idea to do a home safety assessment at the same time, and this can be best done by using the Consumer Product Safety Commission's "Safety for Older Consumer's Home Safety Checklist."[51]

An outcome of the caregiver assessment can be a care plan that helps the care provider to move from point A to point B or begin the process of change in their caregiver role. This embracing of new choices, not being stuck in those generalizations of "I can't," "she won't," and "he never," can trigger change. The care plan can help the caregivers to reduce stress levels, decrease burden, and increase their knowledge of caregiving tasks and stresses. Caregivers can build their competency through a good care plan and learn new caregiving skills. A care plan can lead the caregiver to learning needed skills through training. A good care plan for the caregiver can educate caregivers in what increases their stress levels, what spirals them out of control, and how to avoid extreme reactions such as unnecessary placement or elder abuse.

Unfortunately, there are few documented studies that systematically explore the outcomes of a caregiver assessment.[52]

Care Manager Measures the Outcomes of the Caregiver Assessment

Care monitoring will tell you whether these outcomes take place. Care monitoring is simply measuring whether your care plan is working. Consider Ms. Handy. Ms. Helpmate will measure whether the care plan she crafted for Ms. Handy, her family, and father, Mr. Wilson, is working by making care monitoring visits periodically. These visits have to be agreed upon by the client if you are billing for the visits. You should have a signed contract with your client and have care monitoring in the document, if you plan to do this.

On a monitoring visit, Ms. Helpmate takes her care plan with her and asks if Ms. Handy was getting her father to bed at 10 PM and then getting a full night's sleep herself. The care manager will inquire if Ms. Handy's sisters and brother had actually come to the Handy house and done the respite they promised. The care manager could ask if Ms. Handy's child had improved in school as a result of Ms. Handy having more time for her children. Ms. Helpmate could check if Ms. Handy was going to her support group and feeling happier and less stressed as a result of sharing her story and hearing others who had similar problems. Care managers should use a field evaluation to capture these responses. Please refer to Exhibit 4-2.

In your care monitoring visit you can figure out whether your care plan is working and change it as needed. If Ms. Handy's sisters are not coming those two nights to offer respite, it may be time to contact the long-distance brother who said he would pay for respite care. Another solution may be to ask the sisters to contribute money to pay a formal caregiving service to offer Ms. Handy respite during the week instead of doing it themselves. Here the care manager is seeing whether the care plan is being implemented. The best laid plans often fall apart. Care management means not only creating a great care plan but also changing that plan when the solution is not working.[53]

Exhibit 4-2 GCM Field Evaluation/Care Management Service

Date: 11/18/04	**Client Name:** Zeke Zeigler				
Care Manager's Name: Miss Full Charge					
	(1-excellent 5-poor)				
General Home Environment:	1	**2**	3	4	5
Facility was pleasant. Zeke Zeigler was seated in his wheelchair across from the nurses' station next to the lounge. The lounge was busy yet felt organized.					
General Home Cleanliness:	1	**2**	3	4	5
The facility was generally clean and free of odor.					
Supplies:	**1**	2	3	4	5
(food, cleaning supplies, attends, expense $, Ensure, etc.) Provided by the facility					
Client's Physical Condition:	1	**2**	3	4	5
(personal grooming, overall condition, behavior, etc.) Zeke Zeigler was seated on his chair dressed and ready for his doctor's appt. He was neat and well groomed. Overall he was relaxed.					
Client's Mental Condition:	1	2	**3**	4	5
(oriented, moderately confused, very confused)					

Zeke Zeigler was alert although he was not oriented to time, place, and person. When Zeke Zeigler entered The Stroke Institute, he read the sign and clearly said "Stroke Institute." While waiting for Dr. Feelgood, Zeke Zeigler read a few words accurately from a magazine, but could not connect words together. During the doctor's visit, he responded clearly when Dr. Feelgood asked his name but started singing when asked about his age, family, or symptoms.

New Psychosocial Problems:
Julia Nimble, social worker at Agility Skilled Nursing Facility, reported that his humming, singing, and general agitation bothered Mr. Zeigler's roommate. However, this behavior did not impact Zeke Zeigler and his relation to the outside world. No other psychosocial problems were apparent. He was pleasant and interacted with the GCM, the nurse, and Dr. Feelgood.

Exhibit 4-1 GCM Field Evaluation/Care Management Service (continued)

List of Medications:
(include quantity and expiration date)

During this visit, Dr. Feelgood prescribed Seroquel 25mg, 1/2 to 1 tab daily at bedtime to decrease the agitation and allow him to sleep better.

Specific Concerns:
Dr. Feelgood noted that Mr. Zeigler's right hand was contracted and stiff. He suggested botox treatment on his forearm to paralyze the stiffened muscles and decrease the contractures. This will ease the movement of his right hand and also make it easier for a caregiver to dress him. Dr. Feelgood will do the botox treatment at Mr. Zeigler's next appointment.

Actions:
Care manager rode with Zeke Zeigler in Medical Transport vehicle from Agility Skilled Nursing Facility Care to The Stroke Institute.
Care manager sat with Zeke Zeigler during his visit with Dr. Feelgood. Dr. Feelgood took over from Dr. Baseline and spent this visit reviewing symptoms, current therapy, and getting to know Mr. Zeigler.
Care manager waited with Zeke Zeigler until Medical Transport came to pick them up. Due to the time of day, we had to wait for over an hour for transport back to Agility Skilled Nursing Facility Care.

Plan:
Return visit was set for Thursday, February 10, 2005 @ 9:45 a.m. During that visit, Dr. Feelgood plans a botox treatment to decrease the contracture of Mr. Zeigler's hand.

Summary of Visit:
Miss Full Charge, Care manager, accompanied Zeke Zeigler to a doctor's appointment at The Stroke Institute scheduled for 4:30 p.m. Pick-up was scheduled for an hour before the appointment. Zeke Zeigler was seated on his chair dressed and ready for his doctor's appt. He was neat and well groomed. Overall he was relaxed. Zeke Zeigler was alert although he was not oriented to time, place, and person. When Zeke Zeigler entered The Stroke Institute, he read the sign and clearly said "Stroke Institute." While waiting for Dr. Feelgood, Zeke Zeigler read a few words accurately from a magazine, but could not connect words together. During the doctor's visit, he responded clearly when Dr. Feelgood asked his name but started singing when asked about his age, family, or symptoms.

Source: Cresscare, Case Management for Elders, Cathy Cress, Director, 2006.

FAMILY SYSTEMS APPROACH TO CAREGIVER ASSESSMENT

Caregiver assessment should have a family systems approach to care. The care manager needs to see the family as a whole, not individual parts, with the caregiver as part of that larger system. Aging families deal with relational stresses around loss. It is not just the mental or physical decline of the aging parent but also the loss of relationships within the family members. These losses are rarely seen ahead of time by the family, and when they occur the whole family can be thrown off balance. In the case of Ms. Handy and Mr. Wilson, when Mrs. Wilson died, Ms. Handy moved her father into her home. She coped with the loss of the mother for the whole family. But, as no one else in the family shared the caregiver burden with her, Ms. Handy lost her grip on her own family, her free time, her standing in her job, and her health in the form of sleep. This created a whole new family crisis besides the feelings of loss. The caregiver assessment opened up Ms. Handy's view of her stuck, lonely caregiver situation; she could see that she could ask the whole family for help. Her sisters and brother came through without disagreements. But many families need a caregiver assessment and a care manager to help because the siblings' approach to parental crisis is sibling disagreements. These disagreements are often based in old parent–child conflicts. For example, Ms. Handy's brother has never gotten along with his father, but in the family meeting he agreed to pay for formal care rather than do it himself. The geographical location of siblings in a parental care crisis can also cause upheaval. In this case, the one long-distance daughter agreed to fly in every 5 months for respite, where the long-distance son agreed to pay for care. Many times these geographical pressures are not that easily solved.

Family systems theory says that each family is an emotional unit, and behavior in the system is reciprocal and reactive. The family is a living system, and each member is an interdependent part. When you change one part of the system the whole system changes.[54] Ms. Handy almost placing her father in a nursing home brought the whole family system to a crisis. With the help of a caregiver assessment, the family dynamics changed. This is an important theory for care managers to understand when working with family caregivers. Their collapse brings on a family crisis. However, assessing them with a caregiver assessment can prompt a care plan that can deal with the family crisis and avert the caregiver from being overwhelmed and breaking down.

The care manager also needs to see the unit of care within the family system. The dyad within the family system that the care manager focuses on is the family caregiver and the care recipient. This is not to the exclusion of the entire family system. But in assessing the family caregiver, the care manager is assessing the caregiver's relationship with the care receiver. This minisystem within the family system leads the care manager to work with the family system as a whole. We can see this in Ms. Helpmate first assessing Ms. Handy and then performing a psychosocial and functional assessment on Mr. Wilson. The daughter and father dyad—the unit of care—prompted the solution to many of the caregiver's problems because Ms. Helpmate used the entire family system to solve Ms. Handy's, and thus Mr. Wilson's, problem of being moved into a nursing home. Here Ms. Handy and Mr. Wilson are the unit of care that the care manager focuses on. This unit of care theory is adapted from the palliative care movement.

WHEN TO ASSESS THE CAREGIVER

A caregiver assessment can be triggered by many client or family events. As stated, after the care recipient's care plan is in place and implemented is a good time to assess the caregiver. Before that the focus of the care manager and all services will be on the care recipient. It can be prompted by the care manager's intake, where the caregiver is obviously under stress. It can be triggered by a discharge of a client from care management services where the care manager understands that other services may have to be put in place. For example, if you think that potential elder abuse may occur after you stop services because of caregiver stress or an old child–parent conflict, the care manager may have to report this to adult protective services. A caregiver assessment can be triggered by a hospital admission where it is clear that the caregiver needs assessment to deal with the increased level of care of the client upon discharge. It may be triggered by discharge from the hospital where the caregiver must be assessed because he or she does not have the skills to render the new level of care and either the discharge planner did not arrange for help or a different level of care must be arranged. The care manager may find the caregiver should be assessed on a care monitoring visit if the care manager finds that the caregiver is under enough strain to affect his or her health or the care receiver's health or care situation. Any change in the caregiver's health status should trigger a reassessment, especially before, during, and after hospitalization of the care receiver.

Caregiver assessment could be triggered by a professional referral. Pharmacists, clergy, physicians, parish nurses, social workers, home care workers, adult protective services, or the courts could find problems or stresses with a family caregiver that would prompt a family caregiver assessment. For the care manager this underscores the reason to perform a psychosocial intake at the beginning of the case and determine all available informal and formal resources. This way the care manager knows who supports the client, and those people will know to contact the care manager if they spot trouble.

The caregiver assessment should be done periodically as a reassessment, if the family and client, if mentally competent, agrees to do so. The care manager can update information as needed and discover changes that have occurred in the caregiver's and care receiver's situation. If the care manager is monitoring care on an ongoing basis, he or she will note changes in the care receiver that may require new skills of the caregiver or place new stresses on the caregiver. All this should be recorded in the care receiver's care monitoring file. For example, if the client begins to have falls and a walker is ordered, then the caregiver will need instructions on how to best help the older client use the

walker. The care manager can arrange for this training. If the family caregiver gets a new diagnosis of a medical illness, such as macular degeneration, then this will prompt a care manager's reassessment of the caregiver's skills. The care manager may have to, at that point, suggest additional formal care. Other reasons that might prompt a reassessment might be a complaint of the care recipient, caregiver workplace issues, or concerns verbalized by another family member or friend.[55]

WHERE TO ASSESS THE CAREGIVER

The optimal place to assess the family caregiver is in the home of the care receiver where the daily assistance is taking place. In the home the care manager can get a clearer picture of exactly what the caregiver does beyond the ADLs, such as socializing with the care receiver, talking to other relatives, and the minutiae that take up the family caregiver's day. The caregiver assessment should optimally be done out of earshot of the care receiver so that the caregiver can feel free to talk openly. This ensures the care recipient's dignity. If the care manager assesses the caregiver separately, he or she will also build a better level of trust with the caregiver. Because the caregiver could be experiencing significant levels of psychological distress, or physical or mental health issues, privacy in the caregiver interview is crucial.[56]

But the care manager also needs to be flexible as to where the caregiver assessment takes place. The National Center on Caregiving suggests that the simple answer is that the assessment should take place in a setting that is convenient to the caregiver. The assessment could be in the home. But it may be best for the caregiver if the assessment was done in a coffee shop, local restaurant, a community agency, or at the caregiver's home after work, on weekends, or together with the care receiver, if this works best for the caregiver. If the only choice is with the care receiver present, it is a good idea for the care manager to arrange respite so that the caregiver can be assured of privacy.[57]

TECHNIQUES IN CONDUCTING A CAREGIVER ASSESSMENT

The National Center on Caregiving at the Family Caregiver Alliance suggests specific interviewing skills are necessary to assessing the caregiver, including the ability to give the caregiver room to tell his or her story. Offer a relaxed and confidential place and atmosphere. The care manager must use relaxed and open body language and a calm voice. Each question should be clear, and the caregiver should be told the clinical relevance of each question. So, if you ask, "Are you getting enough sleep?" make sure you relate this to the care of the older family member, not just a curious and inappropriate question from a stranger. The care manager should always explain the purpose of the assessment to the family caregiver; it should always be a face-to-face encounter unless distance and special circumstances intervene. This includes long-distance caregivers or a caregiver who cannot leave the older family member alone, thus leaving the phone as the best choice. The care manager must convince the caregiver that the purpose of the assessment is to meet their needs. This requires a trustworthy attitude on the part of the care manager. The care manager needs to show the caregiver through body language, voice, and interviewing skills that the care manager values the caregiver and recognizes him or her as the expert in caring for their aging family member. Care managers also need to make clear to the caregiver that the

assessment is a means to an end, not the center of the process.[58]

ASSESSMENT TOOLS FOR A CAREGIVER ASSESSMENT

The National Center for Caregiving at the Family Caregiver Alliance tells us there is no set protocol to follow in a caregiver assessment and no single approach that is optimal in all care settings. The center suggests the form and the content and process of the caregiver assessment be tailored to the caregiving context, services setting, and program.[59]

There are seven domains that should be measured in any caregiver assessment, according to the National Center on Caregiving. The seven domains are the following:

1. The context of the caregiving rendered by the caregiver
2. The caregiver's perception of the health and functional status of the care recipient
3. The caregiver's values and preferences
4. The well-being of the caregiver
5. The consequences of caregiving
6. The skills and abilities and knowledge needed to provide care
7. The potential resources the caregiver could choose to use[60]

Feinberg suggests that there are six pieces of information that should be included in any caregiver assessment. These are the following:

1. Type and frequency of the current care provision
2. How able the caregiver is to continue with care
3. Whether additional responsibilities or stressors affect care provision
4. The degree of informal support provided
5. What formal services are required
6. The caregiver's overall health status

Morano and Morano suggest that a care manager gather the information needed to assess the caregiver based on narrative information at the time of initial intake of the older client. Pearlin's stress and appraisal model of caregiver assessment can be used by a care manager as suggested by the Moranos. They also suggest the care manager could use standardized screening instruments that have been empirically validated through research. They suggest the appraisal of burden and appraisal of satisfaction scales by Lawton and colleagues.

We have included a suggested care manager caregiver assessment tool at the beginning of this chapter (see Exhibit 4-2). This tool has not been empirically validated through research, but it is a beginning point for developing a care-manager-based caregiver assessment tool.

HIPAA AND THE CAREGIVER ASSESSMENT

To perform a caregiver assessment the care manager must make sure he or she is HIPAA (Health Insurance Portability and Accountability Act) compliant before he or she assesses the caregiver. At intake the care manager should have the client or family member (if client lacks capacity) sign a release of information form, giving the care manager the right to share client information. It is also a good idea to have a release of information form signed at intake by the family caregiver, if he or she is present at the time. If not, get the HIPAA-compliant release of information signed by the caregiver when the client assessment is in place and the care manager can focus on the caregiver. The care manager should also have a HIPAA-compliant shared database of the patient's information. (See Chapter 1 for HIPAA compliance and care management.)

TRAINING THE CARE MANAGER TO ASSESS THE CAREGIVER

The National Center for Caregiving and the Family Caregiving Alliance have called for professional education and training curricula for family caregivers be developed by all professions who interact with older individuals and their family caregivers. This includes physicians, social workers, physical therapists, registered nurses, and occupational therapists. Care managers need to integrate this into their training and curricula. The National Association of Professional Care Managers (GCM) and the Case Management Society of America (CMSA) will, it is hoped, begin to offer workshops to train care managers to assess caregivers as well as offer continuing education credits and student training programs. College courses and degree programs in care management should also include how to assess a family caregiver in their curricula. San Francisco State University's master's program in gerontology offers an emphasis in geriatric care management that does include this subject now.

One training point that needs to be included in any curriculum is a change in the care manager's point of view. According to a United Kingdom report, a care manager who assesses a caregiver must have a specific mindset. They term this a "caregiver-in-partner approach." The attitude taken in the United States has been to look at caregivers as dehumanized "resources" or "informants." This new partnership approach means the care manager recognizes the caregiver as an equal partner in rendering the type of appropriate and highly skilled care to the client that the care manager strives for. Adding caregiver assessment training to care manager academia and association training will take a big step toward helping care managers reframe the unequal partnership they have had with family caregivers.

Beyond a team approach in the care manager's mind the care manager must have training or expertise in other areas. This includes interviewing skills, knowledge of human behavior, family and caregiving dynamics, aging and disability, the continuum of care in the community, and caregiver skills. These skills include such things as lifting the patient or giving injections, something caregivers are now asked to do as older family members come home from the hospital "sicker and quicker."

CONNECTING THE CAREGIVER AND THE CARE RECIPIENT'S ASSESSMENTS

Care managers are in a unique and excellent place to link the caregiver's assessment and the care recipient's assessment. Care managers are already highly skilled in creating care plans and have always included caregiver directions and needs in the care plan. The two assessments are linked in the care plan in the problem section of the care plan and in the solution sectier assessment of Ms. Handy, is exhaustion from lack of sleep from getting her father to bed at midnight. The solution in the care manager's care plan after assessing the caregiver, Mon of the care plan.

For example, in the case of Mr. Wilson and his daughter Ms. Handy, the care manager knows that the burden of Mr. Wilson staying at home squarely falls on the shoulders of Ms. Handy. An initial problem in the care plan, gleaned from the caregivs. Handy, is to have the care manager coach Ms. Handy to change her father's bedtime to 10:00 PM, set up a family meeting to get siblings involved in respite, and to get the daughter involved in a support group. The care manager subsequently changed this care plan as care monitoring visits were made; interventions were

implemented (family meeting occurred, siblings started to offer respite). The key to linking the care recipient's assessment to the caregiver's assessment, for the care manager, is the ongoing care plan.

Another question to ask is how much responsibility the care manager gives the caregiver when it comes to setting priorities. The care manager should give the caregiver equal weight in the decision, along with the opinions of other professionals, the care manager in this case. However, the care manager is the ultimate arbiter and decision maker. He or she must listen to everyone's opinions and needs—professionals, family, and caregivers. After hearing everyone's point of view, the ultimate creator of the care plan is the care manager. The care manager needs to treat the caregiver respectfully but use his or her own opinions to forge the best care plan for the care recipient.

For example, Ms. Handy wanted to place her father in a nursing home. The care manager listened to her politely and heard her point of view. However, after the care manager assessed the caregiver, she was able to understand why the caregiver could not cope and was ready to place her father in a facility. Mediating factors were not yet arranged such as social supports of family respite and community services. After these were in place, the family caregiver could cope, and Ms. Handy could keep her father at home. The care manager respected not only the family caregiver's opinion but heard her pain and was able to bring in solutions to help her cope. This can be likened to a care manager who respectfully hears a physician who says, "I can't treat this patient any longer; they never show up for appointments." The care manager would respectfully hear the professional point of view and then cobble together a care plan that had solutions to help get the patient to the physician.

ETHICAL ISSUES AND A CAREGIVER ASSESSMENT

One of the ethical issues in adding a caregiver assessment to a care manager's repertoire of assessment tools is the conflicts that may arise between the rights and needs of the care recipient and the caregiver. (See the "Who Is My Client?" section of this chapter.) The care manager must see the caregiver as a client as well as the care recipient. But ultimately, when balancing the needs of both, the care manager must defer to the needs of the care recipient. Ultimately, as has been discussed in this chapter, meeting the needs of the caregiver will result in the needs of the care receiver being met. However, if that process is not effective, then the care manager must defer to the needs of the care receiver.

Confidentially is another ethical issue. Care managers must strive, as they always have, to protect the confidentiality of every source in the care receiver's informal and formal support system. Privacy issues must be addressed ethically. This is reflected in following the legal requirements of HIPAA, as has been addressed in this chapter. There are potential conflicts between the subjective perspective of both the care recipient and the caregiver that will arise. Again, meeting the needs of the caregiver often results in meeting the needs of the care receiver. However, care managers are hired to meet the needs of the care receiver; the needs of the care recipient take priority over the needs of the caregiver. For example, if a caregiver needs time off for a personal appointment on a regular basis and the care receiver cannot be safely left alone, then the care manager has to arrange respite or the family caregiver cannot leave. As this is a new perspective and assessment tool in a care manager's toolbox, the ethical issues will be discussed and resolved in future dialogues and research.

BARRIERS TO CAREGIVER ASSESSMENT

There arc many barriers to implementing a caregiver assessment that care managers have to overcome. One barrier that looms is whether the family or client will pay for this new assessment. The care manager is almost always contracting with a payment source, and that payment source must approve a service. The care manager will have to request this new assessment and get approval from the payer source to expend the time to perform the assessment, devise solutions to the caregiver's problems, and then implement those solutions. This means the care manager will have to clearly explain the link between the needs of the care receiver and the caregiver. This harkens back to the need for the care manager to have a mindset that the caregiver's needs are very important to meeting the care receiver's needs. You can't make a sale without believing in your product. So a major barrier remains, will the payer source reimburse the care manager for assessing the caregiver and then meeting the caregiver's needs? Care managers should be trained to make this shift in thinking: it is their responsibility to convince the payer source at intake that this is a needed service, or when taking an inquiry call about services to explain that caregiver assessment is a major goal of care management.

Another barrier is the need for an organizational shift in thinking. Accepting the addition of a caregiver assessment tool would also take a major shift in thinking up and down the care management agency whether it be a small care management agency or very large corporate one. All administrators, supervisors, and in-the-field care managers must be in full agreement that this shift can and will occur. This requires care management agencies to rethink and build consensus around this issue; it requires rewriting of business plans from mission statements down to procedures, and then writing those procedures and training staff in their use. Training, then, is key to implementing a caregiver assessment in a care management agency. A training program is critical to a care management agency that wants to implement a caregiver assessment tool.

A care management agency should evaluate the implementation of a caregiver assessment tool within the agency to determine its effect on operations of the agency. These effects can be measured in terms of client records, policies and procedures, caseload size, and the budgetary and organization effect of all these changes.[61] The National Center for Caregiving at the Family Caregiver Alliance states that the length of the caregiver assessment tool results in one of the biggest barriers to implementing a caregiver assessment. The issue of time comes up in almost all discussions on caregiver assessment. One mediating factor to control this is a care management agency adding a brief but effective caregiver assessment tool.

Another barrier is the family not seeing themselves as caregivers but as kin. Family members may recoil from the term *caregivers* because they never conceived of themselves as caregivers. The cultural understanding that caregiving is what a family does is itself a barrier to getting help, especially when the caregiver begins collapsing under the burden of care. This harkens back to the problem geriatric care managers have. The general public had no idea until very recently that such a thing as a geriatric care manager existed and so could not call upon the profession for help. Education and outreach on the part of aging agencies have to be continued to help family members identify themselves as caregivers so that they see their own needs. This would follow the outreach and education that has been done over the years by the Family Center on Care Giving.

Another barrier is the multicultural composition of the American caregiver population. Multiethnic families have different cultural values around care and caregiving, and this can be a barrier to caregiver identification and assessment. Language is another barrier because both caregiver assessment tools and the care managers themselves must be fluent in the caregiver's language or get an interpreter. Care managers must strive to be culturally sensitive and learn cultural norms, use the language of the caregiver, get interpreters, and put assessment tools in the language of both the care receiver and the caregiver.

The family caregiver—those relatives, friends, neighbors, or life partners—are a primary solution to the care manager's quest to keep the older client at the safest, most optimal level of care possible. But at the same time the care manager must learn to see them as human beings, not as anonymous solutions. These family caregivers, unpaid, unrecognized, and unrespected by the larger healthcare system, are relied upon in the effort to shorten hospital stays. More often older clients come out of the hospital "quicker and sicker," landing in the arms of these untrained, accidental nurses, social workers, and home health aides. The care manager is on the proverbial cutting edge to recognize them for what they are to the client and the care plan—a salvation. Second, the care manager should respect them for what they do so lovingly for their kin. Third, the care manager must be able to answer to their needs by hearing them in a caregiver assessment, a new but vital tool in the care manager's toolbox.

SUMMARY

The caregiver is the glue that holds the aging family altogether. The family caregiver is the spine of long-term care. However, that back will break and that glue will lose its bond if we as care managers do not offer support to the family caregiver. The beginning of that support is assessing the caregiver and finding out what he or she needs. Too long care managers have held the coin of caregiving yet not been able to spend it because, as a profession, we only saw one side of the coin—the care receiver. Now seeing a two-sided coin, care managers will have much more capital to spend to meet the needs of the entire aging family. The United States will join other countries that already assess the caregiver and see the clear holistic picture. Much like care managers need to see not just the health needs of a care receiver but also the psychosocial needs in order to do a geriatric assessment, we need to do the same for the family caregiver. By seeing all sides of the care receiver and the caregiver we will truly be able to see the big picture and begin to meet the aging family's needs.

REFERENCES

1. Family Caregiver Alliance. *Caregiver Assessment: Voices and Views from the Field. Report from a National Development Conference.* Vol 2. San Francisco, CA: Family Caregiver Alliance; 2006:97.
2. Feinberg LF. The state-of-the-art caregiver assessment. *Generations.* 2003–2004;Winter:24.
3. Family Caregiver Alliance. *Caregiver Assessment: Voices and Views from the Field. Report from a National Development Conference.* Vol 2. San Francisco, CA: Family Caregiver Alliance; 2006:39.
4. Family Caregiver Alliance. *Caregiver Assessment: Voices and Views from the Field. Report from a National Development Conference.* Vol 2. San Francisco, CA: Family Caregiver Alliance; 2006:39.
5. Family Caregiver Alliance. *Caregiver Assessment: Voices and Views from the Field. Report from a National Development Conference.* Vol 2. San Francisco, CA: Family Caregiver Alliance; 2006:61.
6. Levine C. Family caregiving: Current challenges for a time-honored practice. *Generations.* 2003–2004;Winter:2.
7. Levine C. Family caregiving: Current challenges for a time-honored practice. *Generations.* 2003–2004;Winter:2.
8. Family Caregiver Alliance. *Caregiver Assessment: Principles, Guidelines and Strategies for Change. Report from the Consensus Development Conference.* Vol 1. San Francisco, CA: Family Caregiver Alliance; 2006:5.
9. Family Caregiver Alliance. *Caregivers Count Too: A Toolkit to Help Professionals Assess the Needs of Family Caregivers.* San Francisco, CA: Family Caregiver Alliance; 2006:2.1.
10. Levine C. Family caregiving: Current challenges for a time-honored practice. *Generations.* 2003–2004;Winter:1.
11. Zarit S, Knight B. *A Guide to Psychotherapy and Aging, Interventions with Family Caregivers.* Washington, D.C.: American Psychological Assoc. 1996:141.
12. Zarit S, Knight B. *A Guide to Psychotherapy and Aging, Interventions with Family Caregivers.* Washington, D.C.: American Psychological Assoc. 1996:141.
13. Family Caregiver Alliance. *Caregivers Count Too: A Toolkit to Help Professionals Assess the Needs of Family Caregivers.* San Francisco, CA: Family Caregiver Alliance; 2006.
14. Family Caregiver Alliance. *Caregiver Assessment: Principles, Guidelines and Strategies for Change. Report from the Consensus Development Conference.* Vol 1. San Francisco, CA: Family Caregiver Alliance; 2006:13.
15. Morano CL, Morano B. Applying stress and appraisal, and coping framework to geriatric care management. *Geriatric Care Management Journal.* 2006;17(1):3.
16. Family Caregiver Alliance. *Assessment of Family Caregivers: A Practice Perspective, Report from the Consensus Development Conference.* Vol 1. San Francisco, CA: Family Caregiver Alliance; 2006:49.
17. Family Caregiver Alliance. *Assessment of Family Caregivers: A Practice Perspective, Report from the Consensus Development Conference.* Vol 1. San Francisco, CA: Family Caregiver Alliance; 2006:10.
18. Family Caregiver Alliance. *Caregiver Assessment: Principles, Guidelines and Strategies for Change. Report from the Consensus Development Conference.* Vol 1. San Francisco, CA: Family Caregiver Alliance; 2006:14.

19. Feinberg LF. The state-of-the-art caregiver assessment. *Generations.* 2003–2004;Winter:24.
20. Thompson L. *Long-Term Care: Support of Family Caregivers.* Washington, DC: Georgetown University Long-Term Care Financing Project; 2004:7.
21. University of Maryland Center on Aging. Cash and counseling: Demonstration and evaluation of a consumer-directed model for long-term care services. Available at: http://www.hhp.umd.edu/AGING/CCDemo/overview.html. Accessed May 2008.
22. National Center on Elder Abuse. *Preventing Elder Abuse by Family Caregivers.* Washington, DC: National Center on Elder Abuse; 2002: 8–10.
23. Family Caregiver Alliance. *Assessment of Family Caregivers: A Practice Perspective, Report from the Consensus Development Conference.* Vol 1. San Francisco, CA: Family Caregiver Alliance; 2006:63.
24. Family Caregiver Alliance. *Caregivers Count Too: A Toolkit to Help Professionals Assess the Needs of Family Caregivers.* San Francisco, CA: Family Caregiver Alliance; 2006:2.3.
25. Feinberg LF. The state-of-the-art caregiver assessment. *Generations.* 2003–2004;Winter:25.
26. Family Caregiver Alliance. *Caregivers Count Too: A Toolkit to Help Professionals Assess the Needs of Family Caregivers.* San Francisco, CA: Family Caregiver Alliance; 2006:2.2.
27. Family Caregiver Alliance. *Caregivers Count Too: A Toolkit to Help Professional Assess the Needs of Family Caregivers.* San Francisco, CA: Family Caregiver Alliance; 2006:2.2.
28. Family Caregiver Alliance. *Caregiver Assessment: Principles, Guidelines and Strategies for Change. Report from the Consensus Development Conference.* Vol 1. San Francisco, CA: Family Caregiver Alliance; 2006:8.
29. Thompson L. *Long-Term Care: Support of Family Caregivers.* Washington, DC: Georgetown University Long-Term Care Financing Project; 2004:4–5.
30. Family Caregiver Alliance. *Assessment of Family Caregivers: A Practice Perspective, Report from the Consensus Development Conference.* Vol 1. San Francisco, CA: Family Caregiver Alliance; 2006:16.
31. Family Caregiver Alliance. *Caregiver Assessment: Principles, Guidelines and Strategies for Change. Report from the Consensus Development Confer-*
32. Cress CJ. *Handbook of Geriatric Care Management.* 2nd ed. Sudbury, MA: Jones and Bartlett; 2006:229.
33. Family Caregiver Alliance. *Caregivers Count Too: A Toolkit to Help Professional Assess the Needs of Family Caregivers.* San Francisco, CA: Family Caregiver Alliance; 2006:3.9.
34. Family Caregiver Alliance. *Caregiver Assessment: Principles, Guidelines and Strategies for Change. Report from the Consensus Development Conference.* Vol 1. San Francisco, CA: Family Caregiver Alliance; 2006:19.
35. Family Caregiver Alliance. *Caregivers Count Too: A Toolkit to Help Professionals Assess the Needs of Family Caregivers.* San Francisco, CA: Family Caregiver Alliance; 2006:3.1.
36. Family Caregiver Alliance. *Assessment of Family Caregivers: A Practice Perspective, Report from the Consensus Development Conference.* Vol 1. San Francisco, CA: Family Caregiver Alliance; 2006:42.
37. Hikoyeda N, Miyawaki C. Ethnic and cultural considerations in geriatric care management. In: Cress CJ, ed. *Handbook of Geriatric Care Management.* 2nd ed. Sudbury, MA: Jones and Bartlett; 2006:99.
38. Family Caregiver Alliance. *Caregiver Assessment: Principles, Guidelines and Strategies for Change. Report from the Consensus Development Conference.* Vol 1. San Francisco, CA: Family Caregiver Alliance; 2006:30.
39. National Center on Elder Abuse. *Preventing Elder Abuse by Family Caregivers.* Washington, DC: National Center on Elder Abuse; 2002:12.
40. Morano CL, Morano B. Applying stress and appraisal, and coping framework to geriatric care management. *Geriatric Care Management Journal.* 2006;17(1):3.
41. Family Caregiver Alliance. *Assessment of Family Caregivers: A Practice Perspective, Report from the Consensus Development Conference.* Vol 1. San Francisco, CA: Family Caregiver Alliance; 2006:21–23.
42. Morano CL, Morano B. Applying stress and appraisal, and coping framework to geriatric care management. *Geriatric Care Management Journal.* 2006;17(1):3.
43. Bandler R, Grinder J. *The Structure of Magic.* Palo Alto, CA: Science and Behaviour Books; 1975:80.
44. Family Caregiver Alliance. *Caregiver Assessment: Principles, Guidelines and Strategies for Change.*

Report from the Consensus Development Conference. Vol 1. San Francisco, CA: Family Caregiver Alliance; 2006:16.

45. Family Caregiver Alliance. *Assessment of Family Caregivers: A Practice Perspective, Report from the Consensus Development Conference.* Vol 1. San Francisco, CA: Family Caregiver Alliance; 2006:14.

46. Thompson L. *Long-Term Care: Support of Family Caregivers.* Washington, DC: Georgetown University Long-Term Care Financing Project; 2004:4.

47. Newquist D, Rosenberg C, Barber C. Functional assessment. In: Cress CJ, ed. *Handbook of Geriatric Care Management.* 2nd ed. Sudbury, MA: Jones and Bartlett; 2007.

48. Morano B, Morano C. Psychosocial assessment. In: Cress CJ, ed. *Handbook of Geriatric Care Management.* 2nd ed. Sudbury, MA: Jones and Bartlett; 2007:25.

49. Cress C, Barber C. Care planning and geriatric assessment. In: Cress CJ, ed. *Handbook of Geriatric Care Management.* 2nd ed. Sudbury, MA: Jones and Bartlett; 2007.

50. Family Caregiver Alliance. *Assessment of Family Caregivers: A Practice Perspective, Report from the Consensus Development Conference.* Vol 1. San Francisco, CA: Family Caregiver Alliance; 2006:26.

51. Newquist D, Rosenberg C, Barber C. Functional assessment. In: Cress CJ, ed. *Handbook of Geriatric Care Management.* 2nd ed. Sudbury, MA: Jones and Bartlett; 2007:58–70.

52. Family Caregiver Alliance. *Assessment of Family Caregivers: A Practice Perspective, Report from the Consensus Development Conference.* Vol 1. San Francisco, CA: Family Caregiver Alliance; 2006:26.

53. Cress C, Barber C. Care planning and geriatric assessment. In: Cress CJ, ed. *Handbook of Geriatric Care Management.* 2nd ed. Sudbury, MA: Jones and Bartlett; 2007:82–84.

54. Cress CJ, ed. *Handbook of Geriatric Care Management.* 2nd ed. Sudbury, MA: Jones and Bartlett; 2007:342.

55. Family Caregiver Alliance. *Caregiver Assessment: Principles, Guidelines and Strategies for Change. Report from the Consensus Development Conference.* Vol 1. San Francisco, CA: Family Caregiver Alliance; 2006:17.

56. Kaszniak AA. Techniques and instruments for assessment of the elderly. In: Zarit S, Knight B, eds. *A Guide to Psychotherapy and Aging, Interventions with Family Caregivers.* Washington, D.C.: American Psychological Assoc. 1996:174.

57. Family Caregiver Alliance. *Caregivers Count Too: A Toolkit to Help Professionals Assess the Needs of Family Caregivers.* San Francisco, CA: Family Caregiver Alliance; 2006:3.1.

58. Family Caregiver Alliance. *Assessment of Family Caregivers: A Practice Perspective, Report from the Consensus Development Conference.* Vol 1. San Francisco, CA: Family Caregiver Alliance; 2006:46.

59. Family Caregiver Alliance. *Caregiver Assessment: Principles, Guidelines and Strategies for Change. Report from the Consensus Development Conference.* Vol 1. San Francisco, CA: Family Caregiver Alliance; 2006:16.

60. Family Caregiver Alliance. *Caregiver Assessment: Principles, Guidelines and Strategies for Change. Report from the Consensus Development Conference.* Vol 1. San Francisco, CA: Family Caregiver Alliance; 2006:16.

61. Family Caregiver Alliance. *Assessment of Family Caregivers: A Practice Perspective, Report from the Consensus Development Conference.* Vol 1. San Francisco, CA: Family Caregiver Alliance; 2006:48.

CHAPTER 5

Tools to Support Family Caregivers

Steve Barlam and Bunni Dybnis

INTRODUCTION

The focus of this chapter is to discuss how the care manager can provide the tools, resources, and support for family caregivers. To do so, it is important to look at the needs of the older adult in the context of the family unit. How do the needs of this person affect the family? How can family members gain or maintain a sense of balance? What are the tools that the care manager can offer family caregivers to assist them in the process? How can care managers engage family caregivers effectively?

Barbara, 52, is a family caregiver. Mrs. Kaufman, her 84-year-old mother, was born in Poland and survived the Holocaust. She was orphaned at age 16, losing her parents, siblings, and other close relatives in the war. She was married 50 years to a fellow survivor and has three adult children, two sons and her only daughter, Barbara. Her eldest son, Steve, is a successful investment banker who lives an hour from Mrs. Kaufman. He calls weekly and visits infrequently. Mrs. Kaufman's youngest child, Michael, is single and is a person who has a mild developmental disability. He lives semi-independently in a group home and works in a subsidized job. For now, Michael is able to live modestly on government entitlements. Although he can't assist his mother financially or physically, he and his mother are very close and he visits her weekly.

Mrs. Kaufman, who had been widowed 10 years prior, had been managing independently until 6 months ago when she began to be unstable on her feet. She had fallen twice in the last month and has had some difficulty in managing some of her household chores and self-care needs. She recently received a diagnosis of Parkinson's disease.

Prior to the recent changes in her mother's functional abilities, Barbara would have described her life as extremely busy. Barbara is married, works full time as an attorney, and has a son in high school. Barbara had been told from early on about the trauma of her mother's life. She has repeatedly been reminded of the sacrifices her parents made so that Barbara could enjoy the advantages they never had. She also has understood the expectation that she as the only daughter was responsible for her mother's well-being. Barbara feels the weight of the increasing demands on her time and anticipates it only getting worse. Recently she has made daily visits to her mother to assist with her personal care needs. The complaints from Barbara's husband regarding her neglect of him and their son, as well as the raised eyebrows from her colleagues due to time off from work, all contribute to Barbara's feeling that she is at the breaking point. In addition to exhaustion, she experiences the overwhelming guilt that she is letting everyone down.

At the suggestion of her mother's physician, Barbara engages a professional geriatric care manager. During the initial contact, Barbara only wants to talk about her mother's needs. Barbara gets impatient when the care manager asks about how this is impacting her. In spite of Barbara's brief annoyance, she agrees to have the care manager come out to meet her mother to assess the situation.

Aging is a family affair. The aging process does not only affect the older adult, but it is felt by the entire support system.[1] Family members, friends, neighbors, involved professionals, as well as the community at large are all affected. Family caregivers take the brunt of the stress of managing the needs of an aging senior:

> A substantial body of research shows that family members who provide care to individuals with chronic or disabling conditions are themselves at risk. Emotional, mental, and physical health problems arise from complex caregiving situations and the strains of caring for frail or disabled relatives.[2]

Care managers strive to understand the changing needs of the older client and how they affect those involved in the aging person's life. With this understanding, care managers can create successful interventions to help not only the senior client, but the entire family system.

The common starting point that care managers employ is the assessment. Although an entire chapter has been devoted to assessing the family caregiver, it is important to discuss the role of assessment of the family system as it relates to the tools care managers use to provide support for family caregivers.[3]

ASSESSMENT

Many cherish the idea of traveling. When traveling as part of a group, it is crucial to take into account the individuals' personal preferences, personalities, expectations, and limitations. Without doing so, this seemingly positive experience can be fraught with disaster. Not only must the care manager assess the concrete needs, functional abilities, and resources of the elder, but equally important are the extenuating circumstances and family dynamics that are essential to any assessment. An understanding of generational issues, family history, and the quality of the ties must be part of the assessment. Like the vacation that is ruined by disagreements about the itinerary, so too are the best laid plans for the senior made without evaluating the entire family situation. Often, the unaddressed family caregiver's issues may result in resentment, premature placement, burnout and, at times, even abuse. Like the successful traveling experience, a thorough assessment can set the stage for a successful care management experience.

During that initial evaluation, the care manager was sensitive to the fact that Mrs. Kaufman did not yet understand how her needs and preferences affected her daughter. The care manager was careful to frame her questions focusing on Mrs. Kaufman's needs, while obtaining information about what was expected from her children. Asking Mrs. Kaufman about all her children as well as how her elderly relatives were cared for in past generations afforded the care manager information about the demands made on her only daughter Barbara. When Mrs. Kaufman excused her sons from any direct role in her care, Barbara was quick to interject her feelings that, in spite of their good intentions, she felt alone in this process. Barbara was relieved with the line of questioning, and appreciated the fact that the care manager was able to identify the needs of her mother as well as her own.

Prior to this meeting, Barbara had thought that the only solution to her present situation was to place her mother in a senior facility. The anxiety of having to move her mother against her wishes was untenable. After all her mother had been through, didn't she deserve to stay in the home she loved, cared for by the daughter for whom she had sacrificed so much? The care manager's questions regarding the role of her brothers, socialization with peers, and the mention of non-family care providers gave hope to Barbara that the care manager also understood her concerns. By the end of the initial assessment, the groundwork for a plan for both mother and daughter was set. Barbara was feeling much better about the care manager and agreed to set up a follow-up telephone meeting to fill in the gaps.

The care manager, using the adage, "begin where the client is at," identified the daughter as an essential element of this family unit. The care manager integrated the daughter's needs into the assessment process and aligned herself with Barbara's pace, which set the stage for the entire process.

The primary focus of the care manager is that of understanding. Without an objective understanding of the situation, it is impossible to provide the necessary support, guidance, and recommendations that are at the core of most care management interventions. Through observations, asking questions, and review of records, the care manager gathers and analyzes information to formulate a thoughtful plan based on the facts.

The Whole Person Approach

Historically, the goal of the assessment process is to understand the needs, problems, and issues facing the client. Care managers invest in understanding the issues beyond the physical needs of their client. With the use of multidimensional assessment tools, they look at the "whole person." The assessment tools incorporate questions pertaining to health care, mental health, social history and needs, formal supports, informal supports, spiritual needs, functional abilities, risk factors (medication, behavior, falls, nutrition, cognition, abuse, substance misuse, etc.), strengths, preferences, and values.

The Whole Family Approach

If a stone is thrown into the center of a pond, ripples emanate from the point where the stone first touched the water. Consider that touch spot as the senior with care needs. The perceived ripples are the effects of those care needs on the family caregivers close to the center all the way to the greater society toward the edge of the pond. From the onset, investing in understanding the impact of the senior's needs on the family affords the care manager the ability to create more sustainable plans that help balance the needs of the senior and family caregivers.

Who Is the Family?

In the last three decades in the United States, there have been significant changes in the concept of family caregiving.[4] Some of these changes are due to the lack of availability of the traditional nuclear family including increased divorce rates, new blended families, and more acceptance of same-sex relationships. These factors contribute to changing attitudes as well as definition of *family*. With divorce there often comes the possibility of remarriage, often adding additional familial responsibilities. It is now common for an adult child to have more parents and step-parents alive than they do children. Additionally, geographic mobility, economic realities, and increased women in the workforce all help define the new family caregiver.

Care managers, when assessing families, must embrace a broader definition of family. This should not be limited to biological ties, but rather to ties of choice.[5] This expanded definition of family includes extended families. Care managers work not only with spouses, siblings, and adult children, but with friends and partners, as well as distant blood relatives. When older adults are estranged or separated from their nuclear family, often they create families of choice with whom the care manager needs to be working. The care manager must not make assumptions about who is family, but rather, ask the question and be open to the answers.

Who Is the Family Caregiver?

Within any family structure, there are some individuals who have assumed the role of family caregivers. They have taken on the responsibility of providing the required care for a family member in need. For some it is a calling or it relates to their personality; while for others, they feel that they are the only one available to provide the needed care. There are some who are groomed from a very early age to be a family caregiver. The scripts are well rehearsed, making the message loud and clear. "Most caregivers for aging parents remain adult children, although their spouses provide a good deal of the care."[6] When working with family caregivers, it is always important to understand what has led them to this role. What works for them to be the family caregiver, or what function does it serve? Through insight gained by understanding the underlying motivating factors, the care manager identifies strategies to connect, acknowledge, and provide support in a way that will nurture the family caregivers.

Who Else Is Involved?

As part of the assessment process, care managers identify those professionals involved in the client's life who comprise the formal supports including physicians, attorneys, financial planners, accountants, and therapists. It is equally important the care manager identifies the informal supports including relatives, friends, and community organizations with whom the senior is affiliated. The ties, extent of the ties, and the quality of the support system depend on characteristics including age, gender, number of years known, relationship, and proximity of these supports.[7] Studies show families provide more hands-on support while friends more emotional support.[8]

What Affects the Role of the Family Caregiver?

As care managers assess the family caregiver's needs, the following issues should be considered (see Chapter 4, "Assessing the Caregiver"):

- Severity and duration of situation—The severity or extent to which physical, cognitive, and behavioral decline is prevalent in an aging relative along with the duration of the caregiver experience will greatly affect the family caregiver experience.
- Level of burden or stress—Stress is defined as the strain felt by the caregiver, and burden refers to the management of tasks, which depends partly on the coping skills and other supports available.[9] The energy needed to provide for the caregiving needs of a senior relative compared to an individual's own reserves must be examined. Additional responsibilities, stresses, and individual personality characteristics will help determine the burden of specific caregiving situations. The highest levels of stress and depression occur among caregivers when there are severe behavioral problems or memory loss.[10]
- What has changed or been compromised in the family caregiver's life because of the senior's needs? The family caregiver's responsibilities to his or her nuclear family, job, personal health maintenance, and other community activities all need to be considered when evaluating the impact of

the senior's needs on the family. As Jill Quadagno explains, "Marriages may be strained by the loss of time couples have for each other when one spouse is caring for an aging relative."[11] Care managers must ask themselves "why now?" and what has changed in the family unit that has created the need for the family to take action at this point in time?

- Past history or trauma—It is important for the care manager to identify critical events in the history of the family and during the aging member's life, including psychiatric episodes, health issues, and other life-changing events. Wartime experiences, political upheaval and displacement, childhood abuse, neglect, and abandonment are just some of the issues that may influence the family caregiver's response.

- Sandwich generation issues—Many family caregivers have multiple generations requiring their attention and care. In 1981, Dorothy Miller coined the term *sandwich generation* to refer to inequality in the exchange of resources and support between generations.[12] Specifically, Miller was referring to a segment of the middle-aged generation that provides support to both young and older family members yet does not receive reciprocal support in exchange. Miller emphasized the unique stressors of multigenerational caregiving and the lack of community resources available to assist the middle generation. Because multigenerational caregivers are most often women dealing with the complex role configurations of wife, mother, daughter, caregiver, and employee, some researchers use the phrase *women in the middle* interchangeably with the *sandwich generation*.[13]

- Religious and cultural issues—Expectations based on religious or cultural practices, rituals, and differing belief systems between family members all need to be considered. Are the expectations of the children and the parents consistent? Often conflicts emerge because of differing life experiences. As intermarriage becomes more common, the attitudes within the family toward religious and cultural differences have created new challenges, particularly among the different generations. For some family caregivers, their religious convictions provide them with a sense of meaning of the caregiving experience.

- End-of-life issues—These issues can be complex and emotionally charged. They may be connected to cultural, religious, and moral beliefs. When important end-of-life decisions need to be made, the stress of the responsibility and the seriousness of the situation can cause great discomfort. Care managers are often engaged to help facilitate the discussions and help family members come together to work as a functional unit. Understanding the differing viewpoints is critical. Knowing what a parent wants and does not want during the last days and hours of life help define and simplify the role of the family. It relieves the family of the burden of having the responsibility of making decisions that may not be what their parents want. Knowing what the aging parent wants can also avoid family conflicts when adult children may have differing values.[14] Proactive discussions and legal planning can help to reduce some of the potential conflicts (see Chapter 9, "Dying, Grief, and Burial in the Aging Family").

- Quality-of-life issues—What is important to the senior? What is important to the involved family caregivers? The care manager can assist families by opening up the dialogue to facilitate open discussions on preferences and values. Attention to the individual's need for social interaction or privacy, the importance of physical environment, value of family, proximity to cultural stimulation, and adaptability to change are just some of the many quality-of-life considerations. When values and preferences differ between individuals, it is important to identify how the differences may affect all involved in the process.

• Relationship to money—Values concerning spending, saving, and inheritance often affect the family caregiver. The circumstances for those who lived through the Great Depression have made many adults fearful of spending and taking any financial risks. Raised in a relatively secure environment, this can be very difficult for the adult children to understand:

Talking to parents about money is difficult, especially if the money you are talking about is theirs. They belong to a generation that was taught to keep their information private, and not to share their concerns openly. Even if they need help, they may not be willing to talk to you, because it's "none of your business," or because they are afraid to give up control over their financial affairs.[15]

It is incumbent upon adult children to bring up this difficult topic of money before a crisis hits. This can ensure that the emotional aspects of spending, the differing relationships to money, and the objective realities are resolved. All too commonly, when financial issues are ignored, a situation of inappropriate spending, withholding of services, or fiduciary misconduct arises. There are other situations in which family members may question expenditures for the senior, out of concern that future inheritance may be depleted.

• The family unit—Care managers assess the quality of relationships, expectations of individuals, proximity, availability, and the willingness to be involved; in addition, they assess both past and present conflicts among family members. Sibling discord often surfaces due to the unequal division of caregiving duties. Generally, one sibling takes on the primary role of caring for a loved one. This may be because he or she lives closest to the parent, is perceived as having less work or fewer family obligations, or is considered the "favorite" child. Regardless of the reasons, this situation can lead the overburdened caregiver to feel frustrated and resentful and other siblings to feel uninformed and left out.[16]

• The degree of involvement—Utilizing their clinical skills, care managers can evaluate the level of involvement of family members by evaluating the tasks and amount of time that is invested. This assessement helps the family to objectively consider in which of the current tasks they want to participate. This process assists to identify others both within the formal and informal support systems who may be able to provide support. Additionally, the tool helps family members identify gaps in service provision.

• Special needs in the family—When there is a child of an aging parent who is disabled or otherwise dependent there are additional stresses on the family unit. For the parents, there is the concern of who will take care of the dependent child when they cannot. For the siblings, this question is often of equal concern to that of taking care of any older parents. Financial, emotional, and logistical issues as well as the specific responsibilities need to be considered by these families, due to the fact that the duration of the care often is longer than the care required for a senior family member.

Assessing the Family Caregiver

Not all family members are equally willing or able to participate in caring for an aging relative. Several factors must be considered when considering how family members can be involved. There are numerous tools described in the chapter on assessing family caregivers that the care manager can employ to better understand the needs of the family caregiver. The assessment should include the following components:

- Ability to provide the physical care
- Mental health: burden, stress, depression, and satisfaction
- Willingness to participate
- Understanding, literacy, or mastery of the issues and tasks involved

Using the Modified Caregiver Strain Index[17] (www.hartfordign.org), the care manager can help determine to what degree the caregiving responsibilities are negatively affecting the family caregiver.

The care manager had a strong sense of the needs, values, preferences, and strengths of Mrs. Kaufman. The care manager needed more information on how her current needs affected the daughter. The care manager observed Barbara's posture and facial expression change from tense to more relaxed when the discussion turned to maintaining her mother at home. Reflecting that observation back to Barbara created an opportunity for her to identify the underlying fear around placement. Barbara went on to discuss her belief that because of her mother's wartime experience, the regimented environment of a senior facility would be traumatic for her. "My mother says she doesn't want to be a burden; however, she wants me to take care of her, and I just can't." Barbara felt stuck. In the course of their conversation, the care manager gathered important information and insights that later helped her in formulating a plan. The care manager understood that Mrs. Kaufman would need more assistance than Barbara could reasonably provide. She would now identify other outside supports to fill in the gaps.

PLANNING

The care planning process can provide family caregivers with a sense that there is a light at the end of the tunnel. Many family members are going through this for the first time. Care managers can provide reassurance from their experience of working through the beginnings, middles, and ends of many different kinds of similar situations, and they can knowledgably outline the best possible options.

During the care planning process, care managers work closely with the senior client and involved family caregivers. Care managers lay out the identified issues, concerns, problems, and needs based on the professional assessment. The care manager then prioritizes the issues and identifies the possible outcomes. Following the identification of goals, the care manager identifies appropriate services and resources to help the senior and the family achieve their agreed upon goal. The care manager concurrently confirms that both financial and human resources (formal and informal support networks) are available to assist the senior. The care manager assesses the informal and formal support networks as to skill sets, level of involvement, availability, and willingness to assist.

Care managers must identify why and by whom the request for services was initiated. Although the presenting problem is almost universally focused on the older adult, for a plan to succeed it must address the goals of the other parties involved. Often unstated, the plans must address the underlying issues of family caregiver burnout, guilt, anger, financial agendas, and threats or challenges to the well-being of those involved. Without considerations to each individual's stake in the plan, the implementation may never occur.

If the care manager only focused on Mrs. Kaufman, responding to her need for personal assistance, the plan of care would have most probably listed Barbara as a resource for assistance. After all, from Mrs. Kaufman's perception, Barbara would be the most logical person to provide the needed care. Due to the guilt and ambivalence that Barbara experiences around her role as a family caregiver, if asked to provide the needed care for her mother, she more than likely would have agreed to the plan. As a result, she may have resented both the mother and the care manager for placing this demand upon her. Without understanding the daughter's perception of the current situation, the care manager could be setting up a plan that most probably would not be able to be sustained. Additionally any alliance with the daughter would be compromised due to the request from the care manager that did not take into account her willingness to participate in specific tasks.

One common pitfall for care managers to remember: Before the care manager presents the plan of care, the potential obstacles must be identified.

When perceived needs aren't aligned with objective needs:

- Mrs. Kaufman's perceived need is for minimal assistance with her activities of daily living including cooking, laundry, bathing, and getting undressed in the evening.
- The objective needs identified by the care manager are for moderate assistance with cooking, shopping, housekeeping, bathing, dressing, and laundry. Additionally, due to her unsteady gait, Mrs. Kaufman is a fall risk and would benefit from ongoing supervision. Last, Mrs. Kaufman had lost 10 lbs in the last 4 months and has not been eating properly.

When the senior's desired outcomes are not aligned with those of the family caregiver:

- Mrs. Kaufman's desired outcome is "for my daughter to come by nightly, to bring in some food, do a little laundry, help me with a bath, and get me ready for bed."
- Barbara's desired outcome is "for my mother to improve physically and, if that can't be achieved, I want to be assured that my mother is assisted with her daily needs—but by someone other than myself. Also, I don't want my mother to fall and have to go to a nursing home."

When prioritizing the needs, the senior and family caregiver cannot agree:

- For Mrs. Kaufman, her primary needs include help with a bath and having food brought to her.
- For Barbara, her primary needs include having someone with her mother to help avert another fall, and to make sure her mother is eating, and to monitor that her mother's hygiene is maintained. Barbara also does not want to continue neglecting her husband and son.

When options for interventions cannot be agreed upon:

- Mrs. Kaufman's solution was easy, "My daughter who lives nearby can stop by and provide the minimal assistance that I need. *I don't want a stranger in my house*, and *I definitely don't want to move to a facility!*"
- Barbara's solution, too, was easy but not the one that her mother would easily accept: "I know that my mother would not do well moving and that she truly needs more care than what she is currently willing to accept. While I know that she would prefer for me to provide the care, I just do not have the time to commit, nor do I want to have to be there every evening. Having a paid caregiver come daily sounds like the best option."

- Parents may resist paid caregivers for a variety of reasons. They may cherish their independence and privacy, be unaware of how dependent they are, may fear being robbed or exploited, have racial attitudes, or worry that they will lose contact with their children.[18]

When the needs of the family caregiver are in conflict with the needs of the senior:

- Barbara's relationship with her husband was becoming strained; her son required her time and attention; and since her legal practice was growing, her partners needed her to be focused on work. Barbara needed to find a solution that would balance her desire to be a good daughter while not neglecting her other responsibilities. At the present, she had less time as opposed to more time to spend with her mother, and this was in direct conflict with her mother's needs.

When there are differing views on how to allocate resources:

- Mrs. Kaufman feels that she is not able to afford to pay for any additional care if it means that she will have to tap into her savings. It is important to her that the principal remain intact as well as her home remain free from debt. Her desire is that her estate should be left to her family. Her son, Michael, must have a home once she is gone and have money to ensure his future needs will be met.
- Barbara feels her parents worked hard for their money and her mother should spend it on herself. Although Barbara could use the money, she would rather see it spent on her mother's own needs. Steve has expressed to Barbara that he feels that their mother has the money, and so he has not felt the need to offer support. She knows,

however, that her brother could and would be willing to contribute if the need arose. Barbara feels some resentment toward Michael, who has always been the primary focus of her mother's attention. She feels the state supports him at the present, and will continue to do so.

During the care planning stage, when conflict arises, the care manager must employ the best communication, consensus building, and interpersonal skills to help the senior and family caregivers reach an acceptable level of agreement. This can include assisting family caregivers in recognizing that behaviors are often based on emotions and past experiences that may not always be rational. By helping family members communicate openly and honestly, without blame, the care manager can help families get beyond some of the impasses.

The care manager coaches Barbara to help her clearly articulate her dilemma to her mother without anger, guilt, or resentment. "Mom, I hope you know how much I love you and care about you. I am sure you also realize I have a full-time job, a husband, and a son…so unfortunately, I am not able to give you the time you need to assist you in staying at home safely. We will just have to look for other ways of keeping you at home."

The desired outcome of the care planning process is for care managers to secure agreement to the plan of care. Time is needed to engage the senior and the family caregivers in the process in order to help them understand the rationale of the plan. This is a critical stage in the process because in spite of the care manager's skill in developing and presenting a quality plan of care, it can all fall apart if those involved do not genuinely agree to it.

Mrs. Kaufman now understood that she did need some additional help. She was fearful that if she accepted care from an outside source, her daughter may step away from the situation and not be involved. The care manager had heard Mrs. Kaufman mention during the assessment that she did not want to be a burden to her daughter. Helping the mother and daughter reach consensus, the care manager had coached Barbara to articulate the other responsibilities that she was facing at the present. Given Barbara's reality, the care manager had her identify how much time during the week she has available to spend with her mother. Barbara committed to seeing her mother twice during the week and once on the weekend. Having that commitment articulated allowed Mrs. Kaufman to let go of some of her fears that her daughter would disappear if she accepted outside care. Reinforcing her desire not to be a burden on her daughter, the care manager discussed options on how Mrs. Kaufman could get the care she "felt" she needed during the week. A compromise was agreed upon that included a paid care provider available to her three times a week for 4 hours a day as a starting point. The care manager stated that she felt Mrs. Kaufman may need more care at the present, due to the fall risk, but both Barbara and Mrs. Kaufman needed to start off slowly, understanding both the potential risk and the ability to adjust the plan as required. Additionally, Michael could be more actively involved in assisting his mother by being responsible for some of the concrete daily tasks, including laundry and light housekeeping.

When family members have shared values, the planning process is much more likely to succeed. Care managers identify the values in common and use these to strengthen the plan. With a focus on the shared values and common goals the care manager can help families weather the strains that naturally occur when dealing with competing preferences.

Barbara and her mother shared the common value of aging in place, agreeing that Mrs. Kaufman remain at home for as long as possible. While they both had the same desired outcome, they had different ideas of how to get there. Underscoring the commonalities the care manager was able to create a safe environment that allowed each participant to hear each other's ideas with minimal defensiveness.

When Mrs. Kaufman minimized her own needs, the care manager was able to use objective information obtained from the assessment. This helped the process stay on track. The care manager pointed out that despite Mrs. Kaufman stating "I'm just fine," Mrs. Kaufman had, in fact, fallen several times in the past several weeks. Just last week she was found on the bathroom floor by her daughter during an evening visit. Mrs. Kaufman was not able to pick herself up. Mrs. Kaufman reluctantly admitted that she did get a little nervous when her daughter did not get there daily. At the end of the meeting Mrs. Kaufman acknowledged that she would be willing to consider outside care.

IMPLEMENTING THE PLAN AND ONGOING INVOLVEMENT

Care managers partner with seniors and their family caregivers to implement the recommendations and provide ongoing monitoring of the plan. They bring to the relationship a unique set of CORE skills that help the family caregiver achieve greater success in their roles:

C—Containment
O—Objectivity
R—Resources
E—Expertise

Containment

By the time a family caregiver is introduced to a care manager, she or he often has experienced a great deal of stress, burden, or anxiety about the situation. The need is explicit. "I must take action," or "There must be a better way." There is most often some confusion as to what is the best way to proceed. Most family members want to do "the right thing" but struggle with determining what it is. This can lead to additional emotional strain and a feeling of being out of control.

Many of the decisions that family caregivers face are complex. They are affected by the often conflicting preferences, values, expectations, and needs of the senior, other family members, and others in the informal and formal support systems. There are family rules as to what family members are "supposed to" do for other family members.

There are situations in which family caregivers feel compelled to act, feeling the weight of the responsibility of being a "good" family member, yet they have no authority to take action. Family caregivers may be told by others "you really need to do something," yet when stepping in to intervene, the senior family member flatly refuses the assistance. Assuming the senior has capacity, the family caregivers often have their hands tied. As seniors lose capacity and poor judgment puts them at risk, family members often must face using the legal system or other aggressive measures to go against their loved one's wishes. The complex nature of family relationships further complicates these situations. Care managers can play a pivotal role in assisting these families to understand the dynamics involved and create a plan to help them achieve their objectives.

It is not uncommon for family caregivers to be overburdened and overwhelmed with the task of caring for a senior. Family caregivers may experience feelings of frustration, resentment, anger, and sadness. There are many different reasons for these emotions to surface: the family caregiver may not be acknowledged by the senior or by other family members; they may not be getting support from others; they may be criticized by others for either not doing things correctly or not doing enough; they may be neglecting other parts of their own life; or from sheer exhaustion.

Family caregivers often describe feeling "stuck," which creates an additional sense of discomfort. Care managers often serve as a container in which the family caregiver can deposit some of these uncomfortable feelings. For family caregivers, knowing that there is a care manager accessible with whom they can talk and who will respond with empathy can help relieve some of the burden and stress.

To contain the anxiety for their clients, active listening techniques help care managers stay focused. This technique involves listening with a purpose. It is used most effectively to gain information, understand others, solve problems, see how another person feels, or to show support. Using specific phrases to clarify, encourage, restate, reflect, summarize, validate, and empower helps the care manager to stay engaged in a meaningful way.

Objectivity

Everyone who goes through the caregiving experience is viewing that experience through their unique lenses. These lenses are always tinted based on past history with the care recipient, life experiences, personal values, and religious or cultural background. Most family caregivers want to do the right thing, but the right thing is not always easy to identify. When a family member is in the midst of the caregiving situation, it is not easy to achieve objectivity. Partnering with an objective third party can afford the family caregiver a unique vantage point, allowing them to get feedback that can assist in managing the caregiving situation well. Utilizing facts obtained from the assessment, observations, and discussions with involved parties, care managers synthesize a professional unbiased understanding of the situation and can be instrumental in assisting families in reaching a blame-free resolution of conflict.

Resources

Family caregivers turn to care managers for education on resources. They seek information on available resources, appropriateness of resources to their specific needs, and how they are accessed. Specific resources to support family caregivers must be included in the plan of care. A list of resources can be found in Figure 5-1.

Emotional Support Resources

Family caregivers often strive to better understand, cope, and come to terms with both longtime family conflicts as well as their new and changing roles. Services that support the emotional well-being are provided in several venues and can be paid for in a variety of

---

Emotional Support for Caregivers

Online discussions and support:
Family Caregiver Alliance—www.caregiver.org
Help guide for caregivers—www.helpguide.org

Support Groups

Caregiver support groups are available in most areas for families that are confronting Alzheimer's disease or other debilitating illnesses. National Web sites will have links to local branches.
Alzheimer's Association—www.alz.org
American Diabetes Association—www.diabetes.org
American Cancer Society—www.aca.org
American Parkinson's Disease Association—www.APDA.org

Individual Counseling

American Association of Marriage, Family Therapists—www.aamft.org
National Association of Social Workers—www.nasw.org
American Psychological Association—www.apa.org

Psychiatric Interventions

American Association of Geriatric Psychiatrists—www.aagpgpa.org

Legal and Financial

National Academy of Elder Law Attorneys—www.NAELA.org
National Guardian Association—www.nga.org
Certified public accountants—www.aicpa.org
Elder mediation, Association for Conflict Resolution—www.acr@acrnet.org
Certified Financial Planning Association—www.cfp.net
American Bar Association for Specialists in Estate and Probate—www.aba.net

continues

Education

National Council on Aging—www.ncoa.org
Alzheimer's education and support—www.Alzinfo.org
AARP: Information, advocacy, and service—www.aarp.org

Advocacy

National Senior Citizens Law Center—www.nsclc.org
Center for Healthcare Rights—www.healthcare.rights
National Caregiver Alliance—www.caregiver.org
Caregiver Resource Centers—www.caregiverresourcecenter.com
Alliance for the Mentally Ill (also support groups)—www.nami.org
The Arc of the United States—www.thearc.org/NetCommunity/Page.aspx?&pid=183&srcid=-2
The American Association on Intellectual and Developmental Disabilities (AAIDD)—www.aamr.org

Public Benefits

Medicare—www.medicare.gov
Public benefits— www.benefitscheckup.org
Medicaid—www.cms.hhs.gov
Family Medical Leave Act—www.dol.gov
Social Security—www.ssa.gov

End of Life

American Hospice Foundation—www.americanhospice.org
Five Wishes—www.agingwithdignity.org.

Home Safety

Home Modification Resource Center—www.homemods.org

Figure 5–1 Online Resources for Family Caregivers

---

ways. There are government or grant-funded support services often provided for low or sliding scale rates by not-for-profit agencies, services provided at no cost to employees by employee assistance programs, and services that accept third-party insurance reimbursement for services rendered by professionals. Care managers can make recommendations based on availability and affordability criteria.

- Support groups—Professionally or para-professionally led groups can offer psychological support, resources, and sharing of common experiences and thus provide family members with great comfort and relief. These groups are often provided by condition-specific or other not-for-profit organizations as well as by private therapists on a private-pay, sliding scale, or free basis. Support groups are generally geared toward those who are experiencing a normal adjustment reaction to the caregiving situation. When there are complex underlying stressors and/or a psychopathology, a professionally led group by a psychotherapist is generally indicated. Care managers can locate senior-specific resources by contacting the Area Agency on Aging office in their local community.

- Individual counseling or psychotherapy—One-on-one sessions can provide individuals the support they may not be getting elsewhere as well as the opportunity to delve into unresolved personal conflicts involving parents, sibling(s), or caregiving topics. Depending on the nature of the situation, sessions can either be facilitated by a licensed professional, trained paraprofessional, or peer counselor. Sessions can either be short or long term depending on the issues and the therapeutic framework employed. To locate a licensed therapist, care managers can refer to Figure 5-1 for professional, discipline-specific Web sites.
- Family meetings—Sessions with some or all of the family members present can help resolve family conflicts. It is important to make sure there are guidelines set up to ensure that everyone is heard and treated with respect. This venue allows for all involved participants to hear information, recommendations, and concerns all at the same time, therefore eliminating possible miscommunications.
- Psychiatric interventions—There are times when family members suffer from long-term mental illness or psychiatric symptoms brought on by the stresses associated with assuming the caregiver role. In such situations a psychiatrist may be necessary to provide medications and medical oversight. With over 71% of family caregivers experiencing at least one symptom of clinical depression, these professionals are underutilized. See Figure 5-1 for the American Association of Geriatric Psychiatrists Web site. Care managers would benefit from receiving personal recommendations from allied professionals.
- Biofeedback, hypnosis, and other related modalities—Any of these may help to reduce stress for the family caregiver. Re-

ferrals to professionals licensed by their specific discipline would be recommended. Licensure requirements may vary by state.

Self-Care Resources

Stress management can be accomplished by individuals in a variety of settings based on the individual preferences of family members. Often, these resources are overlooked, since the focus of the family caregiver tends to be on the care recipient. Resources that positively affect the care recipient are generally embraced, while those resources specifically for the family caregiver are seen as a nicety as opposed to a necessity. Helping family caregivers understand the direct relationship between self-care and quality of care provision is an important task for the care manager. Stress management techniques include the following:

- Massage
- Nutritional consultation or counseling
- Exercise
- Regular medical care
- Yoga or meditation
- Acupuncture or acupressure

Educational Resources

Care managers strive to help family caregivers master the tasks at hand. One important way this can be achieved is through education. Care managers can contribute to the care and healthcare literacy of the family caregiver by providing access to applicable resources. Family caregivers have the opportunity to better understand the caregiving situation through reading as well as attending lectures, workshops, and trainings. With more information, they can feel more confident in their decisions and actions. There is a growing number of resources that support the various challenges of family caregivers:

- Books and periodicals—Includes *Who Is the Family Caregiver?* guides and training for family caregivers as well as conflict resolution and how-to books on communication with seniors. See the list of additional reading at the end of the chapter.
- Online resources—Web sites abound on both family caregiving support and disease-specific information. These can offer education and resources.
- Workshops and conferences—Local as well as national organizations understand the unique needs of the family caregiver. Annual retreats, symposia, and conferences are available in many cities.
- Libraries—Many public libraries carry an inventory of books, periodicals, and audio and videotapes that focus on family caregiving and disease-specific topics.
- Disease- or condition-specific organizations and associations—There is a myriad of both national organizations as well as local chapters whose missions are to provide education and resources to individuals and family caregivers who may be compromised by specific conditions.

Legal and Financial Resources

- Estate planning attorneys—This specialized professional can provide assistance in creating documents such as wills and trusts to ensure appropriate transfer of the senior's estate at the time of death. Additionally they can assist with creating advance directives to ensure appropriate transfer of decision-making authority at a time of incapacity or death.
- Legal documents
  - Wills
  - Trusts
  - Power of attorney
  - Durable power of attorney for health care
  - Durable power of attorney for finances

- Living wills
- Do-not-resuscitate orders
- Attorneys specializing in elder law—This emerging field of law is composed of attorneys with an expertise in Medicaid planning, conservatorships, special needs situations, and end-of-life decision making. Many have expertise in estate planning. These professionals are trained to look at an elder's needs in the context of the family. See Figure 5-1 for the National Academy of Elder Law Attorneys Web site information that provides a comprehensive list of attorneys that specialize in this area of the law.
- Financial planners—These professionals assist with long-term planning and investment management. This is particularly important when a family member obtains financial control over the finances and needs a qualified professional to assist with budgeting and asset management. See Figure 5-1 for contact information for the Financial Planning Association.
- Accountants—Certified public accountants can be helpful in the creation of budgets, paying of taxes, consulting with the estate planning attorneys when documents are being created, and the management of income and expenditures. They often have access or can provide bookkeeping and daily money management services.
- Elder mediation—A relatively new field is emerging of trained neutral parties to assist families in resolving conflicts. This can be a useful tool to be used to avoid conservatorships or avoid the chaos that often occurs when there are disagreements between contesting parties. To ensure the appropriateness of the resource, care managers need to obtain information as to the mediator's professional background, experience, training, and areas of expertise. See Figure 5-1 for contact information.

- Insurance professionals—Private insurance brokers and companies can be of assistance when considering products to help finance health care, disability, long-term care, and estate tax needs. The care manager can refer to the HICAP program in their local community for detailed insurance information and advocacy. See Figure 5-1 for contact information.
- Professional Who Is the family caregiver? —Bank and trust companies, as well as professional conservators and guardians, can assist family caregivers in managing the finances for a senior adult who lacks the capacity to manage independently. There are built-in protections that ensure oversight. When looking for a professional conservator/guardian, the care manager can turn to the National Guardianship Association. See Figure 5-1 for contact information.
- Mortgage brokers—There is a growing number of real estate and mortgage brokers who have expertise in senior issues. There are situations in which families want to keep a senior at home, but to do so the family must access assets tied up in a home's equity. Reverse mortgages, equity lines, and traditional loans may be options for families who cannot otherwise finance their parents' needs. Conferring with trusted real estate agents or other trusted financial professionals can assist the care manager in identifying appropriate professionals.

Respite Resources

Over 85% of families are caring for elder relatives by themselves.[20] Family caregivers going it alone can experience detriments to their physical, emotional, and financial well-being. Enjoying a break for even the most devoted family members can improve the quality of life for all involved. Two important resources for both the care manager and family caregiver are the Family Caregiver Alliance (FCA) and the National Center on Caregiving (NCC):

> They work to advance the development of high-quality, cost-effective policies and programs for caregivers in every state in the country. Uniting research, public policy, and services, the FCA and the FCC serve as a central source of information on caregiving and long-term care issues for policy makers, service providers, media, funders, and family caregivers throughout the country.

See Figure 5-1 under advocacy for contact information.

Respite comes in many forms:

- Facility-based respite—When vacancies permit, many community facilities can provide weekend, weekly, or even monthly accommodations for families that could benefit from a weekend away or for a more extended vacation. Care managers can refer to their local office of the Area Agency on Aging or the ombudsman program to help identify appropriate resources.
- In-home care respite—Paid caregivers can provide relief to families for as short as 4-hour periods up to full-time around-the-clock relief. Getting a break from caregiver duties, even once a week, can help family caregivers regain a sense of balance.
- Care management—Some family caregivers have not considered taking time off from the responsibilities of tending to the needs of the senior. Who could or would fill in for themselves? Care managers can help arrange for care, while providing the oversight to ensure that all goes smoothly, while a family caregiver takes time away from the caregiving responsibilities.
- Social day care centers—These activity centers provide seniors with meaningful

social stimulation and activity, while providing family caregivers with needed respite. Consulting with the local office of the Area Agency on Aging and the local senior information and referral services (both generally housed in local senior centers) will provide the care manager with available programs.

Spiritual Resources

The caregiving experience can provide some family members with a great sense of fulfillment and meaning. For others they may be searching for the meaning in the acts of caregiving. There are many family caregivers who receive great comfort from their religious or spiritual communities. Care managers should become familiar with resources that can help nourish the spirit of the family caregiver.

- Literature
- Clergy
- Activities within the spiritual or religious communities
- Yoga or meditation

Advocacy Resources

There are many resources available whose shared missions are based on amplifying the voice of family caregivers in order to make policy changes on the federal, state, and local community levels. Most of these organizations rely on volunteers and staff to educate lawmakers and community leaders as to the issues that are most important to family caregivers. Besides providing family caregivers with educational information, resources, and referrals, they also provide a venue for family caregivers to get involved.

- Family Caregivers Alliance
- HICAP: local branches in most major cities
- AARP http://www.aarp.org

- Caregiver Resource Centers: http://www.caregiversresources.org
- National Alliance for the Mentally Ill: http://www.nami.org

Care Management Resources

Because adult children often live at a distance from their parents, being familiar with a network of care managers can provide access to resources within the local community that might benefit out-of-town families. One such organization is the National Association of Professional Geriatric Care Managers (www.caremanager.org), which provides contacts from their network of qualified professionals.

Public Benefits and Governmental Programs

Although care managers are well versed on public benefit programs, it is always important to empower family caregivers with knowledge about applicable benefit programs.

- Medicare—A federal health insurance program for individuals who are 65 and older and who have contributed to the program during their working years (or their spouse has). Additionally, Medicare is for those under 65 who suffer from qualified disabilities or other specific situations. This program is administered by the US Social Security Administration, which reimburses hospitals and physicians for medical care provided to qualifying individuals, as well as other medically oriented benefits.[19]
- Medicaid—This is the US health program for individuals and families with low incomes and resources. It is jointly funded by the state and federal governments and is managed by the states. Among the groups of people served by Medicaid are eligible low-income parents, children, seniors, and people with disabilities. Medicaid is the largest source of funding for medical and

health-related services for people with limited income.[21]

- The Family and Medical Leave Act of 1993—This is a US labor law allowing employees to take a specified amount of unpaid leave to care for a sick or aging "first-degree relative" without risk of losing their job.
- Social Security—This program encompasses several social welfare and social insurance programs funded through dedicated payroll taxes.
- Benefitscheckup.org—A Web site of the National Council on Aging that assists individuals to identify all public benefits to which they may be entitled based on specific criteria including age, location, disability, financial resources, veteran status, and other information (see http://benefits checkup.org).

Resources for the Kaufman Family

Financial Planning Resources

The discussion around financing Mrs. Kaufman's long-term care needs is one that Barbara would prefer to avoid. Mrs. Kaufman owns her own home worth $700,000, as well as having another $800,000 in savings. Her income is ample to cover her current expenses but in order to pay for additional care, Mrs. Kaufman would have to dip into her principal assets. Mrs. Kaufman has not been willing to do that, since after all, she and her husband worked very hard so that they would not have to be dependent on others. Additionally, Mrs. Kaufman wants to be able to leave a legacy to her grandchildren and make sure her son Michael will always be taken care of. Just thinking about how she will approach this topic with her mother contributes to Barbara's procrastination. Understanding this dynamic, the care manager customizes the recommendations.

Mrs. Kaufman admits she can no longer take care of her finances. Her eldest son Steve stepped in at the time of his father's death to manage her finances. With Steve's agreement, the care manager recommended a certified financial planner (CFP) who has worked with similar families to help Steve devise a plan. The goal is to ensure that additional revenue is generated to help pay for the needed care without having to touch the principal or equity in the home. The plan also included providing his mother, in the form of a loan, with a monthly stipend to ensure that she will have enough to pay for the appropriate level of care. His siblings understand that although Steve is willing to "lend" his mother a monthly stipend, once she dies, he will be repaid by her estate.

Steve and Barbara understand the expenses involved in long-term care. While it is too late for their mother to take advantage of the value of a LTC insurance product, both Barbara and Steve may benefit from learning about their options. The care manager provided them with referrals to qualified long-term care insurance agents.

Estate Planning Resources

The care manager next referred the family to an attorney with a background in estate planning and the experience working with special needs situations. The attorney can assist Mrs. Kaufman by reviewing her current estate planning documents as well as creating documents that may include a will, a living trust, a special needs trust, or advance directives.

The attorney encourages Mrs. Kaufman to discuss her estate plans with her children. This not only serves as an assurance that they will perform the roles she may request of them in her estate plans, but moreover, it can help mitigate the potential conflict that arises within many families after a parent's death.

Home Care Resources

The care manager educated Mrs. Kaufman and her family on the available in-home care options. The family all agreed that the care manager should help in the interviewing and selection process. The care manager worked with the family to ensure that they each have a role in the process. The care manager arranged to set up the caregiver interviews and offered to be involved in helping to orient the chosen caregiver and oversee and monitor the care situation. Steve agreed to handle the financial aspects of the care. Barbara volunteered to be involved in the initial interview process and remain the primary family contact. Michael wanted to be involved by helping the caregiver feel comfortable with his mother, as well as being involved in assisting with some household duties.

Home Safety Resources

It is not easy for Mrs. Kaufman to accept some of her physical limitations as well as her vulnerability to falling. Thinking about her mother on the floor was an image that created undue stress for Barbara. She wanted to learn about fall prevention resources. The care manager suggested to the family that they remove the shag carpets from the floor and several electrical wires that could cause a fall. Additionally, she recommended an occupational therapist to conduct a thorough home safety evaluation at no cost to Mrs. Kaufman, paid for by Medicare. Steve agrees to pay for an emergency response system that the care manager recommends. All three children appreciate the suggestions made.

The Three Ps

Besides knowing the appropriate resources, care managers must know how to present them. This should be done in a manner that ensures that the family caregiver will be able to take the information in and act upon the recommendations. Following the three *Ps*—*P*lanting the seed, *P*rioritizing, and *P*artnering—can help care managers ensure successful outcomes.

Planting the seed (proactive approach). Accepting resources is not always easy for family caregivers. Often, they feel that they should be able to manage the demands on their own. Care managers can introduce specific resources employing a proactive approach. "You may not need these resources right now, but I thought it may be helpful if we could just take a few minutes to review a couple of them that may be of help in the future. My goal is for you to know that specific resources exist and the value that they have provided for others who have been in similar situations." By following this process, the family caregiver can be introduced to the resources, without feeling pressure to act now. When the resource is needed, the care managers can refer back to the resource, which should sound familiar.

Prioritizing. When presenting a laundry list of resources to family caregivers, the list itself can seem overwhelming. In most hospital settings, discharge planners have preprinted lists, with multiple providers on each list for skilled nursing facilities, assisted living communities, and home care agencies. Instead of providing relief, the family often feels overwhelmed. With these extensive lists, the family caregiver can become debilitated by the choices, resulting in inaction. Care managers can help clarify the options.

Care managers must be sensitive to the pace of the family caregiver. If the care manager perceives that the caregiver is overwhelmed, discussing one or two select resources may be the best intervention. The care manager should help prioritize what the most critical issues are for that family caregiver. Knowing where to start can be the most difficult task. The care manager helps to set a course of action identifying first steps tied to the priorities.

Barbara's primary goal is to reduce the time she spends caring for her mother and at the same time ensure that her mother will be able to stay in the home she loves. The care manager recognizes that, ideally, Mrs. Kaufman would have around-the-clock care, but realizes that she would not readily accept that recommendation. Taking into account Mrs. Kaufman's needs, Barbara's time constraints, Barbara's willingness to participate in the required tasks, Steve's financial contribution, and the newly created budget, the care manager synthesizes a plan. This creates a starting point that acknowledges the priorities of all involved.

Partnering. Many family caregivers have a difficult time reaching out for assistance. This is most often due to one of five reasons: not knowing about the available assistance, not feeling comfortable asking for help, needing to be in control, feeling that they should be able to do it by themselves, and not recognizing the need.

Knowing that these obstacles exist, care managers should be sensitive to these issues when working together with family caregivers. Once a family caregiver makes contact with the care manager, there is a unique opportunity to help work through these challenges.

Taking the first steps to engage a new resource is not always easy. Having a partner, someone who can serve as an objective third party to discuss the pros and cons of initiating self-care or planning resources, can be invaluable. The care manager can work closely with family caregivers to help them take the necessary steps. Family members often describe feeling so alone in the caregiving experience. Having a professional partner can ensure successful outcomes. Like any good partnership, the roles and expectations must be well defined.

Care managers often help family caregivers stay on task, within the agreed upon time frame. Through follow-up calls and meetings, monitoring how the situation is progressing, adjusting the plan as needed, and providing support, the care manager can partner effectively to help ensure that the family caregiver will be successful.

Change did not occur overnight for Barbara. Yet, over a relatively short period of time, the professional relationship got stronger. Barbara knew early on in the relationship that the care manager was interested in not only her mother, but also in her, and how she was managing the situation. She appreciated the brief phone calls made by the care manager "just to check in" with her. The care manager was not only able to identify appropriate resources for her mother, but she also introduced Barbara to ways in which she could take better care of herself. Once her mother's condition stabilized, the care manager helped Barbara think about what she needed to do to take care of herself. Barbara was interested in attending a yoga class and going to the gym twice a week. The care manager was able to partner effectively with Barbara to identify what tasks Barbara could let go of in order to make time in the week for the gym and yoga classes. With the introduction of a paid homecare worker, and one visit per week by the care manager to monitor the situation, Barbara felt she would indeed have the time to take care of herself so that she could care better for her mother.

Once Barbara started her routine of self-care activities, the care manager then planted the seed of a monthly teleconference with her siblings. Barbara initially didn't embrace this since she had built up some negative feelings toward her brothers due to their lack of involvement and support. When the time was right, and when Barbara was feeling stronger, the care manager reintroduced the idea, offering to help facilitate the first meeting so that Barbara could feel supported while all could be updated on the mother's status and tasks and responsibilities could be discussed.

The care manager also recommended that Barbara attend a support group for adult children of Holocaust survivors. In the community where Barbara lives there are also other support groups that support family caregivers. Barbara was not used to sharing her feelings with others, but after a few sessions began to bond with several of the members. This meeting became a highlight of Barbara's week. In spite of spending more time on activities than she had prior to the change in her mother's condition, she was feeling better and stronger. Her husband and son noticed the difference too.

Expertise

Based on training, education, experience, and professional discipline, care managers afford the family a unique perspective that can help bring clarity to a complex situation. Having access to someone who has gone through many similar kinds of situations can help reduce anxiety and stress for involved family members. Having an expert available is extremely reassuring for family members who may feel less than confident as they navigate through new territory.

There are times when family caregivers understand the care managers' role solely in the context of the concrete services that are requested. It is the task of care managers to demonstrate their professional expertise in the delivery of these services. As the relationship grows, the unique expertise of care managers should become apparent.

Expertise Around Conflict and Family Dynamics

Additionally the care manager, as the expert, can assist family caregivers in resolving conflict.

Resolving conflicts is challenging work. But ignoring the difficulties in a caregiving situation can create greater challenges. Ultimately, strained family relationships can impede a family's capacity to provide quality care for a parent. Care managers can empower families by providing the following practical tips to assist them in resolving conflicts:

- Express your feelings honestly and directly. Let your siblings know their help is both wanted and needed.
- Keep family members informed regarding a parent's condition.
- Be realistic in your expectations. Allow siblings to help in ways they are able, and divide tasks according to individual abilities, current life pressures, and personal freedoms. Assistance with errands, finances, legal work, or other indirect care may be the best option for some family members.
- Express appreciation to your family for the help they are able to provide.
- Accept siblings for who they are, and expect differences of opinion.
- Try to respect others' perceptions and find opportunities to compromise.
- If communication is particularly contentious, arrange a family meeting that includes an outside facilitator, such as a care manager or other qualified professional who can ensure that everyone's voice is heard.[22]

Expertise Around Communication

Dan Sullivan, the Strategic Coach, Inc., has said:

Aging parents do not know how to discuss their economic, medical, psychological, emotional, and lifestyle requirements with their adult children, and their children are not confident about broaching any of these subjects. This is causing an expanding number of family-stressful maladies including neglect, estrangement, bankruptcy, poverty, guilt, resentment, and depression.[23]

One important area of expertise that the care manager can offer is as an expert communicator. The value to family caregivers is that the care manager can facilitate hard-to-raise issues, opening up the conversation. Family caregivers often feel compelled to take action prior to discussing the situation with the senior. The results are often disappointing. Family members may have different agendas, while moving at different paces with differing needs to maintain control. With the care manager's expertise, they can offer family caregivers insight to the differences. The care managers have the expertise in helping family members communicate in a manner that respects all parties. This process can create better understanding, enhanced empathy, and compassion between family members.

Expertise in Gerontology

Care managers have professional training that enables them to assist their senior clients and the families with whom they work. They should have the specialized experience in understanding the geriatric population as well as the medical conditions that are associated with this population. Since most family caregivers don't have the experience or training in geriatrics, they look to the care manager as a source of valued information and support. Care managers increase the family caregiver's care and healthcare literacy (discussed later in the chapter).

Barbara had little success in keeping up with the status of her mother's changing medical condition. She felt guilty that she had to work and

couldn't accompany her mother to the doctor on a regular basis. Due to her professional demands she often wasn't available when the physician took calls. She felt relief when she realized that the care manager could take her mother to the doctor and keep the family informed of her medical condition. Because of the familiarity of the care manager with Parkinson's disease from her work with other clients, the family came to understand that her mother was actually being monitored more appropriately by the care manager, due to her expertise. The care manager also spent time with the family helping them to understand the issues and conditions that faced their mother. As an added bonus, the care manager's longstanding professional relationship with the neurologist gave her access that the family didn't have. Barbara learned to appreciate the multiple areas of competency that the care manager brought to the relationship.

HELPING FAMILY MEMBERS REACH THEIR GOALS

Many family caregivers experience stress related to their role as a caregiver. The leading causes for this include:

- Feeling unsupported and unacknowledged in their efforts to provide care
- Feeling of having no control or choice
- Feeling overwhelmed with all of the responsibilities that are added to the preexisting responsibilities
- Feeling guilty that somehow "I'm not doing enough" or "I'm not doing it right"
- Feeling stuck when conflict arises within the family on how to move forward
- Feeling exhausted (emotionally and physically) from the sheer weight of the tasks

The care manager, throughout the entire care management process, can provide family caregivers with specific tools that can help address these issues and help them feel and care better. Beyond providing the concrete resources tied to the identified needs, care managers can assist family caregivers to master essential skills, tasks, or knowledge. Care managers often assume roles as coaches as they strive to empower family caregivers to achieve the desired outcomes that they deserve. Through skill training, education, and modeling the care manager can assist families with the following issues.

Communication Skills

Helping family caregivers communicate their needs and desires in an open and honest fashion is an essential task in order for the family caregiver to get his or her needs met. Asking for help is not easy. The care manager can help by doing the following:

- Coach the family caregiver in ways to reach out to other family members for financial support, telephone communications, social visits/outings, running errands, assistance with managing the logistics, and emotional support. Create opportunities for all family members to contribute in a fashion that works for them. The coaching process may include role playing to help the family caregiver expand his or her repertoire of ways to engage others.
- Facilitate family meetings (in person or via telephone) in which the care manager can model for the family caregiver how to create an environment in which everyone is heard. This can become a venue in which the primary family caregiver can articulate how he or she is feeling and then with other family members make a balanced plan that will meet his or her needs.[24]
- By modeling for family caregivers, care managers can offer alternative means to resolve conflict.

Consensus-Building Skills

Consensus is a decision-making process that equalizes power over a group of people. Instead of simply voting for an item, and having the majority of the group get their way, the group has to sit down and get a solution to a problem that *everyone* is okay with. People introduce options and await the responses of other paticpants. The solution that the group thinks is the most positive gets chosen, unless a member of the group finds the solution totally unacceptable. Consensus is based on compromise and the ability to find common ground.[25]

- Family caregivers often get stuck when there is a conflict within the family on how to best move forward. This can be a conflict between the caregiver and the senior, or it can be more complex when siblings can't agree on a plan.
- In any situation there are those who have the authority to make the decisions, those who feel the responsibility to make the decisions, and those who have power to derail the decisions.
- "Acknowledging values and preferences of all involved can assist in reaching consensus. The first step in exploring the options is to be sure to understand what is important." [25]
- The care manager can provide support to family caregivers by using or providing them with 12 basic consensus-building steps:

  1. Set a time frame for the process— "Because of the urgency of the situation, I would recommend we come to an agreement by the end of this week. Does that sound reasonable?"
  2. Review the consequences of not resolving the issue—"Without regular supervision, Mrs. Kaufman could fall

or suffer from dehydration and mal-nutrition."

3. Secure buy-in from participants to an agreement in a reasonable time frame—"The family agreed to Barbara maintaining her present schedule until paid caregivers are hired, Steve and Michael will each visit weekly."

4. Present your position as lucidly and logically as possible, but listen to other members' reactions and consider them carefully before you press your point. Avoid arguing solely for your own ideas—"The care manager worked with the entire family to help them understand each other's perspective."

5. Identify the common goals—"All agreed that Mrs. Kaufman should remain safe in her home."

6. Identify the many roads to the agreed upon common goal(s)—"The care manager explored the informal and formal support systems for acquiring caregivers, and all family was encouraged to share possible contacts."

7. Identify who holds the authority, the responsibility, and the power—"Steve has the financial authority to pay for the care. Barbara has the responsibility to ensure her mother's well-being. Mrs. Kaufman has the power to accept or reject the recommendations."

8. Provide a safe venue in which all involved can be heard—"The care manager recommended that she facilitate regularly scheduled family meetings including Mrs. Kaufman and all of her children."

9. Differences of opinion are natural and expected. Seek them out and try to involve everyone in the decision process. Disagreements can help the group's decision because with a wide range of information and opinions, there is a greater chance the group will hit on

more adequate solutions—"In spite of Barbara's aversion to confrontation, the care manager encouraged her to voice her needs. This helped her entire family look at alternative solutions."

10. Keep coming back to the common goal(s)—"Keep Mrs. Kaufman safe at home."

11. Are there ways to combine ideas?—"The care manager suggested for Steve to pay for some of the care at the present, while ensuring that he be paid back after his mother's death provides a creative strategy to address his mother's resistance to paying for care."

12. Provide positive feedback throughout the process and acknowledge all of the hard work everyone is doing—"The care manager coaches the family, along the way, letting them know the progress they are making and acknowledging their hard work."

Family Care Management Skills

Family caregivers do many similar tasks that care managers do. The critical differences are that family caregivers don't have any of the formalized training or the professional experience that the care manager does. It is additionally a challenge at best to maintain the needed level of objectivity due to the familial relationship.

As care managers partner effectively with family caregivers, there is value in sharing some of the skills and tools a care manager uses to help them manage better. These include assessment, care planning, organizational skills and tools, and technology:

• Assessment skills—The most important lesson for a family member to learn is that the best decisions are made based on facts. Family caregivers often are responding to the needs that are affected by their relationship with their parent. It is important for the family caregiver to obtain the objective data from the doctors, the attorneys, the financial planners, and from the care manager in order for the family caregiver to be able to make sense of the situation and take appropriate action. Care managers can partner with family members to create customized assessment documents specifically for them to use. This provides them with a fresh way of viewing the situation and empowers them to play a vital role in the ongoing reevaluation process.

- Care planning skills—Family caregivers are often juggling multiple responsibilities and tasks. Having a plan in hand that has identified the needs, problems, and issues with the associated goals and interventions can help the family caregiver stay on track. The care plan is a living document and can be updated as often as needed. Helping family caregivers understand its value and actually use the care plan provides them with a tool to reduce their anxiety level that somehow they are not doing enough or are doing it wrong. If the plan isn't working, it can be changed. Actively engaging family members in not only the care plan creation process, but most importantly the ongoing revision process, helps build critical thinking skills for the family caregivers. It additionally can strengthen the commitment to the care manager and family partnership.

- Organizational skills—Keeping track of all the information pertaining to caregiver responsibilities can be daunting. Care managers can work with family caregivers to help them organize the information in a manner that will be useful by creating a binder that ultimately can save family caregivers time and reduce their anxiety knowing that the information needed is accessible. Information that may be included:

- Calendars to track appointments and social engagements
- List of regular recurring appointments (hair dresser, dog groomer, hearing, vision, dental, classes, etc.)
- Phone lists including contact information of those within the senior's formal supports as well as informal supports
- Physicians
- Hospital
- Therapists
- Attorney
- Accountant
- Financial planner
- Bookkeeper
- Veterinarian
- Home health agency
- Durable medical equipment company
- Pharmacy
- Home repair (electrician, plumber, painter, handyman)
- Gardner
- Hairdresser
- Clergy
- Friends
- Family
- Emergency contacts
- Insurance information with policy numbers included
- Health history including current diagnoses, past major surgeries, allergies to medications or foods
- List of medications
- Location of important papers and legal documents
- Health exams and screenings—Keeping track of these events will allow family caregivers to stay on top of follow-up appointments with physicians and specialists.
- Burial information
- Phone trees can be helpful to family caregivers who want to communicate with others in the senior's support network, allowing them the ability to broadcast

information by assigning people on the phone tree list with the responsibility to call others.

TECHNOLOGY RESOURCES AND ADAPTIVE DEVICES

Communication Devices

There are a number of devices that have been developed to assist both family caregivers and older adults in the facilitation of better communication. These devices can be accessed through retail specialty stores or through occupational therapy evaluations.

- Phones—Telephones with large buttons, photographs, and amplification and clarity functions greatly help communication between family and older adults.
  - www.lighthouse.org—Products for those with visual impairments
  - www.deafresources.com—Products for those with hearing impairments
  - A selection of telephones that include large buttons, amplification, and clarification
- Cellular phones—www.jitterbug.com: Jitterbug cell phones are easy to use with large buttons and include access to specially trained operators who can patiently assist seniors in making calls and provide general information. These telephones are available both in dial-up or emergency one-touch models.

Other Adaptive Devices

There are a number of adaptive products that have been developed to assist families who care for elders with reduced functional abilities. Most products can be accessed from the Internet. Under certain situations these devices and products may be covered by

Medicare with physician orders with the feedback of a home health physical or occupational therapist or a care manager.

- Alzheimer's Store (www.alzstore.com) Adaptive equipment and gadgets to assist individuals with memory impairment:
  - Safety and wandering products (floor mats, bed pads, door alarms, antiscalding devices, knobs for stoves, etc.)
  - Memory stimulation
  - Activities and entertainment
  - Educational materials for caregivers
- Buck and Buck (www.buckandbuck.com)
  - Adaptive clothing
- The ElderEdge Company (www.elderedge .com) Adaptive products for seniors:
  - Magnifiers
  - Easy grip knobs
  - Reachers and grabbers
  - Nonslip mats
  - Easy grip utensils
  - Floor sentry mats
  - Pull cord alarms
  - Bath benches and seats
  - Grab bars
  - Large-print playing cards
  - High-visibility computer keyboards
  - Large display clocks

Monitoring Technology

New technology is being developed all the time to provide peace of mind for families who worry when their older relatives are unattended or need assistance in an emergency.

Personal Emergency Response Systems (PERS)

This home-installed electronic device summons helps in an emergency. A small radio transmitter in the form of a button or pendant is carried or worn by the user. It is connected to the user's telephone and an emergency response center that monitors calls. In an emergency, the PERS user presses the help button that then contacts the response center. They will notify emergency contacts or paramedics or fire or police departments. The around-the-clock availability to an emergency response team can be a great reassurance to families when face-to-face oversight is not indicated or possible.

There are many reputable companies that have provided this service for many years. For some low-income or socially isolated individuals certain senior centers with funds from the Area Agency on Aging will provide these units. (See www.benefitscheckup.org.)

Private companies include Response Link (www.responselink.com, [866] 809-4057) and Lifeline (www.lifelinesys.com, [866] 714-5297).

Motion Detectors

Providing another level of monitoring, some systems provide sensors that are placed throughout the home. Each sensor transmits information about an individual's activities of daily living and potential emergencies to a central operator. This information is updated around the clock. Family caregivers are notified of any concerns. The value of this system can vary. It can provide reassurance to family caregivers of an older adult's ability to remain safe unattended in the home. It can also provide notification in an emergency and supply objective information on when an older adult needs additional support or assistance. Providers include Quiet Care (http://quietcare.com, [877] 822-2468) and Healthsense, a comprehensive system that can monitor sleep patterns; note opening of the medicine cabinet, refrigerator, and front door; and send out emergency alarms if anything is out of the ordinary (www.healthsense.com, [800] 576-1779).

Nanny Cams—Hidden Security Cameras

Nanny cams are another option for caregivers who are concerned about their parent's well-being. These small, virtually hidden cameras are integrated into everyday objects for discretion and allow caregivers to remotely monitor their parents to provide the peace of mind of knowing that an elderly relative is living safely or being provided with appropriate care from a home care provider.

- www.nannycameras.com—Provides a large variety of monitoring cameras, recording telephone devices, voice monitor devices, and other security products.
- AT&T Remote Monitor—Webcams will monitor living areas, plus a system of sensors track movement (www.att.com/remote monitor).
- GrandCare—Sensor system tracks movement, plus a dedicated TV channel that is hooked up to the Internet (www.grancam .com).

Smart Products

In addition to motion detectors there are a growing number of high-tech devices that can help family caregivers oversee the care of older relatives. There are innovations that monitor medications, keep tabs on medical conditions, as well as provide a running grocery list by inventorying the refrigerator. Every day new devices are on the market to assist families in making sure that older adults are safe and well cared for. Of course, they never replace the human connection and must be evaluated based on the many variables involved in caring for aging family members.

- E Neighborhood: A device, soon to be on the market, takes home monitoring to the next level. Wireless sensors are programmed to detect unusual activity in a senior's house or apartment. This could include a shower running or refrigerator door that has not been opened for a significant amount of time. Operators from a call center will call, and if there is no response, an e-mail will be sent to the identified emergency contact.

- TeleMedicine monitoring devices: In development are in-home devices that monitor the weight, blood pressure, and other vital signs for seniors with chronic diseases and report to doctors or family members. One such device is the Hero Network's Health Buddy that is currently available to specific health providers.

- A smart bed (NAPS) will soon be on the market that can monitor medical information when a person lies on it. There is the need for a caregiver to be able to read and understand data.

- E Health Key by Medic Alert (www.medic alert.org, [888] 253-7890). Computer-generated flash key that enables families to keep pertinent medical information updated and easily accessible for routine and emergency medical needs. Features include records of medical and family history, medication tracking, emergency wallet care, and graphs of lab reports. This service also lets the family obtain automatic reminders of pertinent medical follow-ups and stores medical images.

- Automated telecheck: New programs being developed that automatically call seniors daily, some of which can even deliver customized messages prerecorded by family caregivers. If a senior doesn't answer the phone, the "emergency contact" is notified.

- Medication monitors: Automated pill dispensers can organize, monitor, and remind individuals to take medications. They can also alert caregivers if the medications are not being taken or they are running low.

Three suppliers are MD.2 (877) 563-2632, www.1md2.com, and E Pill at www.epill .com.

Other technical devices to prevent wandering or lost seniors include several different door alarms and tracking devices. An extensive list and comparative ratings can be found on the Technology for Long-Term Care Web site at www.techforltc.org.

Intel's Health Research and Innovation Group is creating gadgets that provide or will provide a safety net for seniors in their homes. One of the products under development is a presence lamp that can be installed in the home of a person in the early stages of Alzheimer's disease as well as in the home of his family caregiver. When the senior is home, the light goes on in the home of the family caregiver and vice versa. Intel is testing a device that provides memory prompts to people with dementia. It connects to the phone and contains information about key people in the elderly person's social network. When someone calls, his or her name appears on the screen, along with their photo and a description of who they are.

The increased use of technology in the home will create a number of questions. Who will pay? Can we demonstrate outcomes that will convince the government to reimburse for charges in order to keep people safe in their own homes? Will home health companies create a fee-for-service division that will "case manage" the information that telehealth systems will provide? Will care managers position themselves as the coordinator of services, information, and follow-through for the senior, family, and professionals? Will families opt-in to care management and caregiving services later in the continuum and choose to use technology instead?

Internet

The Internet is a wonderful tool that enables family caregivers to access information at specific Web sites. By typing in the word or phrase, a family caregiver can obtain specific information on issues of interest or concern through specific search engines such as Google. They can easily retrieve a nearly endless list of resources for specific conditions, medications, professionals, services, resources, products, and support. Although the amount of information available is quite impressive, there is no uniform means for family caregivers to know the validity of the sources. The care manager can be instrumental in helping family members sort through the information and understand which sources may be more trustworthy.

Personal Digital Assistant (PDA)

Treo, Blackberry, and iPhone are just three of the interactive devices that enhance communications between family members. These devices can provide wireless telephones, Internet access in real time, and access to all contact information and personal calendars. Information can be linked from desktop computer programs such as Outlook. These devices are effective tools, particularly for long-distance caregivers who want to stay in the loop regarding communication with other family members and professionals. In addition to the charge for the product there are monthly fees for Internet use. Visit www.pdablast.com for information about PDAs.

FORGIVENESS AND SKILLS FOR LETTING GO

The caregiving experience can bring out the best and the worst in families. When a family member feels stressed by the caregiving experience, many uncomfortable feelings can be triggered including anger, frustration, resentment, depression, anxiety, and rage. There are times that old hurts are relived that pertain to past family conflicts. Without a means of letting go of some of the past traumas, a family member can get stuck in the same cycle of behavior that often gets reinforced by other family members—causing the cycle to continue. To move forward, the care manager can be helpful to family caregivers, reflecting back the value of forgiveness and letting go of the pain. The care manager may recommend readings on the subject, use other client examples, or perhaps refer to a therapist that specializes in this area (see Chapter 12, "Forgiveness and the Aging Family").

CAREGIVING SKILLS

There are times when a family caregiver needs to learn new skills to care for the senior relative. Training on how to give injections or bandaging, learning how to operate new medical equipment, or assisting with baths in a safe manner may not only enhance the competency level of the family caregiver, but also ensure safety for all involved. The care manager can help the family caregiver identify the best source of training for the tasks at hand, while at the same time providing emotional support to address the natural increased stress that accompanies learning a new skill. An important task is to assess not only skill levels but willingness to do the tasks. If it is not the right match, identifying other options is essential.

SELF-CARE SKILLS

There are times when family caregivers feel exhausted, deprived of sleep, malnourished, and they know they are not attending to their own needs. There are a number of things care managers can do:

- Reframe questions—What is important to you? You take care of others; why not yourself? If something happened to you, what would happen to your parent, family, and partners?
- Provide specific suggestions for stress management, time management, and recommendations for self-care resources.
- Partner with family to set goals, plans, and outcomes.
- Explore obstacles and brainstorm to create solutions.
- Help initiate services.

HEALTH AND GENERAL CARE LITERACY SKILLS

One important role the care manager can assume is educator, to enhance the family caregivers' understanding and literacy of the healthcare and general care systems. Greater literacy can occur by suggesting Web sites, books, videos, DVDs, as well as formal and informal training and discussions on the following topics:

- Language and jargon—Use of medical dictionaries, customized lists of abbreviations in elder care, and glossaries can be helpful in coaching family caregivers.
- Basic Aging 101 (topics could include)—Talk to family caregivers about normal aging versus common myths, common medical conditions, common mental health conditions, common issues facing older adults, and the role of finding meaning for older adults.
- Systems—Services for caring for an older adult are often fragmented. Help family caregivers understand the context of how

different senior services delivery systems fit together and how they are funded.
- Roles—Defining and redefining roles of both formal and informal supports helps clarify expectations.
- Conditions—Clear, easy-to-understand material on specific medical conditions can assist families in being educated consumers.
- Treatment options—Care managers can assist families in learning about alternative treatments. With the knowledge, families can make more informed decisions. The care managers can help educate family caregivers on identifying options, where to access care, availability of treatment, where and when to get second opinions, and understanding the risks involved.
- Rights and responsibilities—The care manager can help clarify what family caregivers can expect from other professionals.
- With greater understanding, family caregivers are afforded the knowledge to make more informed decisions. Additionally, it helps the family formulate questions and better understand the responses.
- Suggest disease- or condition-specific materials available online, in libraries, training videos/DVDs, specialty associations, brochures, and pamphlets.

ADVOCACY SKILLS

Family caregivers can gain value from the care manager's involvement to help them get what they are entitled to and what they need:

- Care managers provide family caregivers with information that enables the family to understand their legal rights concerning health care and other systems.
- Care managers provide family caregivers with assertion skills to help empower them.
- Care managers can help family caregivers develop a means of tracking information

in a caregiver notebook or journal; that way information is not lost and is accessible when needed.

CONCLUSION

Senior issues affect the entire family. To respond effectively and create a plan that is sustainable, care managers strive to understand the perspective of the entire client system. The assessment conducted must include not only the needs, but the values, preferences, expectations, abilities, and willingness of those involved as well.

Care managers assist family caregivers by helping them to contain the wide range of feelings that surround the caregiving experience while using their professional objective expertise to identify resources for both the senior and involved family caregivers.

Care managers are most successful when they are *proactive* (planting the seed); able to help with *prioritization*; and when they can successfully *partner* with the family caregiver to provide support, resources, and guidance.

Above and beyond the specific resources to which care managers have access they can help family caregivers develop and master the following:

* Communication skills
* Consensus-building skills
* Family care management skills
* Forgiveness and skills for letting go
* Caregiving skills
* Self-care skills
* General care and healthcare literacy
* Advocacy skills

Providing the education and ongoing coaching in these areas, care managers help to ensure that the family caregiver experience will be the most positive that it can be.

REFERENCES

1. Zukerman R. *Eldercare for Dummies*. New York, NY: Wiley; 2003:37.
2. National Caregiver Alliance, National Center on Caregiving. *Who Are the Caregivers?* San Francisco, CA: National Center on Caregiving; 2003.
3. National Association of Professional Geriatric Care Managers. What is a geriatric care manager? Available at: http://www.caremanager.org. Accessed December 20, 2007.
4. Quadagno J. *Understanding the Older Client*. 3rd ed. New York, NY: McGraw-Hill; 2005.
5. Kingsmill S, Schlesinger B. *The Family Squeeze*. Toronto, ON: University of Toronto Press; 1998.
6. Rein M, Salzman H. *Older and Active*. New Haven, CT: Yale University Press; 1995:238–263.
7. Quadagno J. *Understanding the Older Client*. 3rd ed. New York, NY: McGraw-Hill; 2005:234–235.
8. Bergston V, Parrot T, Burgess E. Progress and pitfalls in gerontological theorizing. *Gerontologist*. 1996; 36(6):768–772.
9. Quadagno J. *Understanding the Older Client*. 3rd ed. New York, NY: McGraw-Hill; 2005:233.
10. Quadagno J. *Understanding the Older Client*. 3rd ed. New York, NY: McGraw-Hill; 2005:14.
11. Quadagno J. *Understanding the Older Client*. 3rd ed. New York, NY: McGraw-Hill; 2005:234.
12. Kingsmill S, Schlesinger B. *The Family Squeeze*. Toronto, ON: University of Toronto Press; 1998.
13. Raphael D, Schlesinger B. Women in the sandwich generation. *Journal of Women and Aging*. 1994;6:21–45.
14. Ilardo J. *As Parents Age: A Psychological and Practical Guide*: Publicon; 1998:211–213.
15. American Institute of Certified Public Accountants. *360 Degrees of Financial Planning*. New York, NY: American Institute of Certified Public Accountants; 2007.
16. Semple S. Conflict in Alzheimer's caregiving families. *Gerontologist*. 1992; :648–655.
17. Hartford Modified Caregiver Strain Index www.hartfordign.org.
18. Ilardo J. *As Parents Age: A Psychological and Practical Guide*.
19. Medicare. www.medicare.gov

20. The Study for the National Alliance for Caregivers and AARP, 2004. Available at www.nami.org. Accessed July 21, 2004.
21. Medicaid. www.cms.hhs.gov
22. Family Caregiver Alliance. *Caregiver and Sibling Relations: Challenges and Opportunities.* San Francisco, CA: Family Caregiver Alliance; 2007.
23. Taylor D. *The Parent Care Conversation.* New York, NY: Penguin Books; 2006.
24. www.msu.edu/-corcona5/org/consensus.html.
25. Family Caregiver Alliance. *Making Choices About Everyday Care (for Families).* San Francisco, CA: Family Caregiver Alliance; 2007.

SUGGESTED READING

Cress C. *The Handbook of Geriatric Care Management.* Aspen; 2007.

Henry SM. *The Eldercare Handbook: Difficult Choices, Compassionate Solutions.* New York, NY: Harper Collins; 2006.

Ilardo J, Rothman C. *Are Your Parents Driving You Crazy? How to Resolve the Most Common Dilemmas with Aging Parents.* Acton, MA: VanderWyk & Burnham; 2001.

Kuba C. *Navigating the Journey of Aging Parents.* Routeledge Taylor and Francis Group; 2006.

Lebow G, Kane B. *Coping with Your Difficult Older Parent.* New York, NY: Harper Collins; 1999.

Silverstone B, Hyman HK. *You and Your Aging Parent.* 3rd ed. New York, NY: Pantheon Books; 1999.

Solie D. *How to Say It to Seniors: Closing the Communication Gap with Our Elders.* New York, NY: Prentice Hall; 2004.

CHAPTER 6

Family Meetings and the Aging Family

Rita Ghatak

INTRODUCTION

This chapter discusses the unprecedented changes confronting families as aging becomes the norm, a few key elements of situations that lead to family meetings demonstrated via case studies, and some important rules of family meetings.

Longevity

If I had known I was going to live so long, I would have taken better care of myself.

—Eubie Blake, famous jazz player, aged 102[1]

Older adults and families are often taken aback at the enormity of what longevity signifies. How many years of life? How many years of caregiving? What about health issues and the ability to live independently? What about the stresses and strains on adult children? What about older adults outliving their resources? It is hard to grasp the many consequences of longevity.

This era has witnessed a most compelling demographic shift in life expectancy. There will be many more people in the world older than 65 in 2050 than ever before—1.42 billion according to the United Nations' projections.[2] That is three and a half times as many as today and over 10 times as many as in 1950. This growth will severely test the ability of families to provide the social, med-ical, and economic infrastructure that older adults need. With declining birth rates and longer life expectancies, countries will have more older adults and fewer young.

Relationships between adult children and their parents are complex and will become increasingly so with the loss of nuclear family structures and the geographic migration caused by employment. Younger and older adults are choosing greater independence in living arrangements. A growing number of middle-aged people do not expect to live with or be supported by their children when they are older. In addition, as the baby boomers retire, the ranks of the middle-aged will also dwindle. Between 2000 and 2050 the share of America's population over the age of 65 will grow from 12% to 21%, while the share of the population aged 40–64 will fall from 33% in 2010 to 28% by 2040.[3] So where will be the reserves of adult children to take on the complexities of supporting older adults?

The *New York Times* reports that with more women entering the workforce, they now have a much longer to-do list than they once did (including helping their aging parents). They cannot possibly get it all done, and many end up feeling stressed. Women provide the majority of informal care to spouses, parents, parents-in-law, friends, and neighbors. They also play many roles while caregiving—hands-on health provider, care manager, friend, companion, surrogate decision maker, and advocate.[4] This goes to the heart of families, family meetings, and the medical and psychosocial correlates of coping with older parents.

With advances in numbers of older adults, the mixed bag of benefits spills on to family relationships. Families differ significantly in ways they cope with this demographic shift. Adult children often report having parents as a support for their growing children and acknowledge the legacy of wisdom and counsel handed to them by parent generations. The other side of the coin holds the many uncertainties and inconveniences that adult children face as they deal with the medical and emotional transitions of parents. How do families cope with the needs of younger generations and still care for their aging parents? There has been growing awareness in recent years of the importance of a family-centered model of care to fully meet the needs of older adults and their families.[5]

FAMILIES

Other things may change us, but we start and end with family.

—Anthony Brandt[1]

As an adult child the author's life was significantly affected by the advanced ages of her parents. Worry about their failing health and potential loss of independence was a constant underlying concern. This anxiety superseded concerns of her own life, and issues around her own career and family often took a backseat. Adding to these endless spirals of worry was the fact that this was a long-distance caregiving relationship, separated by continents. It took years of deliberations and urging till finally, the choices and responsibilities became much easier after the author and her siblings resolved to put aside

their differences of opinions and only focus on what was best for the aging parents.

What is best for aging parents? A simple question and yet wrought with many layers of ambiguities. Who decides what is best for them? Do the medical uncertainties precipitate matters? Do adult children always know what is best? Having witnessed this struggle among her patients and their families as well as in her own life, the author chronicled multiple situations as models for teaching principles for family meetings and caregiver support. During this span the author also realized how important care management and integrated hospital discharge planning was for older adults.

What Is Family?

A family member signifies any person related to the older adult by blood, marriage, or adoption, including but not limited to children, siblings, parents, aunts and uncles, extended family, or cousins.[5] There is also a need here to include a friend or neighbor when the traditional family is not available by circumstance or choice. The number of older adults who are alone and childless and do not have the safety net of the family is increasing. Older adults who either do not live close to an adult child or are childless may be particularly deprived in terms of support and end up relying on friends or community-based support.[6]

Families are defined by relationships, communications, and ambiguities. Being part of a family can become very complex as parents age and move from being in control to becoming dependent. When does this journey take on a new role? Is it sudden or do families see glimpses but never acknowledge the progression of changes? As adult children of the elderly grow older, their own lives take on complexities, some good and some that breed concerns, challenges, and problems. Families that seem to do the best in a crisis or in problem-solving situations are usually families who have good, healthy relationships. Most have someone in their family with whom they have a difficult (at best) relationship. When a family crisis looms, those difficult people can become impossible. The optimal solution would be for families to be in close communication and recognize the strengths and weaknesses of each other so that they are ready to deal with a crisis or new needs of the older adult.

FAMILY MEETINGS

Family meetings help plan interventions and set goals so that an older person, family members, and the multidisciplinary team are all working for the same outcomes. Family meetings are defined historically as being "designed to build and strengthen the natural support and care system for the older adult."[7] The purpose or goal of a meeting is to identify needs, create a plan, and implement that plan. Another good definition posits that the function of the family meeting is to define and establish a plan that provides for the safety, health, and psychosocial well-being of the older adult.[8]

Family meetings have been identified as powerful clinical tools for communication. A successful family meeting gives everyone a chance to talk and be heard. Different members bring different emotions and feelings to the meetings, and they need to feel safe to be able to say what they want. In an ideal world all communication would be mutually respectful and supportive. This, however, is not the norm. When family dynamics dominate the meeting milieu, important issues centric to the older adult often get bypassed. This can lead to two negative outcomes: matters between family members

can get worse, and the needs of the older adult can get neglected thereby leading to an escalation of problems. An enormous responsibility lies on the designated facilitator of family meetings as they greatly aid the process of directing the flow of such meetings and assist with good outcomes.

In a comprehensive 2004 study, three factors were reported as critical to family meetings—preparation, skills, and aftermath. *Preparation* involved preparing the client and family, obtaining consent, and ensuring the key participants were present. *Skills* focused on the ability of the facilitator to summon compliance and attendance and facilitate the meeting. *Aftermath* was listed as dealing with client and family reactions after the meeting.[9] Adherence to these basic principles can assist guiding family meetings. However, despite the importance of family meetings, there has been surprisingly little research into the process around family meetings. Treating the client in the context of their family is increasingly being recognized as vital to positive outcomes for clients, hence paving the way for better attention to the area of family meetings.[10]

What works with one family will not necessarily work well with another. Most often family meetings are initiated by a trigger in the form of subtle changes, illness, or mishap. Families vary in their response time, manner, and intensity of action.[11] Some immediately recognize that all is not well with a parent. Some recognize the frailties or concerns but find it difficult to develop a methodical plan and start using a series of maneuvers to delay action. Some understand the underlying implications of the changes but choose to deny it. Some have already made a decision to step back and passively observe the older adult parent and choose not to participate. Some families have greater emotional resources, some have more financial resources, and some are infinitely better equipped to establish new family communication patterns that will help support the older adult and increase family participation.

One of the best ways to find out more about the family response time and manner would be to start having meetings before a trigger comes into play. Primary care physicians and hospital case managers need to be encouraged to persuade older adults to discuss their health and future status with their families. A friendly meeting before a crisis sets in can be that desirable forum in which everyone gets a chance to come up with an opinion on family procedures and practices.

As per the author's experience, family meetings offer the following benefits:

- Family meetings can be advantageous to opening communication paths by inducing harmony, reduction of conflict, and encouragement to share feelings and action plans with each other.
- Family meetings help adult children and family members pool their ideas and resources toward a common goal, leading to the development of itemizing tasks and goals and developing a schedule so that family members can share tasks.
- Family meetings can become the ideal milieu for sharing the burden of caring for an ill parent by allowing for difficult decisions to be made jointly and bringing creative solutions to the issues at hand.
- Family meetings assist adult children to deal with past conflicts and forgiveness issues.

Often family meetings can be weakened by difficult relationships, emotions, and unsolved issues. Such meetings need a facilitator with the expertise and background to help communication in a professional and orderly manner. Good choices for facilita-tors are social workers from the hospital, clinic, or local agencies; private care managers; ministers; and trained psychologists. Sometimes, if the situation warrants, the physician or a friend or an adult child can take the role of the facilitator.

In conclusion, family meetings (with or without the older adult) provide an excellent time and place for identifying the client's needs, clarifying issues, gathering and sharing information, distributing tasks, proposing a care plan, and implementing it.

COMMON REASONS FOR THE FIRST MEETING

The diverse reasons for a family meeting are dispersed through the chapter as well as noted here. Any significant change in the older adult can be a trigger to call a meeting. Families need to start talking before an acute incident occurs. Done right, family meetings can be a classic picture of consensus in action. Attendance can be voluntary, but those who do not participate need to abide by whatever consensus is reached by the rest of the family. Some noteworthy events that often trigger the need for family meetings are discussed in the following sections.

Health Concerns: A Catastrophic Event or Series of Events

The closer a first meeting is to the acuteness of changes in older adults or a single precipitating factor, the more likely it will be less efficient to create an effective plan or agreement. Planning during an emergency can sometimes cause disharmony and confusion. Often the first visit to the emergency room can count as a catastrophic event and lead to that first family meeting. The following sections discuss the most common reasons for visits to the emergency room and hospital and clinic visits as per statistics being collected for a study at Stanford Hospital and Clinics, Palo Alto, California.

Delirium

Older adults often respond to drug toxicity and infections such as urinary tract infections with delirium. The symptoms of delirium are often misdiagnosed as relating to other conditions. Common symptoms include sudden reduced ability to focus, disturbed consciousness, impaired judgment, and increased or decreased motor activity.[12] Families often confuse delirium for mental illness, and hence it is important to have the older adult clinically evaluated immediately.

Falls

The number of emergency room visits by older adults from falls has increased significantly. Falls are the leading cause of injury-related death for both males and females 75 years and older.[13] The most common injury is a fracture, and this usually heralds immediate changes in the living and caregiving plans of older adults. Families are often summoned to talk together after a fall and look into home safety, adaptive equipment, and rehabilitation options. Older adults often do not return to their prior level of mobility and independence after a fall.

Illness

Diseases such as arthritis, hypertension, cardiovascular disease, sudden altered mental status, cerebrovascular disease or stroke, chronic obstructive pulmonary disease (COPD), vision loss, and urinary incontinence can trigger a need for communications within a family.

Changes in behavior, functioning, or personality due to dementia, such as aggression, combativeness, increased memory loss, language difficulties, difficulty in carrying out motor functions, getting lost, or hurting oneself can be alarming to families. It is common for the older adult to keep coming to the emergency room for these symptoms, and hence it is critical for families to take these seriously and proceed with an evaluation.

Adverse Medication Reactions

Older adults take multiple medications (known as polypharmacy). Common symptoms resulting from an adverse drug reaction include confusion, nausea, decreased balance, changes in bowel pattern, fluctuations in blood pressure, cardiac complications, or sedation. Often these generic symptoms can be mistaken for other illnesses, and occasionally other medications may even be added to treat these symptoms. It is estimated that 3–10% of all hospital admissions for elderly patients are due to adverse drug reactions and often lead to families becoming greatly concerned.[14]

Impaired Activities of Daily Living and Instrumental Activities of Daily Living

Changes in health and living situations affect one of the most important aspects of life for elderly patients—the activities of daily living (ADLs). It is mostly because of these needs that families start rushing to put services and resources in place. It is often the call "Mom cannot bathe, dress, or feed herself" that prompts shifts in living and caregiving options. The day-to-day functioning in an older parent can be affected by disease and illness and result in chronic impairment in one or more activities of daily living and instrumental activities of daily living (IADLs).

The activities of daily living include:

• Bathing
• Dressing

- Grooming
- Eating
- Transferring
- Toileting

The instrumental activities of daily living include:

- Meal preparation
- Housework
- Medication use (preparing and taking correct dose)
- Management of money (write checks, pay bills)
- Transportation

Changes in ADLs and IADLs lead to cycles of emergency room visits and feelings of helplessness in the older adult, as well as cause adult children to give up their time to tend to the older adult. These changes can also cause anxiety among families, as they may see these changes as a precursor to the parent losing independence. Families become very distressed with these changes, and this can lead to increased communications between family members for possible solutions. The author discusses the possibilities of changes in ADLs and IADLs in the older adult during hospital discharge so that families are prepared for changes in the functioning status of older adults.

Subtle Signs of the Older Adult at Risk

Often the reason for summoning a family meeting is to address the common indicators of an older adult slowly displaying signs of becoming "at risk." Adult children often miss these signs. An adult child, a neighbor, a social worker, or someone from adult protective services (the entity responsible for investigating abuse, neglect, and exploitation of adults who are elderly or have disabilities)

may recognize one of these signs and summon a meeting. Some of the signs are the following:

- Untidy appearance, poor hygiene, and body odor
- Dirty, cluttered home with neglected trash
- Depression, disorientation, confusion, and forgetfulness
- Mental illness
- Substance abuse
- Frequent falls
- Possible abuse by hired caregiver
- Financial and social problems
- Frequent visits to the emergency room
- Failing to take medication at the proper time, leading to frequent hospital admissions
- Traffic accidents
- Frequent calls to local police and sheriff for help

Caregiver Stress

Family meetings can become a necessity when the designated caregiver experiences stress, burden, or ill health. Families may sometimes rely on one designated adult child, and this may be the one that lives close by or the one that has been the favorite or the one that is not employed. The adult child experiencing the stress may send a distress call to the others and that may be the trigger of the family to recognize that immediate action needs to be taken.

Acknowledgment by an adult child or spouse that he or she is unable to shoulder the entire burden of the regular or long-distance caregiving usually precedes families getting together to meet and discuss alternate strategies. A family meeting can help analyze the situation to discuss equal responsibilities in the part of family members to prevent physical and emotional breakdown of the burdened adult child.

Finally, caregiver stress can also ensue when sibling rivalry or unresolved conflicts can take front seat and dispel efforts to assist and support the older adult.

End-of-Life Issues

Planning around end-of-life issues is often the trigger for that first meeting or a series of meetings. Families need to consider palliative or hospice care for loved ones facing a life-limiting illness or injury. Hospice and palliative care involves a team-oriented approach to expert medical care, pain management, and emotional and spiritual support customized to the person's needs and wishes. Support is extended to the family members as well. Families can also use meetings to discuss respite services and support groups while going through the end-of-life care for the older adult parents. This is a hard time for most families, and members can find solace and support in meetings.

In the author's experience, families are often unprepared for end-of-life issues, and though they realize the gravity of the parent's condition, discussions tend to be avoided till that sudden visit to a hospital intensive care unit. Families in discussion outside the ICU are common, and a significant amount of research has been done in this area. Physicians and hospital social workers often take on the role of the facilitator at this time and often guide many discussions.

Other Triggers

Other noted triggers for first-time family meetings are:

- Sudden precipitating events like a natural disaster, home emergency like a fire, or an unfit home environment
- An event like a run-in with the law and the immediate need to take away the parent's

driver's license, may be common with patients with dementia
- Request by an adult child, family member, or friend
- Request by the older adult parent or parents
- Request by the hospital, primary clinic, or care manager when they perceive the older adult to be at-risk or needing immediate attention
- Financial concerns or difficulties, involvement in a scam, or being a victim of financial abuse

The triggers listed here are factors that lead to dramatic shifts in the overall functioning of older adults. Presence of any one of the factors can cause uncertainty, cycles of medical or emergency room visits, vulnerability, and failure to follow a purposeful plan of care for the older adult, thereby making family meetings a necessity.

Case Study to Demonstrate Variables Leading to a Family Meeting

Case of Sally Moses

One of the first cases the author encountered was that of Sally Moses. The discharging hospital physician referred Sally, an existing client of the author within the Geriatric Health Services in Stanford Hospital, to a home health agency and a geriatric care manager.[15] (The concept of a Geriatric Health Services (GHS) program is new and does not have much precedence. Hospitals have geriatric departments but hardly any have geriatric health programs. The program created by the author brings to the forefront a model of geriatric perspective to patient care planning.)

The referral by the physician to the geriatric care manager was unprecedented as hospitals rarely consider home health agencies and private geriatric care managers as partners for care planning. Such a process would streamline much of the planning and provide the capability to intervene rapidly if needed. This had been made possible because Sally's family had informed the hospital that Sally was receiving services from the agency.

The case was unique as the daughter Janet was the primary advocate but was unable to participate in day-to-day care planning due to her own progressively deteriorating neurological condition. Sally lived with Janet's son and daughter-in-law, David and Silvia, and their two young children. Silvia had been caring for Sally since January 1998, when Sally experienced a brain stem stroke.

During a routine home visit after the hospital discharge, the author in her role as Director of Geriatric Health Services noticed significant decline in Sally. The care manager was also present, and the visit focused on safety and care planning issues. The care manager had discussed her goals with Janet but was unable to get the attention of David and Silvia. A few days later Janet called the care manager and said that Sally had fallen. There followed a long accounting by Janet that her daughter-in-law had reduced home care hours, the care manager was being shut out, and no one was present during Sally's toileting. In essence the care planning for Sally was not being adhered to. Janet felt bitter and frustrated about her mother not being cared for but could not confront Silvia as she (Janet) could not take on her mother's care. David, the son was ambivalent and felt Silvia was doing her best.

Although Sally was receiving much external assistance from a care management and home health agency, the care was still fragmented. The author and her hospital team felt that the family needed to meet as a group and talk about the overall situation. This was probably the first time the author felt the acute need for understanding the family dynamics and calling on everyone to come together in a meeting. Three meetings occurred in the home setting facilitated by the care manager where a careful plan was developed to utilize Janet's availability to meet the daily care needs for Sally while keeping the harmony between the three women, Sally, Janet, and Sylvia.

WHO ATTENDS THE FAMILY MEETINGS?

If the family meeting is a response to a crisis or an acute change in the client's condition, the meeting can include anyone who is available immediately, such as family, family friend, neighbor, or paid caregiver.

If the family meeting is a planned event, the meeting can be open to all who need to attend. Such meetings can be planned in advance, and members can also take the time to research areas of care planning, obtain information, and even invite experts to address certain health, housing, legal, or financial concerns.

An important and sometimes hard decision is whether or not to include the older adults who are centric to the meeting. In the author's experience this is mostly based on the family dynamics, the level of impairment, and prior stated wishes of the older adult. If the older adult has moderate to severe cognitive impairment and may misunderstand the reason for the meeting, it might be appropriate not to have him or her present. Similarly, terminally ill older adults may have the cognitive capacity to discern what is being discussed, but may be ill at ease with any discussion of severity of symptoms or impending death. A good option may be to consider holding one meeting to focus on important but hard matters, and holding a second meeting with the ill person present.

Every individual that attends a family meeting brings his or her prior perceptions and opinions on how to resolve the issues at hand. Other common influences are emotions, past relationships among family members, and economic and health concerns that may make attendance a difficulty. Once all members are gathered, the passage of the meeting can be difficult or easy based on how quickly the focal point moves from individual issues to issues related to the older adult parent.

A Mix of Diverse Family Meetings

The following are cases encountered by the author and documented to demonstrate how attendees can differ widely in family meetings. They can also give the reader a flavor of the different kinds of family meetings.

Case of Allison Adams. A family meeting was called outside a hospital unit with Nancy (the adult daughter), her spouse, and childhood friend whether or not to intubate her mother Allison, an 89-year-old woman with chronic pain and severe pulmonary complications. Nancy was an only child, and the surgeon had stated that there was a possibility that the intubation could assist with the recovery. On the other hand the primary physician felt that was not a good idea and urged Nancy to consider her mother's overall quality of life. This situation warranted a few meetings, three in total and all outside Allison's ICU unit. The last meeting included the hospital chaplain, and this case ended with the meeting deciding against intubation options for Allison.

Case of Edward Hopkins. A family meeting occurred at the home of Edward Hopkins while he was in the hospital recovering from a debilitating stroke, where John (the adult son) and his siblings gathered together to discuss how to redesign the home to meet Edward's needs. The siblings had very strong desires to keep the father at home (as they recollected "Dad always wanted to stay at home") thereby planning an extensive modification of the home environment. Unfortunately, the wife, Mrs. Hopkins, was against this plan and wanted to relocate him to assisted living. Mrs. Hopkins felt it was too stressful to manage Edward's needs along with having to supervise the home care aides for her husband. The author was asked to be a part of the family meeting, and she in turn also requested a geriatric care manager be present to guide the meeting along. Five meetings occurred, one with the author in the hospital and the remaining with the care manager at the client's home. At the end, the family balanced emotional and economic factors and decided to relocate Edward to assisted living.

Case of Mary Richards. Mary, a 78-year-old woman living alone, called the author to look into options in case she became ill or disabled. Mary also had questions about how much home care would cost. The author connected Mary to a full services agency and a geriatric care manager. The out-of-town children came to be part of two meetings to discuss resources in the area, costs of home care, home safety evaluation, and a general plan of steps to undertake if Mary became ill. The family also had an Advance Directive signed by Mary and discussed long-term care options about where to move Mary if she were unable to stay at home. The author was notified that the outcome was that Mary decided to make her son the proxy for durable power of health care and hired a local agency for a few hours of home care each week to help her with meal preparation and transportation.

The neighbor, family member, primary care physician, social worker, community chaplain, and any other advocate who witnesses any of the preceding situations needs to emphasize the need for family meetings.

Conclusion. A final review of types of family meetings progressing from urgent to nonurgent is outlined here:

- A meeting of family members to discuss current life issues, relationships, past conflicts, or just to see where individuals stand. Such a meeting can happen during holidays when families get together and someone experiences the need to talk. Such meetings can also be triggered if a family member has experienced significant changes in their lives, such as illness, divorce, or loss of a job.
- A meeting to talk to older parents and other family members when health and living conditions are optimal. These meetings can be easy as no crisis looms, and parents feel they are not challenged and forced to engage in immediate action. The problem associated with this kind of meeting is that often the lack of urgency can lead to inaction.
- A meeting when health and living concerns start appearing and families need to come together to discuss minor interventions such as additional help around the home, and planning future legal and financial processes. Again the reasons are nonurgent and may often involve the presence of an external professional such as agency personnel, a friend, a geriatric care manager, or someone called in for specific expertise. Often the meeting is a referral from the physician, a health team member, or an observer of decline in the older adult.
- A meeting that is long distance in nature and convened via telephone or video conferencing. These do have positive results but cannot replace the face-to-face meetings.
- A meeting following an emergency room visit or an acute health crisis, where concerned individuals realize that something needs to be done and usually the hospital team assists in decision making.

- A meeting outside the ICU where possible palliative care, hospice care, or end-of-life issues are discussed. Families usually let the medical personnel take over the initial part of such meetings in the hospital setting. It is then left for the family to meet, talk, and pursue a plan that best fits all present. Here the health team can assist families to call upon a hospital case worker or an external care manager.

The venue for family meetings can range widely and may be selected by the family, hospital staff, or care manager. Common noted venues include the following:

- The family home
- The home of any family member
- The office of the geriatric care manager
- The health clinic
- The hospital
- The local restaurant or cafe

COMMON DISCUSSION THEMES AT FAMILY MEETINGS

Some of the different topics to be covered during a family meeting are spread throughout the chapter but for purposes of clarity are revisited here. Family meetings emerge as a persuasive solution for families facing a crisis with older adults. Several pertinent themes addressing diverse discussion areas are discussed next.

Family Meeting to Discuss and Understand the Older Adult's Health and Its Implications

Families can discuss ways of understanding the parent's health and make sure that one or a few family members accompany the parent for an appointment. The author's program has a specific team that assists families to explore options of accompanying the older parent to an appointment. These are of immense value as they allow the family to understand the progression or limitations of the health condition and help the family work closely with the medical team. Family members are instructed to write down questions so that they don't forget about what they want to say to the doctor. Discussion of physical and cognitive status preferably with the medical team is advisable before a crisis emerges or before the parent enters the cycle of emergency room visits. Families can assist with the following:

• Getting the right diagnosis and understanding the disease or condition
• Getting specialty opinions
• Managing medications and understanding their intentional action and side effects
• Keeping an eye on immunizations, operations, injuries, and hospitalizations
• Helping with transportation to appointments
• Preventing cycling through the emergency room

Family Meeting to Discuss Caregiver Burden and Stress

Caregivers are almost always at increased risk of symptoms of distress: feeling guilty if they think they are not doing enough, frustrated if they feel their individual efforts are failing or being blocked by other family members.

Following are some commonly reported signs of stress that might be discussed in a family meeting:

• Persistent symptoms of depression
• Constant anxiety, irritability, or anger
• Feelings of detachment, exhaustion, self-criticism
• Withdrawal from usual activities
• Negligence or hatred of caregiving responsibilities

• Trouble at work or in relationships
• Substance abuse

Following are some commonly reported activities that can cause caregivers to neglect themselves, their families, and work. These activities can be a source of acute stress that might be discussed in a family meeting:

• Managing medical appointments and medications and supervising caregivers and other home care needs for the older adult
• Being the liaison for the care manager or therapist
• Assistance with remodeling for safety
• Assistance with household chores, such as cleaning, grocery shopping, meal preparation, transportation to appointments or shopping, and house or yard maintenance
• Assistance with all activities of daily living such as eating, bathing, dressing, assistance with coping with losses of vision, hearing, ambulation; more assistance as disease progresses, monitoring ability to drive or live alone

It is important to note that psychotherapists in private practice are trained in family counseling, which may be helpful for caregivers who may be stressed or face issues that emerge during a meeting. Sometimes caregivers participate in support groups to share experiences with other caregivers and these can help ease the feelings and frustrations often involved in being a caregiver.

Family Meetings to Discuss Options When It Becomes Hard for Older Adult Parents to Continue to Live at Home

When parents find it hard to live at home or the home is unsafe, it is important to consider the following topics.

Family Meeting to Discuss Different Options for Safer Housing

- Independent living—For older adults who are self-sufficient and want the freedom and privacy of their own separate, easy-to-maintain apartment or house, along with the security, comfort, and social activities of a senior community
- Assisted living—Numerous kinds of housing-with-services for people who do not have severe medical problems but who need help with personal care such as bathing, dressing, grooming, or meal preparation
- Board and care—State-licensed assisted living for people who need minimal assistance with personal care such as bathing, dressing, grooming, or toileting, but who need or want communal meals and easy access to social contact with peers
- Nursing homes or skilled nursing facilities—Facilities with 24-hour medical care available, including short-term rehabilitation (physical therapy) as well as long-term care for people with chronic ailments or disabilities that require daily attention of RNs in addition to help with personal care such as bathing, dressing, or getting around
- Continuing-care retirement communities (CCRCs)—A complex of residences that include independent living, assisted living, and nursing home care

Family Meeting to Discuss Remodeling as an Option

Meetings can be a forum to discuss products and options that will allow the parent to live safely at home. Common discussion topics include feasibility and affordability of installing durable medical equipment (DME), remodeling of the home, or adding products that can ensure the parents live independently and safely. Families can discuss financial assistance options for the remodeling, as well as investigate if the older adult is eligible for reverse mortgage, insurance benefits, financial aid, subsidized services, or bank loans.

The following are some options to be considered while remodeling:

- Special easy-to-answer telephones
- Ambulatory aids (e.g., walkers, canes, manual wheelchairs, powered wheelchairs, and scooters)
- Remodeling the bathroom for safety to avoid difficulty getting in and out of the shower, slipping in the tub or shower, difficulty turning faucet handles or doorknobs
- Making sure the access to the home is safe and the inside is clutter free with safe walking pathways
- Inadequate heating or ventilation
- Patient lifts
- Hearing and visual aids are in proper place
- Medical alarms, personal help buttons, emergency response system
- Seeking a system that will ensure that all supplies, such as diabetic supplies, nutrition supplies, oxygen, and nebulizer, are readily available

Family Meeting to Discuss Possible Services at Home

Following are various options and services that need to be explored for older adults and can be discussed during family meetings (see www.agenet.com for more information):

- Homemaker services—Can include help with cooking, light cleaning, laundry, grocery shopping, and other household chores
- Personal care—Assistance with a variety of daily living activities such as bathing, dressing, toilet use, grooming, and eating
- Companionship—From daily telephone calls from a "buddy," to a daily

"friendly" visitor, to round-the-clock paid companions

- Home health care—Skilled care that can include nursing; speech, occupational, physical, or respiratory therapy; home health aides; and social work or psychiatric care
- Adult day care—Daily, facility-based programs in a community center setting for seniors who need monitoring or companionship during the day
- Activity groups—Shopping, outings, and other stimulating group activities
- Respite care—A trained volunteer or paraprofessional that stays with the older adult providing brief reprieves for caregivers.
- Live-in help—Home care for older adults who need round-the-clock support. Room, board, and salary is provided in exchange for meal preparation, light housekeeping, and other nonmedical services.
- Hospice care—Medical, social, and emotional services for the terminally ill and their families
- Caregiver support groups—Support for issues about aging, illness-based support, groups for caregivers, grief support, and many others to help people experiencing life challenges with older adult family member

Family Meetings to Discuss Financial and Insurance Options for the Older Adult

Following are varied options, personnel, and resources that need to be explored for older adults and that can be discussed during family meetings (see www.agenet.com for more information):

- Advance Directives—A variety of documents that express healthcare wishes, including a living will, healthcare power of attorney or proxy, durable power of attorney for healthcare decisions, medical directive, or other similarly named documents

- Durable power of attorney for finances (DPA for finances)—A document in which the older adult appoints someone to make financial decisions on his or her behalf
- Elder law attorney—An attorney who specializes in the laws pertaining to the rights and issues of older adults, such as estate planning, wills, healthcare decision making, and financial issues
- Healthcare power of attorney (healthcare proxy)—A special kind of durable power of attorney called a healthcare power of attorney (HCPA) in which the older adult appoints someone to make healthcare decisions should they become unable to do so
- Living will (health care directive)—A legal document that communicates a person's wishes about lifesaving medical treatments should the older adult be in a terminal condition and not able to communicate healthcare wishes
- Bill paying, financial counseling, and insurance:
  - Will and living trust
  - Consumer credit counseling
  - HICAP/insurance form preparation
  - Tax preparation
  - Mortgage loan counseling
  - Balancing checkbooks, organizing tax information
  - Money management
  - Long-term care insurance
  - Medicare, Medicaid, MediCal—applications and benefits
  - Prescription drugs
  - Hiring home care, care management, and therapy personnel

Family Meetings to Discuss End-of-Life Issues

Following are end-of-life issues that need to be explored for older adults and can be discussed during family meetings.[16]

- Palliative care
- Hospice
- Care and equipment (hospital bed, pressure mattresses, etc.) to manage end of life
- Working together to give needed care to older person
- Managing the care of the dying parent and designating who will be the point person for the hospice or palliative care team
- Helping with spiritual support
- Planning the packing, distributing, and clearing of home after the parent's death

WHO DIRECTS THE MEETING—
THE ROLE OF THE FACILITATOR

Although family meetings can be powerful and effective ways to connect with family members, they cannot magically solve all the problems of caring for an ill family member. When families have trouble working together or coming to an agreement or when the family is divided on critical issues, it often helps to invite a neutral outside facilitator to attend. The facilitator is the person in charge of the meeting, someone who moves the meeting along with the obvious consent of the group. Often the facilitator is determined by the one who is immediately available and with the expert knowledge to influence a decision. The person who facilitates should have mediation skills as family issues can be very disruptive, bringing up old issues that keep the meeting rooted in the past rather than allowing for progress on present issues.

Planned meetings often use a social worker in the community or hospital, a private professional geriatric care manager, a clergyperson, or a community advocate. In a clinical setting when matters can escalate and decision making is amidst an urgent situation, the physician, case manager, nurse, or chaplain, or even a family member, friend,

or any person deemed objective by the family can become the facilitator.

Without the facilitator serving in the best interests of the older adult, a meeting may focus on unresolved family dynamics or sibling issues. This can create disharmony and frustration and be a difficult process. An external professional may be an ideal choice, but failing that avenue, the family will need to elect someone as the one who takes charge. It may be the sibling that lives locally, the sibling that has shouldered all responsibility of the parents' care (if it is not about that person being overburdened by care), or the sibling with the strongest personality. Healthcare professionals need to be trained to guide families toward the best choice of a point person or facilitator.

The role and the presence of a facilitator is a critical part of all family meetings. The facilitator can assist with clearing the path to effective planning and help families resolve issues that impede a good plan. The facilitator can also help the family communicate about difficult subjects during the meeting and after the meeting. The author has been part of many impromptu meetings that have been set up within the hour in the hospital and with hospital case managers, physicians, and geriatric care managers.

Functions of the Facilitator at the Family Meeting

A facilitator is someone who accepts the responsibility to assist a family address concerns and issues, develops an agenda, and helps the members discuss options and strategies in the time available to make decisions and plans for their implementation. The facilitator is not the one that actually makes the decisions but helps the group move forward so that all the family members present recognize that they are the ones making the decisions for the parent and it is their task to see that efforts are focused on the parent and not themselves.

Individual agendas and emotions are not the center here, and both facilitators and the family members need to be aware of these at all times.

Following are some key topics to note while facilitating a meeting.

Setting the Agenda and Goals of the Meeting—Defining the Issues and Problems at Hand

This is a complex part of the family meeting process because defining the issues at hand can be a challenge. Common questions raised are: Is it the health of the adult that is the crux? Is it the living situation? Is there financial ability to make needed changes? Are the children on the same page to recognize the primary issues?

The facilitator needs to realize that the identification of the problem and setting of the agenda may take time and expertise.

Case Study in Which the Physician Acts as a Facilitator

Case of Paul Roddick

The author was summoned by a family facing discharge to home with no care services in place. Mr. Roddick lived alone after his wife passed 2 years ago. He was experiencing medical problems, but with no adult child close by, matters slowly escalated. His existing diagnosis was advanced Parkinson's and he had fallen and come to the hospital. The medical team also suspected cardiac issues.

Mr. Roddick was not a good candidate for rehabilitation and could only go home with home care or go to a long-term nursing situation. The family—two sons, Alex and Paul Jr., and a daughter, Becca, flew in, and each had a different opinion about their father's condition and what should have been done in the past. Matters got a bit out of control, and the social worker helping the family finally summoned the attending physician. He came and listened to the diverse opinions. He immediately took control as the facilitator and stated that this was not the time to discuss what measures could have been undertaken in the past, what mattered now was that Mr. Roddick's condition had deteriorated significantly, and he needed supervised 24/7 care that could either be provided at his home or in a facility. If the home option was preferred, someone would need to be designated as the point person for managing the home, the home care team, the multiple medical needs of the father, and so on.

This narrowing of the agenda brought the family to start focusing on matters at hand and seek possible solutions. The family met a few more times with the social worker present and decided to relocate the father to a nursing facility out of state, close to the daughter.

Therefore, the setting of the agenda may involve the following processes:

- Review the current situation.
- Identify the issues at hand clearly—typical examples are "We need to discuss Mom's living situation and its implications," or "How do we all deal with Dad's new dementia diagnosis?" or "X cannot handle Dad and Mom by herself—since we live in different states, how can we all pitch in to help? What areas need assistance and can be distributed?"
- Look at all the immediate needs related to the current situation.

Establishing Procedures During the Meeting—Encouraging and Balancing Participation

The family meeting should be held in an environment that fosters balanced participation. Some key rules that need to be acknowledged before the start of the meeting include the following:

- Everyone listens respectfully to the person that is speaking.
- Everyone understands that good communication skills are imperative if the meeting is to have a good outcome.
- Everyone should feel they can trust each other.
- Criticism, blaming each other, recounting past matters, and sarcasm do not have a place in family meetings.
- Everyone works through the processes of resistance, denial, and hidden agendas and issues.

The facilitator needs to make sure the following rules are upheld during the meeting:

- Everyone is heard.
- Everyone listens attentively and encourages this in others.
- Everyone is honest.
- Everyone speaks to only issues at hand.
- Concerns or topics are not repeated.
- No one overreacts or responds too quickly to what is being said.
- The meeting moves along.

The Case of Mr. Roddick, continued

Using the case of Mr. Roddick—a few statements reflecting key factors of successful facilitating, made by the physician are reported here:

- Being heard—"Alex and Becca have spoken on this issue; however, I have not heard anything from Paul Jr. Is there something you wish to add?"

- Honesty—"Becca, I sense that you are not being very open about the home management issue. Are you sure you are being very honest?"
- Focusing on topic at hand—"Paul, you raise an important issue, but that has to do with situations when your mother was alive. Let's talk about how to deal with the matter now."
- Repetitions—"Becca, we have already talked about the last time you tried to place home care aides in the home for your father. Shall we move to what we can do now?"
- Moving along—"Since we have a time constraint and decisions need to be made, can we move along and go to the next item in the agenda?"
- Taking breaks—"Why don't we take a break and meet after we have had time to think about all this?"

It is important for the facilitator to help family members realize that the need to trust and share is critical during the process of searching for resolutions related to the older adult. To manage the meeting with tact, patience, and fairness and to make sure every voice is heard can be a great challenge, especially when sensitive topics lead to anxiety, sadness, anger, or blame. The goal is to try to get everyone pointed in the same direction and bring people's strengths together to care for the person who is ill or in need of assistance. It is critical to reiterate that goal at the beginning of every meeting.

Identifying Alternatives During the Family Meeting

This part of the family meeting involves looking at multiple options and identifying ways of coping with the issues a hand. Experts may be called in at this time to give information on varied areas under discussion. This may offer different perspectives and solutions to the members. A geriatric care manager or social worker would be well equipped to know diverse creative options and may be a good choice for families faced with this task.

Checking for Consensus, Reconciling Disagreements, and Resolving Conflicts During the Family Meeting

Conflict or disagreements are common in most families. Disputes between members of families can tax the decision-making process and may sometimes involve legal and mediation expertise. Because of the difficult nature of conflict, families trying to rush to a decision may find themselves locked in disagreements about matters not connected to the older adult parent and issues at hand.

Conflict can bring emotions such as anger, frustration, fear, mistrust, hostility, and disruptiveness to the family meeting. Facilitators may try to peacefully resolve the conflict by doing any of the following:

- Persuade members to look at the issues at hand.
- Assist members to look at the processes of collaboration, accommodation, and compromise.
- Move matters toward the common goal of resolving the issues that prompted the meeting.
- Force the members to stay focused on the current issues.
- Move the spotlight to the older adult.
- Encourage the members to seek counseling for the difficult emotions raised during the meeting.

The author has been part of several meetings where emotions have run very high and families have found themselves deadlocked about long and deep-seated conflicts. Such meetings can be difficult and somewhat nonproductive.

Facing challenges of aging can be difficult for both older adults and their caregivers. Problems such as chronic illness, caregiver burden, property despot, residential changes, disagreements among siblings about levels of care for older parents and associated costs, differences of opinion over end-of-life decisions, and management of dementia symptoms of the older adult parent may overwhelm both older adults and their families and cause serious conflicts. It is best to impress on the members that pursuing the conflict will lead to negative outcomes for the older adult and to look for expert counseling and mediation services outside the family meeting.

Facilitators such as physicians, family members, and social workers may need to bring in experts in mediation when the conflicts raised are significant because they can be hugely detrimental to coping with the crisis at hand. Mediation is described as a process in which a neutral third party (the mediator) facilitates the resolution of conflict involving two parties.

Other critical issues that can lead to the need for mediation are conflicts between seniors and their familial and/or professional caregivers, the older adult driving, challenging the living will, estate matters, guardianship, conservatorships, elder abuse, scam, and neglect.

Some useful sites to find mediators are www.ncsmediation.com/adults.html and www.acrnet.org.

A few important steps in mediation as reported by these sites include the following:

1. Introductions and ground rules.
2. Both parties involved present their side of the story.
3. Issues are clarified, summarized, and prioritized. Both parties need to understand each other's needs.

4. Creative brainstorming of possible solutions.
5. Narrow the range of options to the best and most workable solution(s).
6. Document agreement and sign agreement by both parties.

Synthesizing Ideas and Summarizing a Plan of Care During a Family Meeting

After a detailed clarification of ideas and repetition of a formulated plan, it is necessary to start documenting the ideas expressed. Written points are often better adhered to. Many members may notice the similarities of some steps outlined; such similarities can lead to better efficiencies in the planning. Meetings where the plan is documented along with the various responsibilities and timelines have a better chance of success.

The facilitator has the responsibility to make sure the plan for the older adult is cohesive, practical, and safe. This will involve reiterating all steps outlined and summarizing all steps discussed.

IMPLEMENTING THE PLAN DESIGNED DURING THE FAMILY MEETING

Following the family meeting, the facilitator or designated member should provide every member with a brief document including the names of participants, a summary of the significant conversations or issues raised, decisions made, the plan that has been formulated, and who is responsible for each specific action. A written list will lead to focused efforts and stop members from spending valuable time duplicating the gathering of resources or information. Once a plan is in place, members can meet in groups or subgroups to implement various aspects of the plan.

A plan that was developed in one of the author's cases is attached here.

Case Study Demonstrating Best Way to Plan Meetings

Case of Rodney Berg

The family—Mrs. Berg, son Kirk, and daughter Robin—met a few times with a private geriatric care manager to discuss seeking specialty referrals for Mr. Berg for his nonspecific pain, fatigue, and acute scoliosis. Mr. Berg had great difficulty walking and needed a sizable amount of adjustments to be made to his bedroom and bathroom.

The document, handwritten, at the end of the meeting, was handed to all present and looked like the following note. (Sometimes, the facilitator may request all parties to sign similar documents, thereby ensuring responsibility and action.)

Current Problems

- Dad needs a consultation at the pain clinic, possible surgery?
- Mom needs help at home
- They do not have an Advance Directive—who will be the DPOA for health (durable power of attorney)?
- Who takes on what?

Actions to Take

- Kirk will set the appointments for the spinal specialist to consider surgery.
- Robin will talk to the DME consultant for adaptive equipment for ideas for creating a better and safer bath place; the DME consultant would also help Robin with finding a senior remodeling contractor.
- Kirk will discuss home care options with mom and dad for assistance with activities of daily living such as dressing, bathing, meal preparation, medication management, and so on for dad.
- Kirk will help with the ongoing monitoring of the home care aides and pay them

through dad's trust fund, while investigating if insurance will cover any of these costs.
- Mom will meet patient a representative from the hospital to get an advance directive in place.

Case Study Demonstrating the Implementation of a Plan Developed During a Family Meeting

Case of Mary Avery

Mary lived alone and was admitted through the emergency room for a fall. The author made a home visit to evaluate home safety and provided extensive recommendations. Mary continued driving after the fall and was involved in a couple of accidents. The daughter and son called the author for advice, specifying that they were feeling very diffident to approach Mary with this concern. The author recommended a family meeting with a facilitator and gave some names to the family. After some resistance Mary agreed to have a meeting. The family selected a care manager, who spent some time collecting information about Mary's health history, the fall, the accidents, and facilitated the meeting in a nonthreatening manner focusing only on Mary's safety.

At the end of three meetings, the care manager provided the family with a list of actions that had been discussed during the meetings. These included hiring an aide for driving, making the home safe, having routine communications between Mary and the children, and signing up for two local programs (that had been suggested by the author): Lifeline—an in-home emergency response system—and Checking In—a local program that calls daily and checks in with older adults that live alone.

LOOKING AT THE NEW MILIEU OF FAMILY MEETINGS

Family meeting are progressing from the traditional preestablished, structured meetings to the unplanned, impromptu, spontaneous ones. This is often characteristic of the crisis that accompanies situations outside ICUs, emergency rooms, hospital units, and hospital discharge. It is often harder to arrive at a consensus when things are already complicated and getting out of hand.

Case Study to Display the Impromptu Family Meeting in a Hospital Conference Room with a Friend and Adult Children

Case of Jane Shecht

The first time the author got involved in an impromptu meeting was with Jane who lived alone and came into the hospital ER after a fall and altered mental functioning. The ER staff relied on her accompanying friend for Jane's symptoms and chronology of events. According to the friend, Jane had been dealing with her diabetes, kidney problems, and high blood pressure. After a 7-hour wait in the ER, Jane needed to go in for surgery. At that time the friend asked to speak with the physician who informed her that he could only talk to the "family." The friend was irate and reminded everyone with increasing indignation that the children were "never there," and it was she who assisted with the day-to-day activities and was an observer of physical and cognitive decline. The physician also noted that there was no Advance Directive on file for Jane. At this point Jane's children arrived from nearby cities.

The physician met the adult children and friend and raised the issue that Jane was clearly at risk in her present living situation and would need further assistance after her surgery. The author contacted a geriatric care manager at the friend's request and a family meeting occurred in a room next to the ER, with the adult children, friend, hospital social worker, physician, and the author. The physician left after 20 minutes, and the meeting lasted 2 and a half hours with the geriatric care manager facilitating, noting the evolution of the problem, lack of participation from the adult children, the general level of hostility between the adult children and the friend, and the obstacles to a good care plan to support Jane. The care manager acknowledged challenges, managed the rules of a family meeting, and tried to promote consensus and compromise. The final goal was to identify how best to support Jane by first navigating her from the hospital to home, setting up posthospital appointments, linking her to specialty physician referrals, home care, care management, home safety, and transportation resources. Everyone left the meeting with clarity around the various types of roles and tasks each one needed to fulfill.

Planning for older adults is a familywide issue. Adult children play a unique role and serve as a vital support to their parents. Friends can often take on primary responsibilities, but this factor has not been studied significantly. Usually one meeting is never enough to change the negative energies to some positive steps toward care planning. However, it is possible that the severity of Jane's condition and the meeting taking place in a grim hospital environment could have helped everyone shed their underlying assumptions and hostility and work toward a common goal. After a period of 6 months, the author noted significant changes with respect to Jane.

Impromptu family meetings are becoming a norm mainly because of the following reasons:

- Families are not communicating until the situation gets out of hand.

- Families do not live close to each other and hence signs of problems are missed.
- With increases in life span, by the time older adults have significant complex situations, they tend to be older and more frail.

The preceding factors demonstrate the need to start paying attention when problems first begin to appear. Family meetings can help significantly if they are held sooner than later. Medical professionals need to recognize this need and talk to older adult patients to share information about their health and other issues with families. This is a format that has been adopted by the author's program within the hospital and has started yielding very positive results.

FEW FINAL FACTORS TO REMEMBER WHILE PLANNING FAMILY MEETINGS

Understand the Principles of Geriatric Care

Families will need to grasp that older adults have more comorbidities (multiple chronic conditions), see many doctors, and take multiple medications. It is imperative to recognize the need for a big picture approach or a geriatric overview for older adults. Older adults are mostly treated by internal medicine or family practice physicians and not by a geriatrician! Geriatrics is the branch of medicine that focuses on health promotion, prevention, and treatment of disease and disability in later life. A geriatric point of view becomes essential for the following:

- Looking at the big picture
- Supporting complex age-specific needs
- Navigating between multiple subspecialties while seeking treatment
- Looking at different options for treatment and rehabilitation
- Recognizing the care versus cure dilemma

A geriatric assessment done by a geriatrician or an internist that is comprehensive in its scope involves a complete review of the current status of the older person in all of its complex dimensions. The main conditions that need specialized geriatric attention are incontinence, mobility and falls, problems with medications, cognitive thinking abilities and dementia, mental and emotional health, and lack of reserve. A geriatrician will focus on these areas of health and try to find ways to improve a person's situation. Since these kinds of evaluations are so comprehensive, it can only be successfully conducted by a multidisciplinary team of experts. This team might include:

- Physicians
- Ancillary personnel
- Social workers
- Physical and/or occupational therapists
- Dieticians
- Psychologists
- Pharmacists
- Geriatric nurse practitioners

Remembering the Maxim— A Stitch in Time

If interventions are suggested at the right time, families can come together to discuss concerns, possible solutions, and share positive moments. Many families get stuck in this dilemma and choose to ignore signs that predict all is not well. Some areas that families should pay attention to while they still can include the following:

- Assess medical history of older adults and be present during one or two doctor's visits.
- Evaluate the older adult's cognitive status; get neuropsychological testing if the older adult presents short-term memory loss, confusion, distracted behavior, mood changes, or depressive behavior, to name a few.

- Assess financial and physical and cognitive ability for independent functioning.
- Analyze future living and caregiving issues.

Case Study of Family Meetings Displaying the Risks of Ignoring Signs of Emerging Chaos

Case of the Mathews

The care planning process is easier to initiate if meetings begin when illness and frailty are at a manageable stage. A home visit was requested by the primary care physician in 2006 to asses the home situation for Mr. Mathew, a transplant patient with dementia, who appeared to be suffering from malnutrition, and displaying extreme fatigue with occasional falls. The clinic felt Mrs. Mathew was a poor caregiver. Mr. Mathew had worked as an engineer and life seemed "under control" until Mr. Mathew became progressively confused, ill, and eventually underwent a kidney transplant. He was later diagnosed with dementia. The couple had a son and a daughter. The son had an accident and suffered neurological dysfunction with deficits in mood, personality, judgment, and interpersonal behavior. The couple purchased home care for the son and after depleting a great deal of resources had to place him in a facility. The daughter who lived with a boyfriend seemed concerned for her parents, but offered very little in the way of practical help.

The home visit by the author revealed a dirty and cluttered home. The couple ate very poorly. At that time Mrs. Mathew was advised to get help and plan for home care, care management, nutrition, home cleaning, transportation to the hospital, creating advance directives, a financial plan, and possibly moving to assisted living. The community care manager from the local Council on Aging was called in to provide temporary help with resources.

After some difficulties in communicating with Mrs. Mathew, the Council on Aging called a geriatric care manager to intervene, but Mrs. Mathew refused help. The geriatric care manager reported back to the COA, and the case manager from COA called in Adult Protective Services (APS). The APS staff worked on trying to get help to the couple and tried involving the daughter. As per their report, Mrs. Mathew kept reassuring everyone that she would take care of matters and spent most of her time trying to plan care for her husband and son. The COA and APS tried getting the daughter's attention, but as per their notes on the case, the daughter played a passive role through this process.

After a year, Mr. Mathew was hospitalized, and the hospital team noted Mrs. Mathew's sharp change in appearance and cognition. She appeared unfocused and rather agitated. The care manager was called and wanted to refer Mrs. Mathew to her physician to have her needs assessed and bring the daughter onboard as a participant in the couple's care. The care manager felt that Mrs. Mathew could no longer care for her husband and manage her home and that Mr. Mathew should be sent to a long-term care facility. In the absence of any clear planning and the naming of a proxy, the daughter was called as the surrogate to intervene. A couple of family meetings were held in the hospital and at their home to address financial matters, the relationship between the daughter and parents, clear decisions about who would supervise the care plan, and so on. For older adults who do not plan on time, the future is riddled with uncertainty. This case demonstrates the extreme necessity to resolve the chaos and disarray as it starts.

Realizing That Dementia Is a Disease Not Like Any Other

A significant part of the author's energies are directed toward working with families dealing with dementia in conjunction with the hospital neurology department. The most common form of dementia is Alzheimer's disease. The behavioral changes and dangers associated with living alone and driving taxes families tremendously. It is hard to accept the path of decline and the challenges of day-to-day functioning because there is no known trajectory of the exact path of the disease.

Bringing the family together to discuss the symptoms and diagnostic tests can alone take one to two meetings. Diagnostic procedures for dementia and Alzheimer's disease may include scans, blood tests, mental status, and neuropsychological testing. However, the most informative part of the diagnostic process comes from family data on behavior baselines and progression. Taking away the older adult's ability to drive is probably the most difficult consequence of dementia, and families need to meet and discuss best ways to cope with this.

The author provides dementia management tips and resources to interested families because this disease is devastating to families and stresses the family functioning intensely. Many more family meetings are called to cope with this disease than any other. Most adults with dementia will be cared for at home by a family member, who may experience a variety of physical, emotional, financial, and social burdens associated with the caregiving role.[17] Families coping with this disease should seek help and have information about the definition of dementia, the types of dementia, and observable symptoms:

- Memory impairment (short term much more than long term), new forgetfulness, and difficult word finding
- Difficulties in learning new information
- Difficulties in performing complex tasks
- Inability to solve simple problems
- Getting lost in familiar surroundings
- Difficulties in expressing oneself
- Presentation of irritable or aggressive behavior
- Impaired cognitive function

- Difficulty driving or getting lost
- Neglecting self-care and household chores
- Difficulties in managing money
- Presenting judgment and language impairment
- Behavior changes
- Personality change
- Inappropriately friendly or even flirtatious
- Affect shallow or blunted or social withdrawal
- Psychiatric symptoms such as suspiciousness or paranoia, withdrawal or apathy
- Abnormal beliefs or hallucinations

Risks families need to watch for:

- Falling on slippery floors
- Falling down stairs
- Falling from bed onto the hard floor or against furniture
- Starting fire with matches, candles, or cooker
- Scalding with hot tap water or kettle
- Wandering away and spending the night outside or hit by traffic
- Choking
- Unsuitable ingestion of medication
- Abuse from caregiver

Case Study Depicting Family Meetings to Ensure Care of a Dementia Patient

Case of Aunt Lea

Lea was referred to the author by her niece, Eleanor, who was the only surviving family as well as the trustee and lived on the East Coast. Eleanor was shocked at the rapid decline of Lea's language skills, increase in combative behavior, and weight loss over a period of 3 months. Lea lived in the memory support section of a continuing care retirement community (CCRC). Eleanor was concerned whether the CCRC was the right place or whether to move her Aunt Lea close to her. The author assisted Eleanor to make an appointment with a neurologist and connected her to a care manager. Two meetings occurred at the neurologist's office with Lea, the care manager, and Eleanor. Eleanor and the care manager also had a few meetings with the CCRC staff to understand how the facility caregivers responded to Lea's behaviors and health issues.

The goal was to discern whether Lea's decline was caused by the facility not being able to manage Lea or whether it was simply the progression of the disease. After careful deliberations and meetings, Eleanor left her aunt in the same facility with daily home care visits by a trained aide and weekly supervision by the care manager.

CONCLUSION

The health care of older adults is at a crossroads. Although medicine has made significant progress in enhancing the life span and the health of older adults, more needs to be done to meet the complex demands of our aging population. Two important trends that require attention are a look at the big picture while planning health interventions for older adults and working closely with families to develop integrated models of care planning.[18]

Older adults in the community want to stay vital and active in their homes for as long as possible. However, as they age, they face many transitions. While some transitions are predictable, many are unpredictable and require careful intervention, planning, and dialogue between healthcare professionals and their families. But here is the good news—preparation for a transition can begin at any time. Transitional planning involving family meetings may lead to maintaining an optimum level of wellness and social connectedness.

REFERENCES

1. WorldofQuotes.com. Historic quotes and proverbs archive. Available at: http://www.worldofquotes.com. Accessed November 2007.
2. World Population Prospects, the 2002 Revision, 26 February 2003. Available at http://www.un.org/esa/population/publications/wpp2002/WPP2002-HIGHLIGHTSrev1.PDF. Accessed November 2007.
3. Statistics on the Aging Population, Department of Health and Human Services, Administration on Aging. Available at: http://www.aoa.gov/prof/Statistics/statistics.asp. Accessed December 2007.
4. Leonhardt D. He's happier, she's less so. *New York Times*. September 26, 2007. Available at: http://topics.nytimes.com/top/reference/timestopics/people/l/david_leonhardt/index.html. Accessed November 2007.
5. Lederberg MS. The family of the cancer patient. In: Holland J, ed. *Psychooncology*. New York, NY: Oxford University Press; 1998.
6. Dykstra P. Roads less taken, developing a nuanced view of older adults without children. *Journal of Family Issues*. 2007;28(10):1275–1310.
7. Navaie-Waliser M, Feldman PH, Gould DA, Levine CL, Kuerbis AN, Donelan K. When the caregiver needs care: The plight of vulnerable caregivers. *American Journal of Public Health*. 2002;92(3):409–413.
8. Levin NJ. *How to Care for Your Parents*. New York, NY: W. W. Norton; 1997.
9. Hermalin AI, Ofstedal MB, Mehta K. The disadvantaged elderly. In: Hermalin AI, ed. *The Well-Being of the Elderly in Asia: A Four Country Comparative Study*. Ann Arbor, MI: University of Michigan Press; 2002.
10. Tsouna-Hadjis E. First-stroke recovery process: The role of family social support. *Archives of Physical Medicine and Rehabilitation*. 2000;81: 881–887.
11. Chappell N. *Social Support and Aging*. Toronto, ON: Butterworths; 1992.
12. Guze S, ed. *Adult Psychiatry*. St. Louis, MO: Mosby Year Book; 1997.
13. Alexander BH, Rivara FP, Wolf ME. The cost and frequency of hospitalization for fall-related injuries in older adults. *American Journal of Public Health*. 1992;82(7):1020–1023.
14. AARP Administration on Aging. *A Profile of Older Americans, 1999*. Washington, DC: AARP; 1999.
15. Geriatric Health Services at Stanford. Available at: http://www.stanfordhospital.com/forPatients/patientServices/geriatricHealth. Accessed December 2008.
16. The National Hospice and Palliative Care Organization. Available at: http://www.nhpco.org/templates/1/homepage.cfm. Accessed December 2007.
17. Connell CM, Janevic MR, Gallant MP. The costs of caring: Impact of dementia on family caregivers. *Journal of Geriatric Psychiatry and Neurology*. 2001;14(4):179–187.
18. Jarvik LF, Winograd CH, eds. *Treatments for the Alzheimer Patient*. New York, NY: Springer Publishing; 1998.

CHAPTER 7

Working with Couples

Anne Rosenthal

It has been argued that elders have a greater need for human contact than other age groups.[1] Also, the need for intimacy and affection derived from personal relationships continues into old age.[2] For example, data indicate that maintaining close personal relationships is an important factor in good mental health. Marriage improves psychological and physical health and decreases the risk of suicide.[3] Marriage may be conducive to better health because it encourages behaviors that contribute to health and provides support when illness strikes as well as encouraging actions that can prevent disease development. Consequently the need to rely on formal services such as home care and nursing services, a common measure of illness, is reduced.

THE IMPACT OF ILLNESS

When a spouse becomes ill, the nature of interdependence between husband and wife may be altered dramatically. The focus is on the increased dependency of the person receiving care. However, the obligation to provide care can create its own kind of dependency on the spousal relationship, as the caregiver withdraws from other activities in order to meet the healthcare needs of the spouse, creating a basis for symbiotic interdependence between husband and wife.[4] How does the poor health of one spouse affect the marital relationship? Kelley proposes that severe illness or disability creates imbalanced dependence between spouses that leads in turn to rifts between spouses based on the conflict of their interests.[2] The ill spouse has negative feelings about the illness, the need for help, and perhaps more important, the compliance expected in return for care. At the same time, the helper feels responsible to provide care, the need for acknowledgment of the sacrifices being made, and the difficulty of finding time to meet his or her own needs. Although the helping spouse may derive satisfaction from behaving altruistically and performing roles previously assumed by the ill spouse, difficulties in mastering new skills may create frustration. Similarly, the care recipient experiences ambivalent feelings as the help provided by a spouse is both a positive reflection on the marital relationship and an ongoing reminder of the need for help.[5]

The health of one's spouse is related to both marital and life satisfaction. However, the life satisfaction of the older husband is directly related to the functional health of his wife. In contrast, the life satisfaction of the wife is directly related to the life satisfaction of the husband and only indirectly related to her husband's health.[6] Thus, among men, poor functional health of a spouse depresses life satisfaction while, among women, poor functional health of a spouse depresses life satisfaction only if it does so for the spouse.

The division of household tasks is most likely to undergo substantial change if the wife has health problems. In this instance, the husband is expected to carry out tasks traditionally performed by the female.[7] This suggests that a wife's illness is more disruptive to her husband than the other way around. However, a Montreal study found that wives experience greater burden than husbands in providing care to their spouses.[8] Also, a larger percentage of the husbands than wives report that they now feel closer to their cared-for spouse. We can speculate that these differences are because women have greater contact with confidants than men. It has been shown that when women get together with their peers, they tend to exchange feelings in contrast to men who when they engage with their friends, tend to participate in activities together without an exchange of verbalized feelings.

The following is an interesting example of how men approach caregiving differently than their wives: Caregiver husbands appear more concerned about maintaining their wives femininity than caregiving wives are concerned about maintaining their husband's masculinity. For example, a husband whose wife was diagnosed with frontal lobe dementia was diligent about seeing that his wife kept her regular hair appointment and had her nails done as she was accustomed to prior to her diagnosis. In contrast, a wife whose husband had dementia was more concerned about meeting her husband's health needs than maintaining his masculinity through dress or physical appearance, saying, "I just want him to be well cared for."

Another unexpected disparity between the sexes is the greater help husbands report giving to their wives than their wives report giving to them.[4,9] Overall, men perceive that they give a greater amount of help than women. However, it appears this perception is an exaggeration of reality. Given that women are more likely than men to be socialized to fill the caregiver role and that they are more likely to provide health care to their spouse since they live longer and marry men older than themselves, these are curious findings. Why are women more likely to consider the care they provide to a spouse as burdensome, and why are they less likely to report providing health care to a spouse?

There are two possible explanations for the disparity between men and women concerning the perceived amount of help exchanged.[4] First, the larger resource of potential support available to women, such as from friends and relatives, due to their broader social network, heightens the possibility that the support offered by husbands does not compare favorably with that offered by others such as friends and relatives. Women may judge the support provided to a husband in older age in relation to the amount of support offered to children and husband in earlier years and consider it minimal by comparison.

One reason women may experience a greater burden than men when caring for their spouse is the fact they have been caregivers to others for many years, caring for children, parents, and now a spouse at a time when they might feel ready for a respite. Women also give significantly more types of help to their husband than men give to their wives.[9] Another factor that may account for the different perception of the caregiving role as burdensome is the contrast between the sexes in roles previously performed.[10] For women, caregiving is the resumption of a role recently (or never) relinquished, while for men it is newly acquired, following many years of labor force participation. An extreme example from a London study is a mother of nine who also raised two grandchildren, provided concurrent care for her mother- and father-in-law until they died, and was then faced with caring for her husband as he died of cancer. Another widowed mother with five sons tells her story: "After my sons grew up I had my ill husband to look after for seven years. . . . I guess the easiest time that I had was after he died . . . I couldn't get out. I was always there. . . . The only chance that I had of getting out was when the boys (sons) would come to look after him."

Much of the research literature regarding care for an ill spouse reflects the current interest in dementia, a health problem that creates unique challenges to the caregiver. A study in Kingston, Ontario, found that spouses and children are most likely to describe caring for a demented elder as difficult when the severity of the dementia, not the level of physical burden, is high.[11] In another study it was found that over time, both wives and husbands *increase* their tolerance for dealing with the memory loss and behavioral problems of their spouse.[12] And it also appears husbands' and wives' styles of coping become more similar, with women adopting the more instrumental approach of men.[13] An instrumental approach would include an emphasis on activity of daily living tasks rather than a focus on expressive or emotional needs.

Among caregivers aged 50–90, both younger wives and older husbands experience the greatest burden when caring for a demented spouse.[10] The advanced age of the men may be associated with poorer health and a declining ability to take on a new role. The younger women, on the other hand, are likely to be confronting competing obligations.

The following case illustrates such a dilemma: A retired attorney married a nurse 17 years his junior. They had six happy years

traveling, entertaining, and buying income property until a stroke physically incapacitated the husband. His cognitive state was intact; however, after months of rehabilitation it was determined that no additional treatments would improve the husband's physical functioning. He was left with residual paralysis on one side of his body and swallowing difficulties that prevented him from eating a regular diet. He was tethered to a catheter that fed liquid nourishment directly to his stomach. Because of these physical limitations, traveling was not possible. The wife became depressed as a reaction to her new limited living situation. She wanted very much to travel to South America where they had a lovely villa. The husband didn't feel strong enough to make the trip and was resigned to remain at home with his limited activities. The wife engaged a care manager to meet with them to see if their life could be improved. After meeting with the care manager it was determined that the husband would accept help at home while his wife took a short trip to South America. The care manager was able to engage a male law student to serve as an interesting companion and helper to the husband. Additionally some household adaptive recommendations were made: a stairglide was installed that allowed for greater access to the outside and a door to one of the rooms was removed to allow for wheelchair access to the panoramic views of the bay and to a bathroom with a level shower. The wife's trip and the husband's time with the law student were successful and allowed for further discussion about short trips the wife might take for respite. Both developed improved mental states and better coping skills. The Yesavage Depression Scale was used initially as a baseline instrument to determine the level of depression, and several months later after recommended changes were made the scale confirmed the lowered rate of depression in both partners.[14]

Finally, a study of women involved in a support group for caregivers poignantly illustrates the special problems faced by wives caring for severely brain-injured husbands.[14] In these cases the impact of illness on the quality of marriage is profound and resembles having lost a spouse, as is often true in the advanced stages of dementia. It is this feeling that makes adjustment to the caregiving role so hard. Because the spouse is alive, mourning seems inappropriate, but the severity of the impairment limits the spouse's ability to satisfy any of the needs of the caregiver, including companionship. For these women, caring for an ill spouse is in many respects the first step in the transition toward widowhood.

In summary, the interdependence that characterizes most older marriages provides a foundation for adapting to the need for care when one spouse becomes ill. The transition to the roles of caregiver and care recipient heightens the interdependence of older spouses, contributing to a sense of closeness. At the same time, unique forms of conflict, though minimal, sometimes emerge in response to the illness of a spouse and are generally based on the fear of being abandoned through death.[12]

The comments of an 83-year-old childless husband illustrates how his wife's illness isolated them both and underscores the need for respite for the husband: "My wife becomes very nervous if I'm not here at the house. She might panic when I leave for a short time to run errands."

In this case, the care manager was able to engage a nephew to become more involved with his aunt and uncle. An emergency alert system was installed and a cordless phone was available to the wife when she was left alone. The husband was encouraged to join a caregiver's support group offered by a local church, and the nephew arranged to live at the house on weekends, offering respite to the caregiving husband. The care manager encouraged the couple to think of ways they'd like to improve the quality of their life, and they decided to sell their home and relocate to a continuum of care facility not far from their town.

Should illness be followed by death, extreme interdependence can prove debilitating to the surviving spouse. Commitment to the caregiving role may have deprived the surviving spouse of ongoing contact with others. Now widowed, the journey back to involvement with the rest of the world may be long and arduous.

In some cases, the death of a spouse can give rise to feelings of ambivalence, especially when the deceased spouse had a lingering or chronic illness. The comments of an 88-year-old woman whose husband recently died of Alzheimer's a week after she finally placed him in a facility exemplify this:

> My husband and I suffered so much these past years. I know his passing is a blessing, and yet I do miss him. What I miss is the man I shared my life with, not the shadow of the man I had lived with these past 6 years.

The care manager's clinical role in such cases is to encourage sources of support such as attendance in a widow/widowers support group, provide counseling for adjustment to the loss, or refer to clinical resources including hospice if care was provided to the couple prior to the loss.

Additional clinical focus is on acknowledging ambivalent feelings, encouraging the bereavement process to take place, and giving permission for the ambivalent widow to accept her responses as understandable and reasonable.

CASES ILLUSTRATING WAYS THE CARE MANAGER INTERVENED IN SPOUSAL CAREGIVING SITUATIONS

So many spouses have written on the subject of caregiving that one has to conclude this is a profound experience. It has been referred to as a journey, a time of considerable personal growth, and resolution of emotional conflict—as if clarity of thought takes place and frees the individual to focus on what matters. This liberating experience can draw the caregiver closer to the essence of their being and the being of their partner and perhaps even life itself. This is most poignant for caregivers managing with a spouse with a dementia diagnosis.

Spousal caregivers appear amenable to attending support groups and may be eager to meet others who share the same experience and may have ideas and resources to discuss. Some spousal caregivers start therapy for the first time in their lives, or more historically introspective types may return to therapy that ended years earlier.

Still, the doubts of spousal caregivers—wondering if perhaps they could be doing more to improve the quality of life of their spouses, ambivalence about engaging strangers to help in the home, guilt about taking time for themselves, and placement concerns are common issues that the astute care manager will recognize and address.

The care manager is in a good position to evaluate the situation and offer suggestions to make life easier and better for partners, to address outstanding areas of need, and certainly to give weary spousal caregivers permission to care for themselves. Helping spousal caregivers to step back and see all they have accomplished by comparing the current situation to what life was like a week, month, or year earlier can be therapeutic.

Dependent Types: Case of Mary and Glen

Of all types of couples, the dependent partner, one could argue, might have the most difficult time changing to the role of caregiver. This individual might be the husband or wife, and because of their relationship as the primary recipient of nurturance, might not have the range of coping skills necessary to adjust to the role of primary nurturer, organizer, and implementer of care.

For example, Mary, a woman in her late 70s, was the wife of a former Marine pilot who worked as a professor of mechanical engineering at a prestigious university on the East Coast. The couple relished their academic life. The wife, Mary, was comfortable basking in her husband's limelight as the handsome, popular professor. They took interesting trips around the world on sabbaticals. Mary always felt a bit "one down" because she had no more than a high school education. But she was a gracious hostess, very pretty, and had a charming personality. Her husband Glen was dealt a blow when at the age of 78 he had a massive stroke that affected his mobility, speech, and cognition.

Mary was suddenly thrust into the role of caregiver without any preparation. Their two children lived out of state and were not able to provide the support they realized mother and dad required. It was at this point they contacted the care manager for guidance.

The care manager visited the couple at their home and immediately recognized through careful listening and observation of the wife that Mary was not only ill equipped to manage the myriad decisions and organizing necessary, but seemed to have developed an anxiety disorder. Mary's affect was tense as she picked her nails and spoke rapidly and haltingly. The wife confided to the care manager that her primary physician was treating her "nerves" with sedatives. Mary said she was having difficulty sleeping, taking deep breaths, and had been feeling faint since her husband's stroke.

After sharing this information with the care manager, Mary was open to suggestions for herself and her husband and agreed to an assessment of her husband that included cognitive testing using the Cognistat. The Cognistat, or Neurobehavioral Cognitive Status Examination, is a standardized neurobehavioral screening test. It examines neurological (brain and central nervous system) health in relationship to a person's behavior. The care manager determined that Glen had deficits in executive functions that interfered with his ability to write checks, pay bills, and manage his medications. Mary was helping him dress and bathe, but without adequate training she was putting her own safety at risk in doing so.

The care manager contacted the primary physician and requested an order for physical and occupational therapy for Glen. She also asked the physician if he had any objection to Mary seeing a psychiatrist to chemically address her anxiety. The physician agreed to the PT and OT orders and said there was a psychiatrist in his building that he had confidence in and would encourage Mary to see him.

Mary was amenable to seeing a geropsychiatrist and welcomed the opportunity to face her fears. She expressed shame that she had only a high school education and wasn't sure she would have the ability to develop the skills necessary to be a good caregiver to her husband. The care manager offered to continue meeting with her and her husband to support the efforts that were necessary for this to happen and stated her confidence to Mary that she would indeed be able to forge the skills necessary.

The daughter and son were asked by the care manager to increase their contacts with their parents, if only to encourage the progress being made.

As Mary gradually became more confident in her abilities, her anxieties decreased. The physical and occupational therapists worked with Mary and Glen around activities of daily living, and Mary learned how to safely assist him. Durable medical equipment was brought into the home to advance this process, such as a hospital bed with a trapeze, grab bars in the bathroom, and a ramp was built to provide easier access to the house.

A year later much had changed for this couple, and although Glen would never again be the active, vigorous professor he once was, his Mary was a more vibrant partner than she had ever been, and as a result they developed a more mutually satisfactory relationship.

The care manager continued to see this couple for basic monitoring and met alone with Mary from time to time, helping her to acknowledge her progress in her own development and effectiveness and encouraging her acceptance of herself and her husband's chronic condition. The care manager continued to note whether there were any changes in their circumstances, and if so, timely follow-ups were instituted.

The case of Mary and Glen illustrates how the care manager develops rapport by careful listening to establish trust. This allows the couple to accept appropriate services, the help of allied professionals, as well as the assistance of concerned adult children when disequilibrium occurs in the relationship of the older couple.

Domineering and Paranoid Types: Case of Inga and Sven

Another couple who required intervention were living in a small house in a suburb of San Francisco. The couple met in Sweden and moved to the United States in the 1970s. The wife was always domineering in this relationship, and according to their daughter who lived 70 miles away, she wanted her parents to separate years ago because her mother "was such a bully to her husband." Mother, Inga, was 10 years older than her husband Sven and they lived and worked on a ranch for many years.

In the 1990s, Sven was seriously injured when he was run over by a truck on his property. This left him with a significant disability, and he was unable to continue his ranch duties. Inga had always been a squanderer of money and had made many large purchases during their marriage that they could ill afford. After they realized Sven could no longer manage the ranch, they sold it and moved into a small rented house, living in reduced circumstances. Shortly after they moved, Inga was diagnosed with ovarian cancer. It progressed to the point she was on continuous oxygen, quite weak, and using the local emergency room as a clinic. The nurse case manager from the health insurance company contacted the care manager to do a home assessment that included a safety check and to provide recommendations.

When the care manager went out to meet Inga and Sven she was struck by the many expensive looking pieces of furniture and paintings squeezed into the tiny cluttered house. Sven greeted her at the door, saying, "My wife is in a bad mood today; I hope she doesn't insult you." When the care manager sat down to conduct an assessment, Inga took over the conversation, interrupting Sven, correcting his interpretation of their history, and

only wanted the care manager to address how she could get free services. Inga said they could not afford to pay for their medication or hospital bills. When the care manager probed about how much help she needed, she dismissed the question and said, "My husband can help me with anything. I only need help with errands and paying for medication and hospital bills." The care manager asked them to sign authorizations to release medical and confidential information so that she could look into what they would qualify for and they agreed to sign.

The care manager asked about the family constellation and was told about the daughter who "is very busy with her own life and doesn't have time to help us. Please don't bother her." The care manager asked if it would be okay if she phoned the daughter to discuss their situation and both Inga and Sven agreed. The daughter was contacted and said her mother is so suspicious of her, that she will not let her have her social security number or sign a durable power of attorney for health care (DPOA), and her parents had not made out a will. The daughter did not have access to any banking information and expressed concern if anything should happen, she was not sure her father would have the necessary information to follow through.

The next evening Sven phoned the care manager and said he was totally exhausted. His wife had awakened him at 6:00 that morning and demanded his help with cooking, shopping, cleaning, and laundry. He said he had a painful back and wasn't sure he could keep up this pace much longer. He pleaded with the care manager to help and said his wife might be asking him to take her to the emergency room later that evening. The care manager referred the case to Adult Protective Services for abuse of the husband by the wife.

The care manager also contacted the Area Agency on Aging services division in their county and was able to determine that the couple were already on public assistance and had been offered in-home support services, but had declined. They had also been offered to be part of the PACE program and had declined.

The care manager went out again to see Inga and Sven and shared what she had learned. Inga said they didn't need help at home, but she had a stack of hospital bills and bills for medication, and she didn't know how she could pay for them. She agreed to give the bills to the care manager. The care manager mailed copies of the bills to the health plan nurse case manager who worked with the health plan billing department. It turned out a mistake had been made, and the hospital bills were not to be paid by the members. Additionally, the medication expenses would be picked up by the health plan because Inga and Sven qualified for a drug benefit that their health plan offers its indigent members.

When the care manager explained this financial support to Inga, she was so relieved and trusting of the care manager, she was willing to accept the suggestion that she accept help at home through the county in-home support services and enroll with the PACE program. Sven was encouraged to speak up for himself, not overextend, and obtain more help as needed.

Within the month, Sven and Inga were visited by a social worker from the county, had regular subsidized help at home, and were freed from financial woes. Sven was now expressing his needs more readily to Inga who was becoming frailer and too fatigued to be as directive as she once was. A few months later Inga was enrolled in a hospice program and received increased assistance through Medicare.

Meanwhile, their daughter was made aware of this progress and had worked with her parents to obtain a durable power of attorney for health care and finances and her parents wrote a holographic will.

The daughter was tremendously grateful to the care manager who fostered these changes. Their HMO nurse care manager once again recognized the value of sending out a care manager to be the eyes and ears of a system that can't always keep up with its aging members' needs.

The case of Inga and Sven illustrates how necessary it is for the care manager to have knowledge of public entitlement programs and to instruct couples in the importance of legal planning documents. It also illustrates when working with a client's health plan it is important to help with billing questions. In Inga's case, this was the key to building trust with her. Inga's domineering of her husband, denial of her needs, and the toll it took on her husband, combined with her paranoia of her daughter and the system, created a challenging case for the care manager. In this situation where denial was operative, clinical sensitivity and patience are necessary to achieve the desired outcomes.

Gay Couple Issues: Case of Suzanne and Helen

Suzanne and Helen developed a romantic relationship when Suzanne took a political science class from Helen who was a professor of political science at an eastern university. Helen was married to Richard at that time and had no children. Suzanne was in her early 20s and estranged from her mother who she described as an impossible-to-please, manipulative, and spoiled woman. Suzanne and Helen met secretly for many years, and Richard eventually died. It was at that time they relocated to California and moved into separate apartments in the same building. Helen was 25 years older than Suzanne and was used to living extravagantly. Helen "adopted" another young woman, a street artist, and subsidized her living and spent lavishly on herself and others with expensive nights out on the town.

About 10 years after moving to California, Helen developed health problems. She had shortness of breath from emphysema, diabetes, and mobility issues, requiring assistance at first during the day and later into the night. Suzanne provided all of Helen's care until she herself was faced with her own physical decline, due to rheumatoid arthritis.

It was at this time Suzanne was referred by her physician to the care manager. Suzanne told the care manager the story of her life, stating that Helen was controlling of Suzanne, and she was reluctant for Helen to meet the care manager. She also said few people knew of her true relationship with Helen, and they were presenting themselves as good friends. Suzanne explained that her mother was still living and would be appalled if she knew about their lesbian relationship and might even remove Suzanne from her mother's will. She expected to inherit a handsome sum.

Suzanne also explained that Helen had someone organizing her mail and paying her bills and wasn't clear about the extent of that individual's accountability. The bill payer told Suzanne that Helen was spending beyond her means and was dipping into Helen's savings to pay for monthly expenses. She said Helen could be overly trusting and suspicious at the same time, and Helen was dismissing the bill payer's caution. Suzanne said she was becoming distraught and depressed about the situation.

The care manager and Suzanne discussed a strategy that could be used to make Helen amenable to meeting together, deciding to introduce the care manager truthfully as someone who helps older people remain independent as long as possible in their own homes. They arranged to meet at Helen's apartment, and the care manager asked that the bill payer be there at the same time.

When this meeting took place, the care manager was greeted by a commanding woman who walked with a walker, appearing to be holding court in a living room filled with interesting art and sculpture. Helen readily spoke with the care manager and was cooperative and forthcoming about her physical situation. She was clearly a fall risk and was now using oxygen during much of the day.

The bill payer, Jennifer, displayed open hostility to Suzanne and said that Helen was spending too much money supporting Suzanne and others and was running up so much credit card debt that she would be running out of money even with her university pension. The care manager made further inquiries and found out that there was a long-term care policy. The bill payer said a claim had been filed, but the long-term care company was not responding. The care manager inquired how Jennifer acquired the role of bill payer and she stated she was a friend who Helen asked to help. She explained this was an informal arrangement, and when asked about whether she herself was paid to provide this task, she said she wrote out a check to herself every month for the time she worked at the rate of $15.00 per hour. Later Suzanne told the care manager Jennifer was paying herself for not only bill paying time, but time driving Helen as well as time spent when they were out dining together.

With Helen's agreement, the care manager set up help at home for her, relieving Suzanne of some of the daytime tasks. Helen insisted she could manage at night. Each evening Suzanne would check on Helen and find that she needed help getting ready for bed or would be asking for a nighttime snack. Suzanne relayed to the care manager that her arthritis was progressing and she was exhausted from helping Helen at night, but feared having her spend more money on home care.

Meanwhile, the care manager referred Helen's case to Adult Protective Services to investigate whether elder financial abuse was taking place. When the case was investigated, Jennifer resigned and the care manager established the bill paying through a representative payee billing service.

She also reviewed the long-term care policy and contacted the long-term care company to inquire about the claim. It took so long for them to respond, the care manager finally contacted an attorney specializing in long-term care claims to assist, and the company began to pay for help at home.

The care manager remained involved for several years, stepping in to adjust the level of service Helen received at home, helping Suzanne view the situation as objectively as she could, and referring her to a psychiatrist to review whether she could benefit from some chemical support. Suzanne started on an antidepressant with some antianxiety properties and became interested in an analytic approach with her psychiatrist. She began to understand herself and her motives, and shared with the care manager the insights she gained about her relationship with Helen and how it related to her relationship with her mother.

Suzanne's mother eventually died and Suzanne inherited a generous sum. The care manager suggested she meet with a financial advisor and an elder law attorney to assist with long-term financial planning. The first thing Suzanne wanted to do was pay off Helen's credit card balance. She insisted this was the right thing to do.

Helen's health deteriorated, and she eventually moved to a skilled nursing facility where Suzanne visited daily. Suzanne remained in contact with the care manager when difficulties arose and at times for moral support. Suzanne's functional status also began to decline significantly, and the care manager spoke with her about her options. Suzanne's financial picture was very different from Helen's who was now using public assistance to cover her cost of care. Suzanne required assistance but not skilled nursing. Suzanne was willing to consider relocating but wanted to remain close to Helen's facility.

The care manager recommended two facilities that had a continuum of care that ranged from assisted living to skilled nursing and also had public assistance licensure so that if Suzanne's funds were depleted, she would be able to remain in the same facility. Within months, Suzanne made the decision to move to a nonprofit facility not far from Helen. She continued to visit her by cab during the week and called the care manager from time to time regarding resource concerns and updating her on their situation, frequently signing off with gratitude and acknowledging the many areas of support the care manager provided.

The case of Suzanne and Helen shows the need for the care manager to be aware of her or his own issues of countertransference when dealing with issues that may be uncomfortable. In this case where the gender preferences might be different from the care manager's preferences, the core issues and needs for safety, stability, planning, and so on are the same as with any couple.

It is important to maintain an unbiased, nonjudgmental attitude, regardless of how client values conflict or mesh with the care manager's values. This allows the care manager to remain effective and sensitive to client needs and wants.

Husband Stands by While Daughter Is Abusive to Mother: Case of Judy and George and Patty and Jim

Judy was a successful real estate agent whose parents, Patty and Jim, moved in with her and her husband George and 14-year-old daughter Melissa. Patty, the mother, was diagnosed with Lewy body dementia. Shortly after they moved in, Judy's husband, George, was diagnosed with Parkinson's disease.

Patty and Jim, who were both in their 70s, had a long-term marriage with a history of Patty domineering Jim. Patty began to wander and was asking questions repeatedly. When Patty was taken to her doctor's office after a fall, the primary physician referred Judy to a care manager, recognizing they needed more assistance than he could offer.

When the care manager arrived at Judy's house, she was greeted by Jim who explained his daughter Judy would be joining them shortly; she was out showing real estate. He revealed to her that he was troubled by Judy showing hostility and anger to her mother Patty when she repeatedly asked questions or wouldn't shower and an added problem was that now his granddaughter, Melissa, Judy's daughter, was mimicking her mother and treating her grandmother disrespectfully. Jim expressed reluctance to attempt to correct Judy because he felt beholden to his daughter since he and Patty had moved in with her and George.

After a short interval, Judy arrived home and joined the care manager and her father Jim. Judy was forthcoming about the tremendous strain she felt with her job, her mother's needs, and her husband's recent diagnosis. When the care manager asked the question, "What is a typical day like?" Judy said the day was very hectic, never knowing when she might need to leave on short notice to show a house. She disclosed her worries about her husband's illness and had some anticipatory anxiety about his future medical needs. Judy offered that her temper was short, and she felt at a loss how to deal with her mother's behavioral issues and on one occasion she even slapped her mother once out of frustration and felt terrible about her action. She also expressed resentment toward a brother who lived out of state who was not particularly supportive or involved with their parents.

Jim revealed he wasn't sure that the intergenerational arrangement was working out as well as he hoped. When the care manager asked if he had any suggestions to remedy the situation, he said that his wife might be better off in a setting that cared for others with dementia. He said he wouldn't mind remaining with his daughter and her family if a care facility was nearby and he could visit daily.

The care manager determined that a report to Adult Protective Services should be made because of possible elder abuse. The care manager met with George and Judy several more times to offer resource information, counseling, and support, especially around the physical abuse. The care manager explained to Judy, George, and Jim that the impulse to slap derived from Judy's frustration, but it was not an acceptable way for her to deal with her frustration. The care manager explored with Judy what the triggers were that tempted her to slap her mother. Judy said her mother's repeated questions were a particular irritation. The care manager suggested that Judy not respond to every one of her mother's questions, distract her mother, and even leave the room if she felt she might physically strike her mother.

Plans for dementia day care were explored as an option to offer respite to Judy. The care manager modeled responses by responding patiently and appropriately to Patty when she repeatedly asked questions. Judy expressed her shame that she hadn't known how to respond to her mother's new behaviors and now saw there were ways she could redirect her mother and modify her behavior. The care manager said she wouldn't know how to sell real estate without being educated and that managing difficult behaviors was another skill that required education, offering this analogy as a way to diffuse Judy's shame. The care manager suggested Judy share her new skills with Melissa, which she did. Melissa caught on readily that she could communicate with her grandmother in ways that were satisfying for both of them.

The care manager recommended Jim meet with an elder law attorney found through www.naela.org, the National Academy of Elder Law Attorneys, to review their estate, provide them with needed healthcare proxy documents, and address financial planning for the long term. The care manager also provided printed information specifically for caregivers on ways to manage difficult behaviors and directed the family to the Family Caregiver Alliance Web site, www.caregiver.org. This organization has downloadable fact sheets about dementias, Parkinson's disease, how to select a facility, helping children understand when grandma doesn't remember, and so on. They also offer a respite program for caregivers.

A good dementia-specific facility was within 2 miles of Judy's house and appealed to the family; however, the cost was more than they could afford. The care manager suggested to Judy that perhaps her brother would be able to assist financially. This possibility was welcomed by the brother because he was more comfortable helping financially than emotionally.

A few weeks later, Patty was placed in the dementia facility, and after some difficult behaviors were managed chemically by a neurologist, she acclimated well. Jim visited Patty daily, joined a spousal caregiver's support group the care manager recommended, and continued living with his daughter's family in a much calmer environment.

The case of Patty and Jim shows how important it is for the care manager to know the legally required reporting for elder abuse and neglect. In this case the care manager was a mandatory reporter to Adult Protective Services after hearing the daughter slapped the mother. It is also necessary to have working knowledge of when a referral to an elder law attorney is appropriate for spousal impoverishment planning and other future needs. Additionally, it is necessary for the care manager to know when placement is indicated and to be aware of the different levels of care. Finally it is important for the care manager to carefully assess the whole family, not just the caregiving adult child. In the case of Patty, knowing that there was an out-of-town son who could be asked to help with the cost of placement was the key to both placing the older mother and relieving the family stressors.

Spousal Neglect: Case of Mr. and Mrs. Ross

Mr. and Mrs. Ross were in their 80s and lived an active social life until Mr. Ross was injured in a fall and required a long-term orthopedic recovery. Shortly after he was discharged from the hospital to home, his wife developed what their primary physician called a "pseudodementia," a loss of cognitive function related to something other than Alzheimer's, vascular dementia, or another true dementia. Mrs. Ross would spend an average day of 16 hours in bed, would not eat, dress, bathe, or brush her teeth unless she was strongly encouraged. Their daughter, who lived out of state, was appalled at her mother's condition when she arrived to visit. Both parents had lost a significant amount of weight and were clearly neglecting themselves and the house.

The daughter attempted to set up help at home, and it was at this point that she contacted the care manager for assistance. She said her father was indifferent to her mother's need for care. For example, there was an incident when the mother fell into a rose bush and was bleeding and scratched while her husband denied she required any assistance. On another occasion, Mrs. Ross approached her husband holding a pork chop and a pan and asked him, "Now what do I do?" It appeared that Mr. Ross was unrealistic about the extent of his wife's increasing debility and denied the need for help at home.

When the care manager came out to assess the situation, she found Mr. Ross walking with a walker and tripping over throw rugs in the house. Both parents smoked in bed, and there was no smoke alarm in the bedroom. Both Mr. and Mrs. Ross were at risk for falls and took showers, but the bathroom lacked grab bars or benches to make showering safer.

When Mr. Ross was hospitalized for urinary retention the daughter attempted to have her mother placed in a local assisted living facility, but they refused her admission due to her smoking habit.

The care manager listened attentively as Mr. Ross spoke about the life they lived. He expressed pride in the life they made for themselves and spoke about his wife as if she were the way he remembered her from years ago. He dismissed any concerns with comments such as, "Join the club. Everyone is concerned, but we'll do just fine."

The care manager identified several areas for improvement such as removing throw rugs, installing a smoke alarm in the bedroom, and installing a grab bar in the bathroom. Mr. Ross rejected the ideas but agreed to have the care manager remain in contact with him and his daughter.

Meanwhile, the care manager reported the case to the Adult Protective Services because she was concerned about the issue of Mrs. Ross's neglect and Mr. Ross's apparent denial of the problems in the home.

Within 48 hours after first meeting with the care manager, the daughter phoned stating her father had been hospitalized for bleeding from his surgical site and her mother's mental state was fast declining. The care manager met with the daughter again at her parents' residence. She arranged for live-in help through a local home care agency with the caveat that the only person who could dismiss the help would be the daughter.

Mrs. Ross's mental state declined to the extent she was forgetting she was smoking, and the care manager requested that her cigarettes be removed from the house. The local senior center was less than a mile away, and the caregiver agreed to drive Mrs. Ross there during the week where Mrs. Ross received a midday meal and participated in social activities. She soon became the darling of the center, regaling them with stories from her colorful past as a socialite.

Meanwhile, Mr. Ross, who was a large man, required an extended stay in a rehabilitation facility for physical and occupational therapy. He was so pleased to return home that he did not balk at the live-in help. He continued to smoke, but meanwhile the care manager saw that a smoke alarm was installed in his bedroom along with appropriate grab bars and a shower bench in the bathroom.

Prior to Mr. Ross's return home the care manager arranged for the physical therapist to train the home caregivers in safe transfers. The physical therapist also did a home safety check, and additional durable medical equipment for Mr. Ross's bed was delivered to ensure his safety.

The care manager contacted Mrs. Ross's primary physician asking about whether she might benefit from psychotropic medications for her depression and cognitive decline. This treatment was instituted, and she was well established on antidepressants and dementia medication when her husband returned home from the rehab center. Now the husband was more willing to participate in her care. She and her husband regained some lost weight, and the daughter gained great relief.

The care manager remained involved, monitoring the situation at home and following up as their needs changed. Mr. Ross was never really able to admit to his wife's need for help but did not interfere with interventions to keep them both safe at home.

The case of Mr. and Mrs. Ross shows how necessary it is for the care manager to identify spousal neglect, manage it, and evaluate the entire situation to address other outstanding problems. This includes knowing how to do a home safety check and being aware of community resources that support older couples who are living marginally in their homes.

Spousal neglect frequently derives from denial on the part of the well spouse. Feeling overwhelmed, unable to cope with the overarching demands of caregiving and the helping spouse's own needs for comfort and care, spousal neglect is not an unusual occurrence. The well spouse requires help understanding the needs of the care recipient and realizing there are manageable ways to address the safety and well-being of the dependent spouse. Through the care manager's patient,

careful, and nonjudgmental explanation of these areas, the neglectful spouse can become aware of their role in altering the situation and resolving the problem areas and issues. This approach will allow the well spouse to feel more in control of the situation and feel better about how they are conducting themselves. These new, more satisfying ways the well spouse is communicating will give the care manager opportunities to reinforce the well spouse's more desirable behavior. In the case of Mr. and Mrs. Ross, dementia day care, help at home, and recruiting the daughter as an ally of the care manager were keys to resolving this case of spousal neglect.

Case of Cognitively Impaired Husband Who Developed Aggressive Sexual Behavior

Betty was exhausted when she contacted the care manager, stating that her husband had a stroke several months earlier and she needed help with planning. When she arrived in the care manager's office she stated that she and her husband Alan had been married 40 years and since his stroke he has poor short-term memory and an excessive interest in sex that had led to him becoming sexually aggressive. She stated she was exhausted from either fending him off or engaging in relentless sexual relations. Betty stated her adult children and doctor have no idea of the problem but are aware of their father's difficulties with memory. According to the wife, the adult children drove them to see a neurologist for follow-up appointments at a nearby teaching hospital.

The care manager probed to understand more about Betty's interests and personality. Betty was from the Midwest and enjoyed quilting, doing crossword puzzles, and had a generally sedentary lifestyle. Betty also expressed shame that she had gained a significant amount of weight since her husband's stroke. She said she and her husband rarely argued throughout their marriage because she usually gave in when she saw he was upset; now she felt he was bullying her in bed. The care manager scheduled a time to visit Betty and Alan in their home to do an assessment.

The care manager met with Alan and had a conversation with him to determine the extent of his cognitive decline. At the meeting with the husband, Betty excused herself to be in another room. Alan was socially appropriate, appeared to be reading the business section of the newspaper, and took a phone call while the care manager was there.

The care manager engaged Alan in a conversation about current business news and Alan gave vague answers indicating that he might be having problems integrating new information. Later into the interview he became flirtatious, and the care manager terminated the evaluation when she became uncomfortable, and then met privately with Betty.

The care manager scheduled to meet with Betty the following week and at that time encouraged Betty to speak with Alan's neurologist about the behavior problem and inquire about medication that might address Alan's loss of inhibition. She explained that some areas of Alan's brain might have been damaged by the stroke and could be responsible for his inappropriate sexual expression.

The care manager continued to work with Betty regarding ways to manage the inappropriate sexual behavior through respectful and dignified diversional tactics and calm redirection.

After several weeks, Alan's neurologist was able to subdue Alan's sexual aggression through an antianxiety medication, and the care manager began to explore with Betty how her needs for sexual intimacy could be redefined so that she and Alan might be able to enjoy each other's intimate company by including different forms of touch in everyday routines such as holding hands, massage, and cuddling.

Months later Betty made an appointment to meet with the care manager in the office with her adult children. The presenting problem was that Alan enjoyed walking his dog in the evening and became lost. The adult children expressed an equal amount of concern for their father as well as their mother's health and safety. Betty was still exhausted, and Alan didn't want Betty to leave him alone. After a reevaluation of the situation, the care manager recommended an adult day program where Alan could attend during the day and a spousal support group Betty could attend one evening a week. An arrangement was also made for an attendant to come to the house in the evening to walk the dog with Alan while Betty attended a weight reduction group.

Several weeks later Betty called saying how grateful she was for the care manager's creative suggestions and that the quality of her life and marriage was much improved.

The case of Betty and Alan demonstrates the importance of sexuality through the years and how the care manager can be helpful in addressing the abnormal as well as normal expressions of sexuality in late life. The care manager assisted by explaining to the family that a stroke can damage areas of the brain affecting sexuality and referring them to resources that assist with understanding how strokes affect behavior. The Family Caregiver Alliance Web Site at www.familycaregiver.org has fact sheets that can be downloaded and links to support groups. Encouraging appointments with a neurologist if necessary, and explaining that sexuality continues as a normal part of aging is useful for families.

The care manager must be comfortable with her or his own sexuality to be effective with couples who are dealing with sexual behavior.

RESEARCH IN LATE-LIFE COUPLES AND SEXUALITY

A new federally funded study by the University of Chicago helps to refute the notion that sex is only for the young. The study focused on people between the ages of 58 and 85 years in the United States. This was the most comprehensive study ever done on geriatric sex.[15]

The study included face-to-face interviews with 3005 men and women throughout the United States. The researchers also took blood, saliva, and other bodily fluid samples to test hormone levels. They also tested these senior people's senses to see if they could enjoy sex.[16]

The results of the research study were the following:

- Seventy-three percent of the people aged 57–64, 53% of the people aged 63–75, and 26% of those aged 75–85 reported having sex with their partner in the previous year, and the most active said they engaged in sexual activity at least two to three times a month.
- Women were less likely than men to be sexually active, though they also lacked a partner more than the men.
- Healthy people were twice as likely to be sexually active.
- Half the people having sex reported one problem: in men 37% said erection trouble, in women 43% said low desire and 39% said vaginal dryness.
- Of the people that have discussed the topic of sex with their doctors only 22% of men and 38% of women have consulted their doctor after turning 50.

Needs for sexual expression and intimacy continue through late life and should not be ignored or seen as problematic. Many factors affect change in late-life sexuality such as disorders of the vascular, endocrine, and neurological systems; depression; adverse effects of medication; substance abuse; chronic and acute illness ranging from arthritis to incontinence; performance anxiety; obesity; emotional reactions; and stress. Problems having sex can also be a warning of other serious problems such as diabetes, infection, or cancer. If these problems go untreated, many people can fall into depression and social isolation. This subject has been taboo for a long time and has resulted in a reluctance for seniors to talk about sexual problems with each other and with their doctors. Also, many doctors are embarrassed to bring up this subject in consultations. Physicians in geriatric practices should especially consider this problem with senior patients.

Sex needs to remain an important point of interest for the care manager. It should be something that is encouraged and not looked upon as being a taboo subject, but when indicated, an important aspect in a comprehensive assessment. The care manager should maintain an unbiased, nonjudgmental attitude and provide education and guidance to older couples for whom sexual difficulties are an issue.

SPOUSAL IMPOVERISHMENT

A Medicaid program designed to help couples pay for long-term care is available nationwide. Typically it is administered through the department of social services like other Medicaid programs. This program takes a "snapshot" of the finances of the couple when one of them has been admitted to a skilled nursing facility. It then evaluates the financial situation of the couple and limits their financial liability for the institutionalized spouse (the spouse in the skilled nursing facility). This allows the community spouse (the spouse living at home) to maintain the home and a reasonable lifestyle.

The laws vary from state to state regarding allowable amounts, and some states do not offer the benefit. In 2008 the community spouse may keep as much as $104,400 without jeopardizing the Medicaid eligibility of the spouse who is receiving long-term care. The least amount a state may allow a community spouse to retain in 2008 is $20,880. The amount varies from state to state and will change over time. An elder law attorney familiar with local legislation (Naela.org) or a health insurance counseling assistance provider (Hicap.org), frequently found through a local Area Agency on Aging, will be a useful resource for current allowable amounts.

This means the community spouse does not have to give up everything he or she has to take care of the institutionalized spouse.

There are situations when the community spouse can have a higher level of resources. For example, each spouse can have a prepaid burial fund. This is one good way to spend some of the excess money if necessary.

To qualify for the benefit requires an application be completed. To obtain the benefit also requires 5 years of financial records

be proven and a face-to-face meeting with a worker at the department of social services. Additionally, working with a skilled nursing facility social worker to enroll in the program will be the most efficient way to accomplish this task.[16]

The role of spousal caregiving presents its own unique challenges. The care manager is critically instrumental in helping spouses and families cope with the complexities of care and giving them the confidence to manage circumstances that at first might appear beyond their control. How couples react to caregiving depends on many contributing factors such as their unique history; cultural, economic, and gender preference issues; temperaments of the individuals involved; as well as the problems inherent in the condition of the frail partner. All of these factors must be considered in the care manager's approach and continued relationship with the couple.

The care manager must balance the needs and wants of the couple and family, weaving a therapeutic and instrumental service within the confines of the standards of practice and ethical considerations of the geriatric care management profession to achieve the desired outcomes. The care manager needs to take a "whole family" approach with aging couples, responding to the needs of the couple and the family, rather than simply meetings the needs of the initial client referral.

REFERENCES

1. Yarrow P, Marcus L, MacLean MJ. Marriage and the elderly: A literature review. *Canadian Journal of Social Work Education.* 1981;7(2):65–79.
2. Kelley HH. Marriage relationships and aging. In: March JG (ed.-in-chief), Fogel RW, Hatfield E, Kiesler SB, Shanas E (volume eds.). *Aging: Stability and Change in the Family.* Toronto, ON: Academic Press; 1981:275–300.
3. Cumming E, Lazer C. Kinship structure and suicide: A theoretical link. *Canadian Review of Sociology and Anthropology.* 1981;18(3):271–282.
4. Depner CE, Ingersoll-Dayton B. Conjugal social support: Patterns in later life. *Journal of Gerontology.* 1985;40(6):761–766.
5. Connidis IA. *Family Ties and Aging.* Toronto, ON: Butterworths Canada Ltd, 1989.

6. Atchley RC, Miller SJ. Types of elderly couples. In: Brubaker TH, ed. *Family Relationships in Later Life*. Beverly Hills, CA: Sage; 1983:77–90.

7. Brubaker TH. Responsibility for household tasks: A look at golden anniversary couples aged 75 years and older. In: Peterson WA, Quadagno L, eds. *Social Bonds in Later Life*. Beverly Hills, CA: Sage; 1985:27–36.

8. Marcus L, Jaeger V. The elderly as family caregivers. *Canadian Journal on Aging.* 1984;3(1):33–43.

9. McAuley WJ, Jacobs MD, Carr CS. Older couples: Patterns of assistance and support. *Journal of Gerontological Social Work.* 1984;6(4):35–48.

10. Fitting M, Rabins P, Lucas MJ, Eastham J. Caregivers for dementia patients: A comparison of husbands and wives. *Gerontologist.* 1986;26(3):248–252.

11. Kraus AS. The burden of care for families of elderly persons with dementia. *Canadian Journal on Aging.* 1984;3(1):45–51.

12. Johnson CL. The impact of illness on late-life marriages. *Journal of Marriage and the Family.* 1985;February:165–172.

13. Zarit SH, Todd PA, Zarit JM. Subjective burden of husbands and wives as caregivers: A longitudinal study. *Gerontologist.* 1986;26(3):260–266.

14. Yesavage JA, O'Hara RG. The geriatric depression scale: Its development and recent application. In: RM Torres, ed. *Principles and Practice of Geriatric Psychiatry.* 2nd ed. New York, NY: John Wiley & Sons; 2002.

15. *American Care Manger Monthly Newsletter.* September 2007. Available at http://www.american caremgrs@aol.com. Accessed September 12, 2007.

16. http://www.elderllawnews.com Accessed November 2, 2007.

CHAPTER 8

Working with Adult Aging Siblings

Cathy Jo Cress and Kali Cress Peterson

The sound of siblings performing together brings music to many ears. We have the Beach Boys, the Dixie Chicks, the Allman Brothers, the Bee Gees, Stone Temple Pilots, AC/DC, and Los Lonely Boys. There were 11 Bachs composing music. Tommy and Jimmy Dorsey changed the swing era of the 1930s and '40s with their bands, while the McGuire sisters sang. Glen Miller and his brother Herb both had incredibly popular orchestras in the same era. Often siblings in a band share a contentious relationship, but what the audience sees is that sibling connection translated into a musical link. The siblings grow up in the same house, hear the same music their parents play, and start playing instruments at the same time.

Most of their lives siblings get along through thick and thin. The Dixie Chicks twin sisters steadfastly stuck together when President George Bush's country-western fans burned their CDs. Their group was almost destroyed because group member Natalie Maines said she was embarrassed to be from Bush's home state of Texas, voicing her opposition to the war in Iraq. What we see is that the sibling connection translates the similar genetic code into a creative musical splicing. Siblings have that same genetic song to sing, perhaps like the whales that sing eerily beautiful genetically coded whale songs that scientists believe are like auditory fingerprints.

Siblings in a band or group sometimes suffer sibling rivalry. The Wilson brothers, who made up most of the Beach Boys, didn't speak for many years. John and Tom Foggerty of Credence Clearwater Revival didn't talk, even as death claimed one of them. The first murder in history, according to the Bible, was Cain killing Abel. Nature can show us gory cases of sibling rivalry. As baby sharks develop in the mother's womb the largest baby devours the rest of the progeny to ensure that he or she has enough food resources. The first baby eaglet kills all subsequent eaglets by pushing them out of the nest, ensuring its own survival, as the mother will bring all the food to her or him.

Sisters live in history and fiction as loving supports to the passages of time and jealous manipulators of their beautiful siblings. *Little Women*, *Sense and Sensibility*, *Gone With the Wind*, *The Color Purple*, and *The Blind Assassin* give us the fictional representations of the feminine side of both sibling rivalry and the steadfast support of sisters to each other and their family.

At every new developmental phase of the life cycle, the family is the main unit of service. Within the family, the workhorse unit is the sibling dynamic. Care managers have an interest in siblings because they are the strongest alliances in the aging family. Aging adult children call upon the care manager to help with the care of a parent. Those adult children hold great power in the family. Siblings can align against each other to stop another sibling from doing something. For example, if one sibling wants to keep the mother home and the other three siblings don't, the three can line up together against the fourth sibling. What follows are usually family quarrels, legal action by elder law attorneys, and the mother not getting the care she needs when she needs it.

Old–old siblings are a great source of comfort to each other. A care manager can connect an older person with a sibling for visits over the telephone, through letters, in person, or via technology and offer the elder great solace in old age. Older siblings can share reminiscences plus day-to-day comparisons because it is the longest relationship any of us have in life. They have the amazing ability to be both the microscope and a telescope of time. Because siblings have been little studied, especially old–old siblings and young–old siblings, this chapter offers the care manager insight into how the central dynamic of the aging family works and how the care manager can use those sibling dynamics to better care for the aging clients and their family.

WHAT IS A SIBLING?

A sibling is a brother or sister, and this implies a blood relationship. It takes two or more in a family to have a sibling relationship. Sibling relationships can take the form of brothers, sisters, brothers and brothers, and sisters and sisters. Being a sibling is not just a biological fact but also a socially constructed relationship. Researchers Treffers and colleagues have developed up to 26 categories of sibling relationships. Marion and Edgar Head came up with nine categories including full sibling, half, step, and adopted, foster and residential agreements. These were

based to some degree on common genes, common history, family values and culture, and common legal status.[1]

Cicirelli, a major writer in the field of siblings, says that most research has been done with full siblings, ignoring half siblings, stepsiblings, adoptive siblings, or fictive siblings. Fictive siblings are siblings that have been adopted into the family as siblings based on desirability and customs rather than on the basis of blood ties or legal criteria. Most cultures have always had fictive siblings. Think of the concept of blood brothers. In some cultures these fictive siblings are sentimental or honorary yet have all the privileges of full siblings.[2] Gay and lesbian families at times create sibling ties with friends.

Cicirelli believes that a better way to look at siblings and families is from the point of view of kinship—looking at the family through the anthropological lens. With the breakdown of the nuclear family in our culture and the growth of single Mom- or Dad-led families, the concept of extended families is a better model. A kinship perspective seems to fit the family of this century best. This perspective takes in the fact that fictive siblings from the neighborhood and cousins in minority families are often seen as siblings and defined as family. In essence kinship is a better way to examine families because in many families the full biological family members are joined by half siblings, stepsiblings, and adoptive siblings. These stepsiblings and adoptive siblings are connected through the biological parent of the reconstituted family, with whom they share no bloodline.[3] We are moving away from the focus of the vertical parent–child ties and horizontal adult ties of married heterosexual partners of the nuclear North American family. We are looking at siblings through the microscope of social networks where individuals and kin relate to each other over the course of life. Here the study of siblings enlarges into the exploration of family relationships.[4] Families have a contracting and expanding border, and many types of siblings make up this periphery.

This chapter uses Cicirelli's definitions of the various sibling relationships. Traditional full siblings are two individuals who have both biological parents in common. Half siblings are individuals who have one parent in common. Stepsiblings are individuals who have no biological parents in common, but are linked through marriage of biological parents (as in blended families following divorce and remarriage). Adoptive siblings are individuals whose sibling status is established when a child is legally adopted into a family. Fictive siblings are nonfamily members who have been accepted into the family as siblings based on desirability or custom rather than on the basis of blood ties or legal criteria.[5]

Sibling relationships are very important in the study of the family. Eighty percent of the population spends one third of their lives with their siblings, and a 1998 general social survey reported that 96% of American adults have at least one sibling.[6] In spite of their importance to the family in general and aging in particular, the study of adult sibling relationships is a relatively new field. Yet understanding the aging family takes comprehending this lifelong, key part of the aging family.

FAMILY SYSTEMS THEORY AND SIBLINGS

Family systems theory treats the family as a set of separate relationships that are interconnected, and then uses this perspective to try to understand how the family functions. Siblings are a subsystem among other subsystems like parent–child and marital subsystems. Over time, these other systems affect the sibling subsystem, and the sibling subsystem affects them. The uniqueness of the sibling subsystem is that other subsystems may dissolve because of death (grandparents and parents), but the sibling subsystem lives on; it is the longest surviving subsystem. It only breaks down when the family of origin dissolves. The sibling subsystem also moves out into a highly autonomous system in adulthood, away from the interdependent family of origin. These sibling subsystems can be dyads, triads, or larger groups. They wield large power in the family by aligning and exercising their clout based on alliances that meet their needs. Just as the siblings may be able to get together and weasel the mother into lining up with them and getting the father to allow them to go to the movies when they are young, they have similar power in adulthood. A dyad of siblings may align to get the father to leave another sibling out of his will or convince the mother to go into assisted living against the wish of another weaker sibling. They are thus one of the most powerful subsystems within the family system.

What Makes Siblings So Important?

Sibling relationships have the same gene pool. The similar genetic code gives us an inner feeling of coherence. Genealogy views shared genes as invaluable for lines of social descent and shared biological parentages. This common sibling gene pool has come to be a symbol of the naturalness and rightness of biological bonds. This gives us a feeling of inner coherence. Faced with family fragmentation through divorce and the breakdown of the nuclear family, these days many people feel risk and uncertainty. Siblings and their similar genes offer certainly and sameness in a world that becomes more unknown as we move physically away from our family as we age, and farther away from the nuclear family, and the very definition of the family begins to break down its own meaning.[7] Class and race are also something full siblings share. Siblings have the same cultural heritage. They can say of their family's culture that they all came from the family that celebrated Christmas on Christmas Day, or that their mother only made cakes from scratch, or that their parents paid at least $25,000 for each daughter's wedding because the family believes in big family celebrations when joining two families in matrimony.

Beyond the shared cultural background and genetic makeup, siblings share the same secret language and common memory. They have an intimate knowledge that only siblings who were children together will know. For example, all the siblings in a family will know that icy bridge that scared them all when they had to walk over it at age 4 or 5 to get to school and kindergarten. In addition, siblings can share this secret language with each other through a shorthand that might be just a glance or a secret word. They may have different personalities and be separated by years, but this special language and common symbols give them a unique tongue that only siblings can really understand. This ability to reference certain events through one word or gesture comes from their collective life together as children.[8] Gloria Steinem reminisced, "I can say 'Vernon's Ginger Ale' to my sister, and she will understand."[9] Or it could be a sibling saying, "We crawled underneath the coffee table," and the other siblings will know this is the charged phrase for their mother having yet another baby. As adults age there can be huge gaps and distances, but this pivotal beginning of life and intimacy gives them the ability to revive their relationship even if separated by years and miles.

Sibling relationships are also unique because they are the only kind of relationship that lasts a lifetime. In this way they bear witness to all your changes over your lifetime, yet in contrast, siblings age with you as peers. They are also our breeding ground for intimacy and how we deal with it. As little children, we spend more time with sisters and brothers than anyone else. We learn sociability and intimacy by playing with them: joking, bickering, hitting, and making up. This anchors a deep part of our attitudes about social relations with someone very close to us, setting the stage for partners as we grow up. With the divorce rate skyrocketing, there is little attention paid to this petri dish for intimacy—siblings and the very close relationship between them.

Siblings give us the first lesson in sameness and difference as well. Siblings are concurrently individuals yet one in a series. This sets up the conundrum of being separate yet staying connected. Freud said that we wish to belong and be part of the collective, yet this is at odds with our desire to be an individual, unique and free from anyone, especially our families. The social forms of sibling relationships move us toward a need for connections, affinity, and sameness yet at the same time forge our desire for separation, autonomy, and difference from others. Social scientists feel that this connection and separateness born of the sibling relationship creates the dynamic structures of alliance and support and rivalry and conflict that buttress our intimate relations and subconscious social understandings throughout life.[10]

Sibling relationships are also voluntary rather than obligatory, especially as we age and no longer live in our original family. It is a dynamic relationship rather than a static one. This voluntary nature surfaces with age, especially in caring for a parent. Many siblings complain that another sibling was not helping enough, illustrating the voluntary nature of sibling relations.[11]

The uniqueness of a sibling relationship also draws on its ascribed role rather than its earned role. A person is a sibling regardless of any achievement—it can't be earned. It just is because of birth. You remain a brother or sister for life no matter what. It also has the unique quality that in old age, no matter what arguments have separated you or years have dimmed your relationship, a sibling bond can be lit up again with ease, all because it never goes away. It is in your blood.[12]

A relationship with sisters and brothers gives a lateral rather than a vertical psychodynamic perspective. This is very different from the hierarchical perspective you get as a child looking up to your parents. We learn to be deeply affected by our siblings' perspectives instead of just our parents'. Juliet Mitchel, a researcher in siblings, says that those voices we hear in our heads saying "Don't do this" or "Do that," are most often our siblings' voices and not our parents'. Your brother or sister knew you as you really were as a child. They knew the innocent, vulnerable, true self that was there before you assumed the mantle of adulthood—that Teflon protective coating that sealed you when you took on the guise of an adult. Your brothers and sisters have access to the core of you, the person you were before you met your spouse, had children, and joined organizations. They know your secrets, the inner self you stopped showing to the world as an adult.[13]

What Continues Through Early Childhood to Adult Sibling Relationships

The quality of our childhood sibling relationships is thought to continue in our adult sibling relationships. It is believed that our learned patterns of cooperation in early childhood are the cradle for sharing responsibilities in parent care. In addition, attachments that people have with siblings in middle and old age are based on differential parental affection in childhood, early attachment styles, and early interaction patterns based on sibling birth order. The expectations developed in the family in early life foster interactions with siblings over the lifespan and into old age.[14] Patterns of contact with siblings change as we become adults, with many siblings having much less interaction as they marry and start their own families.

Sibling roles are another pattern that continues into later sibling life. Roles are guidelines for socially appropriate behavior. They are usually given to us by parents; we learn them implicitly through telegraphic glances, shakes of the head, or hugs. Roles serve to organize young families and serve to keep domestic chaos at bay. "You take care of your brother after school because I have to work," says the single mother. Without her teenage daughter's role as caretaker, the family could not run smoothly, and children would be left to fend for themselves. Roles also allow the family members to know where they belong in the family activities. The family is the stage, and the role each member takes is part of the family drama. Roles also shape personalities and identity. Siblings begin with large roles, such as gender, with expectations of either masculine or feminine behavior. For example, girls are to be sweet and caring, which obviously endures into later life when women are perceived as better caregivers to their parents than brothers. Roles are also affected by the size of the family, how close in age the siblings are, if a parent was ill, if there was a divorce, or if there was a single-parent family. Roles continue into adulthood, and siblings continue to play out these roles on the family stage, even when the act has significantly changed. A sibling role of "Miss Full Charge" who bosses siblings around because the parents were alcoholics and not there to guide the younger children may not work in later adulthood. If the siblings are all facing parent care in midlife, and they need cooperation to care, not bossiness, the role of Miss Full Charge will not work. Roles do carry over in sibling relationships, but often they inhibit growth and change.[15]

How Sibling Relationships Change in Early and Middle Adulthood

Sibling relationships have remained invisible in adulthood, as scholars have largely studied the nuclear family, not the broader kin relationships where siblings lie in adulthood. By scholars and family researchers focusing on the core nuclear family they have not seen the family panorama that includes adult siblings with no children; adult siblings who never marry; adult siblings who are fictive, half, or stepsiblings, and those who are gay and lesbian. Although transparent to family scholars and practitioners, siblings have a rich life in the family and a place that care managers need to see as well.[16]

Early and middle adulthood is a time when sibling relationships make a major change. Young adult brothers and sisters take the siblings' tasks of nurturing, caretaking, and teaching of childhood and transform them into meeting the needs of spouses and children.[17]

The frequency of contact that we have with siblings changes as we enter adulthood. As we become independent adults our contact changes from intimate contact in the shared living arrangement of a family to contact at a distance maintained by telephone, e-mail, letters, and periodic visits. Contact is less in middle age when we have our own family but increases again as we become old. Cicirelli refers to Bedford in describing this lifetime pattern of sibling contact as an hour-glass, bulbous in childhood, thin in middle age, and bulbous again in old age. These contact patterns can act like rubber bands and be elastic.

Cicirelli believes that affection does not waver and feelings of closeness increase even if proximity diminishes in late adolescence and adulthood, and that those feelings increase as we age more.[18]

Oldest siblings seem to have more contact over the range of adulthood. Adult siblings are more important to unmarried siblings than they are to married siblings. Unmarried siblings have greater contact with their siblings during their adult life. Childless adult siblings have more active sibling ties, based on the interaction of aunts and uncles with nieces and nephews. Having a living parent alive increases contact with adult siblings. Living within a 300-mile radius increases contact and living long distance beyond that decreases contact as could be expected. African-American siblings, according to Cicirelli, saw their siblings less than non-white Hispanics or Mexican Americans. Asian Americans saw their siblings even less. Stepsiblings have contact much less than full siblings in adulthood. Sibling relationships in adulthood reflect the changing family. Siblings have contact over their middle years when they begin to have children themselves, and the cousins become playmates. This increases contact and a common interest that breeds interaction.

In the middle of the family life, the nuclear family (parents, spouses, and children) is called an inner circle of the family. Adult siblings revolve around this inner circle as a second tier of support with contacts coming from the give-and-take of the siblings' relationship with the expectation that there will be an equitable exchange. If the inner circle fails in the midlife family, the siblings can and are called upon to step into that inner circle, offering an increase of support if there is a decrease among the main players.[19] Siblings are like air mattresses. They can be pumped up at any time when you need to call upon them. They become dormant in adulthood and can be activated as needed.[20]

Theories Why Sibling Relationships Continue in Later Life

There are several theories why sibling relationships continue in later life. One theory is based on the norms that our parents teach us. Parents tell us all our life, "You should be kind and loving to your brother or sister," or "Depend upon your brother above anyone else." The second theory is attachment. Siblings feel comfortable in an attached relationship. They like to be with each other and feel happy when they are together and upset when they are separated. Attachment theory tells us that human beings can't survive without a warm, predictable attachment to another person. Early development cannot proceed normally without adequate attachment or contact, especially in the first year. Human beings will take what contact they can get, and they will attach themselves to their siblings, especially when the level of parental contact is not adequate. We all know the phrase *mother figure*. Baby brothers and sisters are often entrusted in part to older siblings, and thus this sibling's attachment begins in childhood and carries on into adulthood and old age.[21]

TYPES OF SIBLING RELATIONSHIPS

The traditional types of sibling relationships are defined in Exhibit 8-1.

Five other types of sibling relationships were identified by Connidis: intimate, congenial, loyal, apathetic, and hostile.

Intimate Siblings

Intimate siblings share devotion, psychological closeness, confidences, love, and empathy. They have frequent and consistent contact, offer emotional and instrumental support, and frequently consider each other best friends.

Congenial Siblings

Congenial sibling personalities are similar to the intimate sibling personality but to a lesser degree on all traits. They are less likely to be best friends, have daily contact, and be empathetic.

Exhibit 8-1 Types of Siblings

Traditional full siblings—Two individuals who have both biological parents in common

Half siblings—Individuals who have one parent in common

Stepsiblings—Individuals who have no biological parents in common, but are linked through marriage of a biological parent of one to another biological parent of the other (as in blended families following divorce and remarriage)

Adoptive siblings—Individuals whose sibling status is established when a child is legally adopted into a family

Fictive siblings—Nonfamily members who have been accepted into the family as siblings based on desirability or custom rather than on the basis of blood ties or legal criteria

Loyal Siblings

Loyal siblings are not completely loyal to each other but are loyal to the idea of being siblings. They illustrate intimacy at a distance. They have a strong sense of family and obligation to each other that is reconstituted during a crisis, but these filial obligations subside when things go back to normal. Loyal siblings are an example of siblings being like an air mattress.[22]

Apathetic or Indifferent Siblings

According to Cicirelli, some adult siblings have little or no contact and are indifferent to each other. They are neither positive nor negative but apathetic, indifferent, or disinterested. Siblings who are apathetic only represent 5–15% of siblings, and there is not much research to indicate the roots of this category. However, it can be intuited that wide age spacing, geographic separation, and failure to develop attachment early may all buttress this adult sibling category.[23]

Hostile Siblings

Hostile is most often used as the descriptive term for this last category of late adult sibling relationship. Hostility, violence, and aggression in siblings, according to Cicirelli, are relatively rare. We can look to Cain and Abel as examples or even to the brothers in *East of Eden*. Cicirelli points out that a good portion of the conflict among siblings in adult and late life that emerges is between stepsiblings and half siblings. Sibling rivalry, treated in a coming section, is a part of this sibling category.

LATE-LIFE SIBLINGS

In later life adult siblings change again and once again reflect the bulbous form of the hourglass. Where the immediate needs of their growing family subside as their chil-dren become adults, siblings in old age reach back out to each other. However, because this is a different act on the family stage they use the deep connections learned in early childhood in different ways to have increased contact and intimacy. The losses of old age can be filled in by sibling relationships. Siblings in later life have four important positive tasks regarding each other: emotional support, reminiscence and the resolution of sibling rivalry, aid and direct services, and well-being.

Positive Aspects of Adult Sibling Relationships in Aging

The relationships of siblings in old age are generally egalitarian. Although power and status differences exist between brothers and sisters and between their various relationships (full, half, step, adoptive, fictive) the majority of aging siblings have an acceptance of each other that allows them to relate as equals. This egalitarian relationship is horizontal rather than vertical (as with a parent–child relationship) for all of the siblings' lives. Siblings in this relationship are relatively equal in power and sociability. Of all family relationships, this most resembles friendship across most of the lifespan and much more so in old age.[24]

Emotional Support

Providing companionship and emotional support is an important function over a sibling's entire lifespan. The phrase "Like a brother" or "My sister in my sorority" captures the cemented closeness that siblings can have. According to Connidis,[25] there are many parallels between emotionally close siblings and friends. Both are age peers, play a broad range of roles, have access to each other, and the relationship is mostly egalitarian. It contains social ability and lacks obligation. The difference is that a friendship is voluntary, while a sibling relationship is ascribed.

Despite reduced contact with their siblings, older siblings report feeling closer to their siblings than younger siblings. In addition older siblings serve as confidants to their siblings in old age. Cicirelli reports that having a sister and having a parent were significant factors in sibling affection.[26] Living closer to the siblings is related to positive feelings about siblings. Living closer to siblings and having increased face-to-face contact increases sibling emotional closeness. Stepsiblings or half siblings were less close. Disruption of the original nuclear system through divorce or death appears to have more negative effects on the sibling relationship over the entire lifespan into old age.

Siblings offer emotional support by bearing witness to the opening and closing of family stages.[27] They are there for marriages, births, and all the rituals that accompany them. In old age, siblings are there for widowhood and death, where they not only participate in the rituals but also are incredibly emotionally supportive through these losses that reflect transitions in old age.

Siblings in old age are rocks to cling to during the many losses in aging. Siblings are generally emotionally supportive during the decline of the parent and are generally supportive during and after the loss or the death of the parent. Siblings are emotionally supportive through the life transition of widowhood. In a 1992 study, Connidis reports that 40% of all comments made by divorced and widowed respondents refer to the strong support they received from their siblings.[28] She quotes respondents as saying, "You don't mind them knowing what you've gone through," speaking about siblings, noting the intimacy that still exists. Siblings are able to build on past closeness to come to the aid of siblings during these life transitions and

losses. Again this is a good example of the sibling relationship as an air mattress, pumped up during death and divorce just when the other sibling needs it.

Closeness in later life does not always require a physical presence. Cicirelli contends that sibling emotional ties in old age are not so much from direct interaction but from memories and the awareness and existence of siblings.

Sibling contacts and sibling activities seem to center around social functions, many times with family. Beyond the family rituals mentioned earlier, the most frequent sibling activities reported were reunions and happy family activities. This was followed by various recreational activities where siblings were involved such as shopping, church, and outdoor and home recreational activities.[29]

If siblings are single women, then the largest part of their companion network is their siblings. Single persons who have a sibling nearby are ranked next to friend as the strongest tie in their companion network. Childless older people list siblings as their companion of choice as well, as reported by Connidis. If you are single and childless in old age, a sibling will probably be your companion of choice.[30]

Late-Life Sibling Reminiscence and Healing Old Sibling Rivalry

The major avenue of communication with elderly siblings comes through reminiscence. Life review, which is a very useful skill of a care manager with the aging family, is another of the four tasks of siblings identified in later life. Life review or reminiscence appears to be both a way to better adjust to old age and to also heal the wounds of early childhood. During reminiscence in later life people analyze, evaluate, and reinterpret their lives in relationship to present events, values, and attitudes. Robert Butler hypothesized that this life review gives us the ability to resolve old conflicts and reach resolution in old age. Siblings are a major part of this resolution. Because our siblings share such a long history with us—actually our longest—reminiscence is something they do at many points in the lifespan. Siblings in old age can use reminiscence to look at early sibling wounds in childhood and see them in the context of the here-and-now. As this is the last stage of life, heralding death, siblings can take this sword of Damocles and through reminiscence learn forgiveness for old gouges dug by sibling rivalry. Gold hypothesizes that sibling reminiscence in old age helped the older people put their current relationships with siblings into a meaningful context, helped them understand present events, and helped them evaluate the importance of sibling relationships. So, the old wound of "Mom loved you best" can be healed in part by the reminiscence of siblings in old age.[31]

Using reminiscence as a tool to heal old wounds may also be a key to solving parental problems. Brubaker suggests that bringing resolution to past sibling conflicts may be necessary to solve parental problems. He suggests that resolving sibling conflicts in a therapeutic setting may be a necessary first step to moving on and coming to terms with such aging filial issues as parental caregiving.[32]

Reminiscence by siblings in old age also gives old–old siblings comfort. Sharing recollections about childhood is a source of warm feelings to the eldest, and speaking about early life with the people who know it best—their siblings—allows older people to have a second feeling of that warmth whether originally real or imagined. Cicirelli tells us that reminiscence occurs more often with siblings than with their adult children. The

fewer remaining siblings in a family, the larger amount of reminiscence that occurs.

Sibling Aid and Direct Services

Among the direct services that young–old siblings provide is care for their aging parents, which is covered later in this chapter. Young–old siblings have to plan collaboratively and cooperatively to arrange or give direct care to their parents. Old–old siblings have the intention to give direct care to their siblings when needed; however, they are often beset by the same frailties of old age as their siblings and cannot provide care.

Another direct support where young–old siblings appear to be very helpful is the dissolution of the family home. Young–old siblings often have to help their parents sort through the memorabilia of a lifetime, family nontitled property, and then pack and move a family member. Moving is a care management task where the care manager can help the young–old siblings sort through the memories and delegate moving tasks to siblings, avoiding bruised brother and sister feelings and family fights. The care manager can then manage the move for the family or find resources in the continuum of care to make the move. In addition the care manager can assist the siblings to locate a place to move where the parent will be in the right level of care and in an economically feasible setting.[33]

A third direct service that young–old siblings appear to give is the support one sibling gives when the other sibling has a disability and needs care after the parents die. If another sibling is physically or emotionally handicapped and has been cared for by the parents, as the parents age they may be unable to care for that handicapped adult child any longer. At times there is always an assumption in the family that the task will fall to the other siblings. Many times this is determined by gender. At times this involves deathbed promises that tend to be honored. If parental expectations about the care of a handicapped adult sibling are not dealt with in therapy and discussed in some way, they may be a cause for sibling conflict.[34]

Siblings and Well-Being

Siblings contribute to their other siblings' well-being in adulthood and aging. This is especially true for sisters. Studies have indicated that having a married sister had positive effects on widows. Seeing a married sister frequently was the strongest predictor of a positive effect to widows. This was not found to be true of men. Cicirelli goes even further to say that the closer women over 65 felt to their sisters, the fewer symptoms of depression they experienced.[35]

Sisters are second only to mothers and daughters in their emotional support. Sister dyads report the greatest degree of closeness, support, acceptance, importance, and contact, and the least envy and resentment. It is also thought that in the five types of siblings noted in this chapter, sister–sister dyads in adulthood and old age report the greatest number of intimate types. Gender enters into this because women have been given the role of kin keepers in our society, especially among siblings.

Elderly men with sisters have been found to have a greater sense of emotional security than those without sisters. Women's emotional expressiveness plus this traditional role as nurturers and kin keepers appear to account for a sister being tied to well-being in old age. Gold found that dyads having a sister had greater involvement than brother dyads.[36]

What Aging Siblings Do Not Do

As they age siblings generally do not help with ADLs or IADLs because they themselves are aging and have similar problems. However, if they have siblings who were never married or who are childless, aging siblings will step up to the plate and offer that care if they physically can. Many things interact to stop aging siblings from giving care: It is not expected of the sibling; in other words, it is not a social norm. Aging siblings may live at a distance, being scattered by age and their own families, thus making day-to-day hands-on care impossible. In later life, many women have cared for elderly spouses, and when asked to care for elderly siblings may refuse because they are unwilling or unable to repeat this daunting task.[37]

Late-Life Siblings' Negative Roles

The positive roles of young–old and old–old siblings seems to outweigh the negative. However there are several areas where siblings appear to put roadblocks in their fellow siblings, lives in old age. These roles include conflicts in caregiving, conflicts due to ambivalence issues with stepsiblings, inheritance, parental remarriage, and sibling rivalry.

Midlife and Late-Life Siblings and Ambivalence

Siblings can be a source of paradox. For some, sisters and brothers are the people they love and whom they can't stand to be around. This ambivalence leads to competition, conflict, and rivalry existing at the same time as love, care, and support. Like the baby eaglets who might have survived had the first not pushed them to their death, siblings compete for their parents' resources, and this can be a source of rivalry in later adulthood.[38]

Conflicts with Stepsiblings

The misery of stepsiblings has played out in all cultures for thousands of years.

Cinderella's horrific stepsisters Drizella and Anastasia represent to us the theatrically mean things stepsiblings can do to each other. The fairy tale itself is meta-myth, shared by cultures all over the world for the trauma of remarriage for families and the suffering of stepsiblings and half siblings.

The term *stepparent* originally referred to a person who replaced dead parents. *Step* in Middle English means *orphaned* or *bereaved*. Historically, remarriages, like the king in *Cinderella,* resulted from the death of a spouse. However, in the 1970s divorce began to tower over death as a reason for remarriage. In this century we are caught between polarities of old and new mythology about stepsiblings. We have the wicked stepmother in *Cinderella* and the utterly wiggy stepmother in the *Brady Bunch,* where the maid, Alice, has to really run the show.

Remarriage, like the king's remarriage to the awful Lady Tremaine in *Cinderella,* is not always filled with nastiness. The dilemma for stepsiblings is this: are they the Brady bunch or just a bunch of children thrown together by circumstances? The effects of remarriage on the aging family means a plethora of steprelations, which negatively affect intergenerational ties.[39] Remarried parents provide less support for their adult children than continuously married parents.[40]

Stepsiblings share with full siblings a struggle for power and a need to balance rivalry with closeness in the family neither of them chose. In the world of their parents' original marriage, children's worlds were safe and tight. Once the remarriage takes place that safe tight place dissolves and the world is never the same again for stepsiblings.

The National Stepfamily Resources Center estimates that although approximately 70% of children live with their two original parents, about 23% live with their biological mother, 4.4% live with their father, and the rest with relatives.[41]

One of the roots of stepsibling conflicts is that they share no family history. When their parents marry, the children of each family come from two different cultures comprising differing customs, values, and family styles. In one remarriage, a young stepdaughter was reported to be horrified because the new stepmother used cake mixes when her real mother made cakes from scratch.

Another hallmark of stepsiblings is their instantaneous relationships. They haven't grown up with each from birth or taken the time to court each other as in a nonblood relationship. A third characteristic of stepsiblings is that they share the common experience of their original family. They share the trauma of their parents' split, the guilt that children seem to have, and the need to relieve themselves of that blame and guilt. How they do this, too often, is to turn that guilt and blame against the other stepsiblings, thus creating real areas of potential conflict with stepsiblings.

This type of conflict embodies different family cultures. In fact with the growing percentage of Americans divorcing, family disolution is so "normal" that blended families can be looked to as a map through uncharted territory. It is an "incomplete institution" with no agreed upon typical behavior and guidelines for solving the problems of family life.[42]

Another area of potential divergence is conflicting loyalties. There are three families: his, hers, and theirs. The stepsiblings have to make room for the present while clinging to their past, their traditions, and their loyalties. Stepchildren find it hard to compromise their beloved rituals, and this is often a source of conflict.

Another line of conflict is the fluid boundaries that stepsiblings grow up with. With the blended family, stepsiblings may be sharing rooms. With parents having joint custody, there may be a constant stream of characters off and on the family stage, with no stability or time to bond.

After being in one family for years and having set roles and set birth positions, in a blended family the youngest may suddenly become the oldest child: Miss Full Charge may be supplanted by an even bigger Miss Full Charge. Siblings may find it very hard to give up these positions and the power they wield in the family and conflict may arise out of this.

Families who are blended take up more space; siblings may lose their room, half of their room, or live on less allowances. Companionship becomes an enemy in many cases with children crowded together.

In the nuclear family, sexual activity outside the husband and wife is incest and taboo. In remarried families, because it is a new frontier in our culture, there are no ingrained taboos. You may have a 17-year-old girl and boy thrown together as stepsiblings, and there are no deeply ingrained rules to monitor that blending. Out of this can come sexual conflicts, especially during adolescence. These conflicts can often be major and explosive.

Stepsiblings as adults can suffer the repercussions of the blending of their families. They have a much more difficult time working together as a result of these wounds. When issues such as parent care and inheritance come up, stepsiblings can both be left out and leave themselves out as a result of not being seen as or feeling like a real part of the family. There appears to be little research on the plight of stepsiblings in midlife con-

flict, but with the surge in divorce that began in the 1960s, we can assume there are many families now suffering with stepsibling conflict in midlife.

Sibling Rivalry

The first murder recorded in the Bible had the bloody handprint of sibling rivalry. Cain, the older brother, was so angry at having to care for his younger brother Abel he posed the now famous question to his parents, "Am I my brother's keeper?" Cain became so enraged that he killed his brother. Cain and Abel's struggle has framed our view of sibling rivalry ever since. We see it through the lens of violence and grappling for power.

The roots of sibling rivalry many times grow from childhood. When siblings experience parental conflict when young, they are unable to direct their anxiety back at their mother and father and often redirect their own angry emotions back at their siblings. The sibling as a foil for angry parents is one root of sibling rivalry.[43]

Favoritism of a parent toward one sibling also seems to foster sibling rivalry. Parents' differential treatment is thought to be another plank in the sibling rivalry bridge. In its most extreme form parents can favor one child by pampering and praising that child and ignoring and punishing another. Rivalry can result in a downward spiral into aggression and violence. This favoritism in the form of greater maternal response and affection has been related to the favored and nonfavored siblings belittling each other, competing with each other, and demonstrations of aggressiveness, rivalry, and lack of affection.[44]

Looking in any family photo album or thumbing through a baby book can give you a snapshot of favoritism. The firstborn will have a museum collection of pictures, and his or her baby book will be filled with almost every first step. The second child has a smaller gallery of pictures and perhaps a less detailed baby book, and subsequent children may have no baby book and all. Go to any grandparent's home and you will see the walls plastered with the first grandchild with the others wedged in.

The last born child just might again have his own album and baby book as the last-born sibling is frequently the mother's favorite. Suitor and Pillemer analyzed mothers' favorites in later life and found they were emotionally closest to their youngest child, the last sibling.[45] Riggio finds in her research with siblings that sibling rivalry does not so much reflect sibling perception of each other but the parent's partiality toward siblings. She also found that this parental favoritism affects the frequency of adult siblings seeing each other if one sibling still lives at home and is deemed the favorite. The sibling who does not live at home may not visit the one who does because he or she may see the biased mother. She found that the main impact on sibling rivalry in adults from favoritism was emotional.[46]

One marriage and family therapist, Patti McDermott, postulates that sibling rivalry can begin even before a sibling is born. She believes that parents have expectations of their unborn children that fulfill unmet needs in themselves. For example, if parents did not feel they were smart, then they might have an expectation that their child will be so. They often have the same expectation for each sibling, thus pitting them subconsciously against each other to meet the parents' unmet need.

Flaring pains from parental favoritism in childhood can be reactivated at any time but especially around parental care in adulthood. Here sibling rivalry over the favoritism can turn into a conflagration once more.

Consecutive siblings and the replacement of a baby by a new baby is an age-old root of sibling rivalry in childhood. A child less than 3 years old does not have the capacity to be reasoned with, so parents cannot convince him or her to love the new baby. The young child feels frustration and anger at being usurped by the offending new infant. The anger can set up sibling rivalry for the rest of the child's life on a subconscious level.

Whether sibling rivalry exists between adult siblings has been debated among scholars and researchers in the field of sibling research. Cicirelli reports that there is a decline in sibling rivalry in aging siblings, and sibling rivalry tends to be low in adulthood and old age. However, based on studies and clinical interviews, Cicirelli hypothesizes that sibling rivalry in adulthood may be higher than anyone thought with little decrease in age. He reports that one study by Bedford reported that 71% of the adults reported feeling sibling rivalry at some point in their lives, and 45% reported feeling rivalrous in adulthood.[47]

Rivalry appears to be highest among brothers. Gold has stated that brothers are compared by parents and society much more than other pairs, especially sister–brother pairs.[48] Gold says that the fundamental development markers—who gets a tooth first, who walks first—are held up higher and louder in comparing brothers. This continues through all of life into who has the better job, bigger income, and more lavish house. She states in our society men are supposed to be achievement oriented, aggressive, and successful. So, this parental comparison may also breed brother–brother rivalry.[49]

Siblings who are classified as hostile and having strong negative feelings toward each other are also seen as having a considerable negative psychological involvement or preoccupations with the relationship. The characteristics of these relationships are resentment, anger, and enmity. Hostile sibling relationships represent only 11% of siblings.

Research indicates that working-class adult siblings are closer and more cooperative with less rivalry than middle-class siblings. Working-class adults are more likely to name a sibling as their best friend. It is thought that working-class families are more connected to extended families than middle class; thus, perhaps caring and connectedness are greater cultural values among working-class siblings, diminishing sibling rivalry. Middle-class families are thought to more highly value individualism and thus feel less obligated to one another. This leads to more conflict when siblings refuse to join in adult tasks such as parent care.[50]

Sibling Rivalry in Adulthood

Sibling rivalry can surface in adulthood around occupational differences. Adult siblings can reawaken sibling rivalry among themselves around time, money, and status in adulthood. Strain and bad feelings can erupt over circumstances from the past that allowed one sibling to advance, go to college, or have greater chances than the other siblings. These educational opportunities can result in the increased financial status of one sibling in later life. Siblings can revisit what they perceive as unequal attention by parents, thus bringing sibling rivalry to the fore of the family stage again.

This sibling guerrilla warfare can be counted in whose time matters more. Siblings with a higher-status occupation can look at another's employment as expendable and worthy of interruptions. This leads to expecting the "lesser trained sibling" to meet unpredictable parental family needs, such as parent care. "I am an attorney, and I can't just take time off from court, while you are a waitress, and you certainly have a more flexible schedule and can care for Mom," are typical statements heard.

The waitress who depends on tips really needs those working hours more than the attorney; thus the sibling conflict erupts again. This also creeps like blood poisoning into the relationship between female and male siblings. Women are often times homemakers and can be viewed by brothers who more typically work outside the home as having a job (or perhaps no job at all) where they can easily meet the parent's needs. Women and men who work at home, more prevalent today, are also vulnerable to this sibling rivalry.[51]

Favoritism in Sibling Rivalry

As stated earlier, flaring pains from parental favoritism in childhood can be reactivated at any time but especially around parental care in adulthood. Here sibling rivalry over the favoritism can turn into a conflagration once more. Wendy Lustbader states that caregiving siblings poke a thorn in the side of the "favorite" when they think that the mother or father is choosing them again around caregiving issues.[52] Lustbader states that what siblings do in reaction to perceived favoritism is retaliate by trying to load the majority of the parental care tasks on the favorite.

Another variation on this theme is when a nonfavorite sibling covets the role of favorite and takes on an overload of parental care, hoping to finally become that sought-after favorite. If parents or other siblings don't recognize this subconscious effort on the part of a seeking sibling, bitterness can arise and parent care can be impaired.

Lustbader also feels that favoritism of one sibling can rear its head in later life over who takes care of the money. If older parents choose one sibling as the money manager of their estate or assign them power of attorney, it can prove to siblings once again that their parents have greater love and trust in one sibling. Parents are usually unsuccessful at showing their other adult children that this choice had to do with money management skills. Indeed, it may not be financial skills but favoritism that led the parent to make this choice. Even if it is better skills with money, adult children remember their childhood hurts and call it favoritism. This usually buys into the fears of the adult children that this favorite will get a greater share of the inheritance.[53]

Sibling rivalry in adulthood connected to favoritism can fade in adulthood because siblings no longer live with their parents or each other.[54]

SIBLINGS AND PARENTAL CAREGIVING

There is an old saying that it takes one mother to care for 10 children yet 10 children cannot care for one mother. This is the picture we often see of midlife siblings and parental caregiving. One of the developmental tasks of siblings is parental caregiving, although few sibling groups are ever prepared for it.

Mid-Life Sibling Conflicts with Caregiving

Family dynamics, especially sibling conflict, are best understood looking over the entire life course. As young children, siblings are asked to care for other siblings or be cared for. In addition in the course of siblings' lives, they may be caregiving for their own children or caregiving for a spouse's parents. A sibling's conflict over participation in parental caregiving can be both a reflection of original family caregiving patterns (young siblings) or other subsequent caregiving of their own children (midlife and older siblings).[55]

Care managers and other professionals have primarily seen parental caregiving through the lens of the primary caregiver. We assess the burden of the primary caregiver and find needed support for the family member. But caregiving should also be seen through the prism of the entire family, and this takes in all the young–old caregiving siblings. We need to look at how other family members, such as siblings, stand in relationship to the primary caregiver and to the other family structures in providing care.

Carolyn Keith, in an article about family caregiving systems, pointed out that researchers who limit caregiving research to the primary caregiver risk underreporting of caregiving contributions of male caregivers. Such studies also leave out what caregiving means to other family members besides the primary caregiver. Keith also adds that to view caregiving only through the aperture of the primary caregiver gives us only one appropriate caregiving choice and may retard the development of other caregiving systems. We also too often look at caregiving in a hierarchical structure and only through the very Western "rugged individualism" point of view. We leave out the possibility of cooperative relationships, which are a much more female caregiving system, reflecting who gives most of the care—daughters.[56]

Sara Mathews has identified five different systems of caregiving that siblings take on when jointly providing parental care. She makes a point that siblings have a choice as to whether they want to take part in parent care or any filial activity. Membership in a family is involuntary, she points out, but whether you participate as an adult is your choice.[57]

Sibling Systems of Caregiving

Routine

This caregiving style allows the siblings to incorporate assistance for the elderly parent into the siblings' ongoing activities. This style means that a sibling is available and can do whatever needs to be done.

Back-Up

This style of care occurs when a sibling avoids giving emotional support or providing actual services but agrees to be counted on by the caregiving siblings to help when asked. These siblings can be counted on to do whatever they are asked to do. An example would be a daughter who lives locally and does not want to provide care but who is willing to spell her sister, who does provide care, when asked.

Circumscribed

The sibling style of caregiving is very predictable but has very narrow boundaries. This occurs when an adult son calls the mother once a week at a certain time but has no other involvement.

Sporadic

This style of caregiving is when siblings only render care to their parents at their own convenience. A daughter might invite her mother over on Sundays when it works out for the daughter but not on any regular basis. A son might take his father to the barber when he himself goes—and when he remembers to do it. However, he can't be counted on.

Dissociation

The sibling who takes on this style of caregiving cannot be counted on to help with a parent's care. In a family of five siblings, four of them may be providing care on a regular basis, but a son who has a long-standing conflict with the father may have distanced himself completely from the father and any care of his aging parent. This does not always mean that the sibling has disassociated him- or herself from the siblings, but it does mean they are disassociated from the parent and caregiving.

Cicirelli tells us that there are stages in caregiving, and siblings enter the caregiving arena at any one of these stages. The first stage is the mother or father caring for the older spouse. There may be occasional help by the adult children, but the primary caregiver is the spouse. When the spouse or other parent becomes increasingly frail, ill, or dies, one or more adult children take over as the primary caregivers. Care at this point is usually done in the older parent's home. As the aging parent becomes mentally or physically more frail, a pattern of caregiving is set up among all of the siblings. When the parents' care exceeds the ability of the sibling system to render that care, usually one sibling takes the older parent into their home or places him or her in a long-term care facility. Cicirelli emphasizes the point that the stereotype of only one sibling as the primary caregiver is flawed. He feels that the problem has been that few systematic studies have been made to examine the caregiving contributions of the sibling system.[58]

Parental care appears to be shouldered mainly by daughters. According to sibling researchers Coward and Dwyer, there is a much higher rate of daughters providing care to parents than there is sons. The highest rate of participation of sons equals the lowest rate of participation of daughters.[59] Daughters are more likely to be the primary caregiver. Sisters share parental caregiving, and the division of labor tends to be equal between them, Cicirelli states, based on the sibling research of Sara Matthews. Matthews tells us that sisters are more likely to use the routine and back-up styles of caregiving. Pairs of sisters offer good parental support. This appears to be because caregiving tasks are culturally based on a gender-based role: women care for the family, and men fix things and handle money. Sisters take the greater burden in care of a parent even if they are employed. Brothers tend to use work as an excuse for not giving care. With long-distance care-givers, sisters reported experiencing more interpersonal conflict than brothers.[60]

Brothers who take part in parent care are less involved caregivers than sisters. Brothers were more likely to offer help that was sporadic or circumscribed. This brother-rendered help was also usually in the area of male domains, such as the parent's home or yard maintenance.[61] Brothers in a family are less likely to do their equal share of care and spend fewer hours in helping their elderly parents than sisters do. Yet when families consist only of brothers, the brothers appear willing to cooperate to meet the parents' needs. Cicirelli postulates that perhaps when sisters are not involved brothers can do what they see as female caregiving tasks.[62]

Lustbader states this gender-defined axiom: caregiving tasks follow gender roles (daughters change diapers, men change light bulbs). A daughter may ask her brother to help with care and may get the response that he is either unfamiliar with care or that it is women's work. Brothers are willing to handle tasks such as bill paying, driving parents to appointments, and expect their sisters to take care of the housework. Lustbader postulates that parents are part of the system that reinforces this. The mother may not ask a son to vacuum, but be angry with a daughter who did not do a good enough job on the rug. Such gender-based roles are deeply embedded in our society. A son's resistance to personal care tasks, toileting, changing diapers, and bathing may also be tied, according to Lustbader, to the societal sexual taboos of parent–son intimate contact.[63]

However, Sara Matthews postulates that if daughters are not available to do the care of a parent, the care often falls to the daughter-in-law. In addition, sons are less emotionally burdened by not taking part in the care of a parent and letting it go to the daughter. Brothers were found to devote less time to parent care and provide fewer services. Brothers also tend to meet their filial responsibilities without consulting each other, which is different from sisters who tend to work cooperatively. They do not mobilize a parent care system like sisters do. Brothers, in fact, wait for parents to ask them for help rather than engaging in "protective caregiving" that daughters tend to do. This is analogous to care monitoring of a care manager.[64]

Sibling Rivalry Around Parental Care

Parental care is a developmental stage in the lives of siblings that at times reawakens sibling rivalry. The family needs to reorganize itself to care for the parent, and if sibling rivalry is reactivated, this can hinder parental care. For example, when one daughter takes over the care of a parent and is not supported by the other siblings, old rivalries may return. If this midlife daughter was an older sister who bullied the younger siblings when they were children, this old wounding situation can be like a hot spot that reignites a forest fire of sibling resentment. This may play out by younger midlife siblings not stopping the sister from providing the care, but sniping at her by complaining she is not making the right decisions or is taking over the resources of their parents. This explodes into a struggle over how the parent care is provided.

Tonti reports that the most common brother–sister conflict is over splitting responsibility for the care of a parent. Brothers tend to be put in charge but at a distance, recalling gender bias in childhood. This sets off a great deal of frustration in the daughter who is stuck with the day-to-day hands-on care of the parents.[65]

Parental caregiving patterns are thought in part to be based on early patterns of cooperation in childhood. When conflicts come up it is thought that such conflicts reactivate early conflicts that arise phoenix-like from childhood ashes to muddle parent care co-operation among siblings.

SIBLINGS INTERACTING WITH FORMAL CARE SERVICES

Cicirelli sees that siblings have two ways of interacting with formal care services. One is mediating with formal health services on behalf on the parent when they remain at home, and the other is providing family support when the parent is in a long-term care institution. Of course, a third way is for siblings to work with a care manager who mediates with formal services both in and out of the home. Cicirelli's research indicates that the sibling who is the parent's main source of overall help, or what we call the main care provider, does most of the mediation activities. Brothers tend to mediate with male role services, such as attorneys and financial services. Sisters tend to mediate with healthcare vendors, such as geriatric care managers

Cicirelli has also studied decision-making beliefs and caregiving decisions themselves among siblings. He found that siblings making care decisions as a group make choices that better respect their parent's autonomy than a single sibling making decisions alone. He feels that a group offers checks and balances together to ensure the parent's view is respected.

So, any formal care service will be better able to represent the older person's autonomy if the decisions about involving such services were made through a group consensus involving young–old siblings. However, too many cooks spoil the soup, so there needs to be one family representative who will speak for the group.

Which Sibling Actually Gives Care?

Cicirelli believes that there are several aspects that determine which adult sibling is likely to give care to an aging parent. These factors are gender, proximity, sibling marital status, effects of sibling employment, coresidence with an elderly parent, sibling status, and level of impairment.

Gender

Gender is the red blinking light framing who provides parental care. Sisters bear the heaviest burden. In families with siblings of mixed gender, sisters provide the greatest care, with brothers giving help only occasionally. Only when there are no sisters and the care must be rendered by only brothers, do brothers take on care. Cicirelli states that most studies show that brothers caring for an elderly parent tend to seek more outside help, like a care manager. They actually provide a different type of hands-on help and abandon their caregiving role much sooner than sisters.[66]

There are few studies on the root of this, but it must be assumed that culturally and historically, women have been the helpers and the caregivers while men have not. When men do take on caregiving they assume tasks that are culturally assigned to males such as home maintenance, financial management, and transportation.

Lustbader ascribes men's avoidance of parent care as a cultural feeling of entitlement. She states that in our culture men come home from work, kick off their shoes, and feel entitled to do that. Women, on the other hand, feel culturally responsible to take care of these men and their parents, even when the women have worked the same amount of hours as the men. Women do not have that cultural sense of entitlement; they work, and then care for the parent and the husband plus the children.[67] Elderly women, many times widows, are the largest group of old–old siblings. Cicirelli hypothesizes that these older women's need for personal care may be largely answered by women (daughters, daughters-in-law, and sisters) tipping the gender scale. This is because of a cultural modesty and wish for women to be physically exposed only around other women. He also feels that a sex taboo in our culture prevents sons from giving intimate care to mothers, and that same taboo may stop mothers from asking.[68]

Proximity

The second factor that determines which sibling gives care is proximity.[69] Brody has found that the gender difference gets wiped out by distance, and siblings who care long distance are simply the brother or sister who lives closest. Studies in siblings seem to indicate that the sibling who gives care is the one closest.

Marital Status

Marital status is the third factor that helps to determine caregivers among siblings. It appears that adult siblings who do not have a primary family (widows, divorced, or never-married siblings) are most likely to assume parent care responsibilities. It has also been found that they receive less help from their other siblings.

Employment

The fourth factor that determines which sibling assumes parent care is employment. Brothers routinely use the excuse that they work and therefore cannot render parent care. Daughters, even if they work, assume the parent care responsibility. Daughters who were employed gave the same types of care as those who were not employed. In one study daughters who were employed reported that they have to give up their job 28% of the time, but it is very rare that a son gives up his job to care for a parent. Pairs of sisters seem to balance work and family very successfully. In a study of 50 pairs of sisters who cared

for an aging parent, Matthews found that when parent care was light, sisters, one working and one not, contributed equally to parent care. However, when parent care became heavy, because the parent was more impaired, the sister who worked contributed less, and the sister who did not work took over much more of the care.

Coresidence

Cicirelli's next factor in determining parent care among siblings is coresidence. He found that when the adult child lives with the parent in need of care, the rest of the siblings give less help. However, since all the caregiving tasks including household maintenance fall on the sibling who lives with the parent, the coresident sibling tends to be overburdened and in need of help. As noted in Chapter 4, "Assessing the Caregiver," coresidence is one of the indicators of elder abuse. The overburdened sibling care provider may resort to fiscal and physical abuse. As was pointed out in that chapter, if the caregiver lives with the parent, the care manager should assess the situation, looking for depression in the caregiver, especially depression that has reached the clinical level. The care manager also needs to do a psychosocial assessment, looking for a history of poor past relationships between the sibling who lives with the parent and the parent. The care manager should see a red flag if there is a history of violence between the sibling who is a coresident and the parent. In addition, coresiding siblings have been found to take fiscal advantage of the elderly parent. In fiscal elder abuse, the care manager needs to assess the coresiding sibling for a history of drugs or alcoholism, a history of sporadic employment, or a history of moving in and out over the lifetime.[70]

Sibling Status

Sibling status is another factor for the care manager to weigh in assessing sibling help with the parent. Unfortunately, there are almost no studies on this. However, the care manager could assume that the stepsibling or half sibling may give less help to the adult parent than the full sibling, especially if there is a history of a poor relationship and the parent gave little help to the stepchild or they had a distant or poor relationship when the stepchild was young. If the care manager sees that stepsiblings or half siblings are the adult children in the care system, the care manager should be alerted to wounded feelings from the past that may be a barrier to care of the elderly parent.

Impairment of the Aging Parent

Cicirelli's last factor that determines sibling caregiving is the level of impairment of the aging parent. He believes that the first stage of parent care is when the parent needs more help, as their care needs increase. He believes that all the adult children usually contribute at this stage. In the second stage of care when the parent's level of impairment becomes more serious, an adult daughter tends to step in as the principal care provider. Then, the load for the other siblings actually becomes lessened. At the third stage of impairment when much care is needed, Cicirelli cites a Matthews study where families tend to hire outside care, like a care manager, to lessen their load.

Cicirelli feels that siblings are fair and patient in general in assessing a sibling's excuses for not doing their fair share of care. He tells us that siblings generally justly assess the entire situation including employment, time, distance, and gender before making a judgment that a sibling is not doing their fair share. But he does state that once

that judgment has been made by other siblings, the sibling relationship suffers among all the siblings.[71]

STRESS AND BURDEN AMONG SIBLINGS IN PARENTAL CAREGIVING

Matthews and Rosner report that over 50% of all families report some conflict over parent care.[72] They also see that the root of the conflict can either be in the present or can hark back to rivalries or wounds from childhood. Sister and brother conflict in the here- and-now seems to rear its ugly head from filial responsibility: are the siblings doing their fair share? Matthews reports that in one study half the families reported conflict, and in most cases the clash occurred in childhood, long before the argument over who took on filial responsibility.[73]

Brody has noted that 50% of the strain over caregiving is made worse by sibling interactions while caring for a mother or father. In this study, 30% of the principal caregivers, 40% of the sisters, and 6% of the brothers reported strain. Friction appeared when the principal caregiver felt a sibling was not doing his or her fair share. It was exacerbated by a sibling's criticisms of another sibling's care of a parent. Main care providers reported these criticisms of their care made them feel guilty. In this study, most complaints came from sisters, who seemed to bear the brunt of the criticisms. In the Brody study brothers seemed not to be held responsible if they did not do their fair share. As the caregiving load increased so did the hue and cry of sibling complaints about each other.[74]

Brody again found that daughters rather than brothers experience the most strain in caregiving. If there is a local sibling, brothers experience the least of the strain and burden. If these siblings were long-distance care providers, the sisters felt the most burdens and the brothers the least. If a sibling lived at a distance, the sister not doing the care received the most complaints from the sibling primary care providers and felt the guiltiest. Judgments are most seriously levied against sisters in care. Brothers again got off the hook.[75]

Gender norms seem to also blind brothers to parental caregiving in their future. When they are called upon to step up to the plate, brothers feel strained and burdened because they feel this is not a "man's role."

When there is a single child doing the caregiving or when there are only brothers or only sisters in the care network, sons and daughters do not differ in terms of stress. But when a daughter enters a mixed-gender caregiving network, she suffers more caregiving stress and burden than the sons in the network.

CARE MANAGERS WORKING WITH SIBLINGS AROUND CAREGIVING

Care managers can now look at siblings as a rich and potent tool in working with aging families. They can also see them as a barrier to the care of an aging family member. But with the understanding that they create a barrier, care managers now have many tools at their disposal to help warring siblings come together to meet the care needs of an elderly parent.

Brody has noted that 50% of the strain over caregiving involves midlife sibling interactions around the care of a mother or father. In this study 30% of the principal caregivers, 40% of the sisters, and 6% of the brothers reported strain. Friction appeared when the principal caregiver felt a sibling was not doing his or fair share. The care manager can help to deliver higher-quality care to an aging adult by reducing conflict among siblings. One tool that a care manager needs to start with is a caregiver assessment tool (see Chapter 4). In the overwhelmed Ms.

Handy's case, the care manager, Ms. Helpmate, found that the family caregiver—the daughter, Ms. Handy—was so overwhelmed that she was about to place her father Mr. Wilson in a facility. By the care manager doing a caregiver assessment, psychosocial assessment, and a genogram, the care manager found that there were siblings who could be tapped for support. She arranged a family meeting and helped organize that care among the siblings. So, a potent care manager tool is a family caregiver assessment to identify the young–old siblings of the aging parent who might support the principal caregivers.

The Use of Family Meetings in Setting Up Caregiving Systems

Care managers can greatly enhance a family caregiving system through setting up a family meeting. Fair is hard in families, and sometimes fair just can't be achieved without some outside guidance, such as the creative work of a good care manager.

Family meetings can help a sibling who is the main caregiver voice feelings of being overwhelmed. Such a speaking out at a family meeting can help all the siblings understand that a caregiving system is much more fair than a hierarchical main caregiver. A family meeting can thus assist the brothers and sisters in dividing up the care more fairly. Lustbader lists the many reasons to have a family meeting involving siblings all connected to sources of unfairness in caregiving. A care manager should consider convening a family meeting if caregiving is being impaired by the following conditions:[76]

- The main caregiver sibling is too burdened
- When daughters are doing all the work
- When siblings are spending money rather than putting in time and effort, generating resentment among the siblings

- When sibling resentment is being generated for various reasons
- When one sibling counts his or her time as more valuable than another sibling's
- When long-distance care providers are involved, and there is friction between them and local siblings
- When favoritism rears its ugly head
- When inheritance is a sore point among siblings and impeding the care of an older parent

Lustbader suggests that the professional, in this case the care manager, phone each sibling before the family meeting to find out which sibling may have not done their share in the eyes of their siblings, what historic resentments are present from childhood between siblings, and how these resentments or rivalries may be preventing siblings from communicating and thus working together to help care for the parent.

Family meetings help siblings plan care collaboratively. Cicirelli's research tells us that siblings who work in partnership while making parent care decisions make better choices that respect the autonomy of the aging parents. So, a care manager encouraging a family meeting over parent care is really advocating for the older client.

By convening a family meeting a care manager can also explore grief in the siblings. Perhaps one brother is not doing his fair share because he has a difficult time seeing his father as he is now. If a care manager can assure the siblings that financial help for the other siblings doing direct care (as in the case of Ms. Handy) and not hands-on care for the parent is also valuable, the care manager may be able to invite that sibling into the caregiving fold.

Many family meetings originate from an inequity among young–old siblings in tasks that help the parents' care. A family meeting among siblings usually involves listing all the tasks that the family must complete to care for the parents. What will result from the meeting, it is hoped, is a task list delegating these jobs fairly among siblings, other family members, partners, and friends.

Referring Warring Midlife Siblings to Therapy

Using reminiscence, as a tool to heal old wounds between brothers and sisters may also be a key to solving parental care problems. As a family meeting is meant to solve problems in the present, it is not the appropriate setting to deal with old sibling issues that may be blocking parental care. However, as a care manager's main tool is using the continuum of care in the community, they should consider referring warring siblings blocking parental care to a marriage and family therapist who specializes in aging and has a background in reminiscence or a psychotherapist who has a similar background. As mentioned earlier, Brubaker suggests that bringing resolution to past sibling conflicts may be necessary to solve parental problems. He suggests that resolving sibling conflicts in a therapeutic setting may be a necessary first step to moving on and coming to terms with such aging filial issues as parental caregiving issues. The care managers who attempt using this technique themselves should be seasoned, highly trained in reminiscence, family therapy and elder mediation or have a degree in marriage and family therapy or psychotherapy.

Coaching Sibling Caregivers to Ask Siblings for Help

Once a care manager has identified other siblings that may be able to join a caregiving system, the care manager can help the main care provider or other siblings by using one-to-one coaching with the adult children on how to ask their siblings to participate in care. The communication between brothers around the care of a parent is usually impoverished. A care manager may have to coach a brother to ask for another brother's help. Mixed sibling systems seem to lean heavily on sisters, and sisters appear to accept that burden. The care manager may have to coach the sister to ask for help from other siblings, including often-reluctant brothers.

Care managers need to not only ask themselves who is the primary caregiver, but also who are all the players in the family caregiver system, which often is populated by many siblings. Seeing the caregiving structure as a system, not a top-down hierarchal army, helps care managers to see all the parts they can draw on to set up a successful family caregiving system for the older client. This takes using a genogram, and the Moranos suggests seeing the family system and its happy , bitter, and reluctant members.[77] Care managers should become fluent in psychosocial assessment and assessment tools like the genogram so they can find all the sibling actors on the family stage and whether their relationships are negative or positive to each other and their aging parents.

Care managers can enhance a family caregiving system, once multiple siblings are involved in care, by coaching siblings to understand the importance of thanking their siblings for helping out. Many times family members assume that because participating in family care is expected, no thank-you is warranted. As has been pointed out in this chapter, participating in a sibling system in later life is a choice. After a sister or brother has made the choice to help out, a care manager can coach siblings on how and when to thank their siblings. Good old-fashioned thank-you notes work fine, as do calls and e-mails. Family members may need that extra

push to see the intelligence of this civility, and the care manager can greatly enhance the family system by encouraging simple but heartfelt appreciation. Even in situations where one sibling is doing much more than other siblings, a simple acknowledgment such as, "I know I come do the bills, but that's about it, Sis. I just want to say a big thanks," can really help a sister appreciate a brother, who may not help as much but at least acknowledges her burden.

Care Managers Assessing a Sibling System of Care

Perceived favoritism of one sibling over another can ignite again in midlife around parental care. The care manager can intervene in the caregiving situation when that perceived favoritism affects the quality of a parent's care and the health of a family caregiver.

An adult child who is seen as the favorite by the other adult children can be perceived as chosen again during caregiving issues. In this case other siblings can "retaliate" just as they did when they were children. In this case the means of getting even can be loading the great majority of the caregiving tasks on to the favorite. This is an example of "Mom loved you best" wars, and the care manager should step in to lessen hostilities.

Stepping in can include a family meeting to look at each task and apportion all items more fairly. It can be speaking out in either the meeting or communicating individually with siblings through calls made by the care manager. It can include sending the family to a marriage and family therapist skilled in aging issues to work out the family history so that it does not negatively affect the present care situation. Again, using the caregiver assessment tool can reveal the inequality in tasks among siblings and give the care manager a place to begin this work with the midlife siblings.

Care Managers Working with Midlife Siblings Around Time, Money, and Status Issues

Care managers can also work with midlife siblings and parent care to prevent sibling guerilla warfare over time, money, and status. If the family history includes one or more siblings obtaining a higher education than other siblings, this can lead to status wars. When a sibling or group of siblings, as a result of their degrees, makes more money, has newer cars, or has a bigger house, words such as these are often heard: "My time is more valuable than yours," with the unspoken meaning of "So you have more time to take care of Mom." This can also be seen in female and male siblings who work at home, whether they are a housewife or a telecommuter. Their being "at home" more hours can be perceived by other siblings as them having more "time," when they may indeed not.

This can be determined in a family caregiver assessment and individual interviews with the sibling caregiving family. Again the use of a family meeting, individual coaching, referrals to marriage and family therapists (MFT) skilled in aging issues can be solutions to this problem. The care manager who is not an MFT or a psychotherapist should not be a therapist but an advocate for the older clients and the caregiver in the interest of increasing the quality of the older client's care. Deep psychodynamic sibling and family problems should only be dealt with by a care manger with an appropriate professional background.

Care Managers Working with Siblings Around Gender Issues

Gender, as you can see in this chapter, is the elephant in the living room of siblings and parent care. The daughter does the bulk of the care, most of the time unequally dividing the caregiving tasks among the brothers and sisters. Gender inequality is rooted in our culture and comes from unspoken cultural assumptions of men and women and brothers and sisters. Parents also contribute to the assumption that only a daughter can give good care. There are also sexual taboos involved.

The care manager again can use family meetings as a way to open up this family can of worms and try to redistribute the care. Acting like a bulldozer among these deep cultural beliefs can be a lethal step for a care manager. As Lustbader points out, men grew up with these traditional roles and suddenly expecting them to wash the mother's urine-soaked sheets or go grocery shopping may be a boot camp approach that may not work.

As Lustbader suggests, men tend to feel "inept and overwhelmed when faced with what they perceived as woman's work." She suggests the professional begin by expressing sympathy with these culturally confusing situations for men. She encourages the professional, in this case the care manager, coach daughters to express their own overwhelming feelings concerning their caregiving tasks. The care manager can help the daughter take the next step and ask a brother for help by acknowledging her own stress. Lustbader also suggests coaching daughters to acknowledge that brothers can feel demeaned by changing soiled sheets or doing laundry and asking the brother to choose between the least demeaning task. This approach, she suggests, fends off resistance on the part of the brother. Using a blunt approach such as, "This is the 21st century not the Dark Ages," will usually not help and tends to make the brother dig in his heels further, according to Lustbader.[78]

Lustbader suggests gently teaching brothers some of tasks of caregiving because they probably never did them. Brothers may have basic household skills, but showing them what is expected may be something the care manager may have to coach the daughter to do. In addition the care manager can become a resource to the brother if he chooses to opt out and pay to hire someone or an agent to do the task he does not want to do. In Ms. Handy's case the brother volunteers to hire respite during the family meeting when the daughter, Ms. Handy, told her siblings she was so exhausted she was going to place their father in a facility.

Care Managers Enhancing Quality of Life Through Involving Old–Old Siblings

Care managers should also use research in midlife and old–old siblings to understand what a vibrant force siblings can be in improving the quality of life of an older person. Herndon and Thorpe show care managers how to optimize an older person's quality of life by using a quality of life assessment tool.[79] Such questions as "Do you have a sibling?" and "Would you like more contact with the siblings?" should be added to the QOL tool. Care managers should ask these questions of old–old siblings. They then can arrange occasions or visits where the old–old siblings can gather together.

Old–old siblings enjoy gathering and most frequently get together at rituals such as weddings, funerals, christenings, or any family passage. A care manager's job is to keep up on when and where all family rituals may be happening and arrange if possible for the client to attend these events and see his or her siblings. If the older sibling cannot attend, arranging telephone calls and e-mail if the client is technologically savvy, are the next best thing. Having slideshows sent on photo sites and shown on the laptops of adult children or grandchildren is another way to engage older siblings in rituals where other

siblings are in attendance. Family reunions are another form of occasional activities where elderly siblings can be paired with sisters and brothers to increase quality of life.

Weekly or even daily activities as well can build interaction with elderly siblings. Various recreational activities such as shopping, church, outdoor barbeques, or any community activity can be arranged with siblings. Even if siblings live in the same town, adult day care, senior center activities, or socialization geared for seniors can be shared by elderly siblings.

Home recreational activities were seen by siblings as very enjoyable occasions to be with their siblings. If your client likes puzzles or watching *Jeopardy,* pair him or her with a visit of a sibling. Assess your client's interest in activities and if possible make sure they attend such events or you arrange the events, like shopping with siblings. As seen by the research here, this is not only going to enhance the well-being and psychological state of your client, but elevate their quality of life. It may be a good idea to add this to the care manager's psychosocial assessment tool and ask these questions on a routine basis of your older client and their young–old family members.

Care Managers Supporting Widows and Single Women by Connecting Them to Sisters

Because women live longer than men, widows predominate in Western culture. Care managers are often faced with working with widowed women. Siblings can be an excellent tool to emotionally support a woman who has lost her spouse. As seen in this chapter, widows who have a married sister to interact with are happier than those who don't. Visits with a married sister is the strongest predictor of positive effects on widows. A care manager arranging visits between widows and their married sisters will enhance the quality of life of that widow. Even if the visits cannot be in person, arranging visits by phone or e-mail, if the client is computer literate, can be an excellent addition to a care plan. Enlisting adult children who can help sisters send photos, CDs, and tapes can be another good solution to a care plan, helping to allay the pain and grief suffered by recent widows.

If a care manager has clients who are single women, whether they are divorced or never married, connecting them with sisters can be a great enhancement to their quality of life.

Women in general when connected to their sisters in middle age or old age show fewer symptoms of depression, according to Cicirelli. Connecting sisters in midlife, but especially in old age, can be an excellent tool in a care plan.

Care Managers Using Siblings with Reminiscence

Reminiscence can be a great comfort to the old–old. Siblings offer the best audiences, prompts, and fellow actors in remembering an older person's past life. A care manager who interjects reminiscence techniques (e.g., story boarding, photo albums, art therapy, and reminiscence groups) and does it in tandem with visits by siblings will increase the quality of life of the old–old.

Late-Life Siblings Reminiscence and Healing Old Sibling Rivalry

As mentioned earlier in this chapter reminiscence is an excellent way to heal the wounds of early childhood. During reminiscence in later life people analyze, evaluate, and reinterpret their lives in relationship to present events, values, and attitudes. Care

manager's coaching on a one-to-one basis for old–old siblings may resolve sibling rivalry. It is highly suggested that the care manager learn forgivenss techniques before doing this (see Chapter 12). If the care manager is highly seasoned and has a family therapy or psychodynamic background, and the old–old siblings are able to get physically together, therapeutic reminiscences could be done between two or more old rival siblings. Siblings in old age, as suggested earlier, can use reminiscence to look at early sibling wounds in childhood and see them in the context of the here-and-now. As death is so close in the lives of these old–old siblings, remembering old feuds while also recalling the better times, old–old siblings can be more eager to learn forgiveness for old gouges due to sibling rivalry. Again as mentioned earlier, sibling reminiscence in old age helped the older people put their current relationships with siblings into a meaningful context, helped them understand present events, and helped them evaluate the importance of sibling relationships. So the old wound can be healed in part by the reminiscence of siblings in old age.

SUMMARY

Siblings are the most powerful subsystem of the aging family. They are the most abiding and long-lived relationship of our lives. They are our mirror and sometimes our enemy. For care managers they are a powerful tool to enrich the life of an older client and get them through the agonizing losses of old age. They are sometimes the air mattress that comes to life when sister and brother needs them and are then tucked away until the next crisis. At times they are our enduring best friends. They are the best time traveler for moving into the past that an older person can have. They not only were there, but they were there from the beginning. Siblings are a great care plan tool for care managers, underutilized yet brought forward as we learn more about their abilities. Fritz Pearls, the 1960s psychologist, used to say

"The obvious is the hardest to get." Care managers through this chapter can see and now use this wonderful source of connection and reassurance for the aging family.

REFERENCES

1. Edwards R, Hadfield L, Lucey H, Mauthner M. *Sibling Identity and Relationships*. London: Routledge, Taylor and Francis; 2006:22.
2. Cicirelli VG. *Sibling Relationships Across the Lifespan*. New York, NY: Plenum; 1995:4.
3. Cicirelli VG. *Sibling Relationships Across the Lifespan*. New York, NY: Plenum; 1995:17.
4. Walker A, Allen KR, Connidis I, eds. Theorizing and studying sibling ties in adulthood. *Sourcebook of Family Theory and Research*. Thousand Oaks, CA: Sage; 2005:167.
5. Cicirelli VG. Sibling relationships in old age. In: Brody G, ed. *Sibling Relationships: Their Causes and Consequences*. Norwood, NJ: Ablex; 1996:47.
6. Floyd K, Morman MT. *Widening the Family Circle, New Research on Family Communication*. Thousand Oaks, CA: Sage; 2006:23.
7. Edwards R, Hadfield L, Lucey H, Mauthner. *Sibling Identity and Relationships*. London: Routledge, Taylor and Francis:25.
8. Hapworth W, Hapworth M, Heliman JR. *Mom Loved You Best*. New York, NY: Penguin; 1993:11.
9. Fishel E. *Sisters, Shared Histories, Lifelong Ties*. Berkeley, CA: Conari Press; 1997:239.
10. Edwards R, Hadfield L, Lucey H, Mauthner. *Sibling Identity and Relationships*. London: Routledge, Taylor and Francis; 2006.
11. Edwards R, Hadfield L, Lucey H, Mauthner. *Sibling Identity and Relationships*. London: Routledge, Taylor and Francis; 2006.
12. Theorizing and studying sibling ties in adulthood. In Walker A, Allen KR, Connidis I, eds. *Sourcebook of Family Theory and Research*. Thousand Oaks, CA: Sage; 2005:173.
13. Lamb ME, Sutton-Smith B. Sibling Relationships, Their Nature and Significance Across the Lifespan, Lawrence Erbaum Asso, London, Cicirelli, Victor Eds. Sibling Influence Throughout Life. Pg 268.
14. Hapworth W, Hapworth M, Heliman JR. *Mom Loved You Best*. New York, NY: Penguin; 1993:10.
15. Riggo HR. Measuring attitudes toward adult sibling relationships: The Lifespan Sibling Relationship Scale. *Journal of Social and Personal Relationships*. 2000;17:710. 707DOI; 10.1177/0265407500176001.
16. Greer J. *Adult Sibling Rivalry*. New York, NY: Ballantine Books; 1993:21.
17. Cicirelli VG. *Sibling Relationships Across the Lifespan*. New York, NY: Plenum Press;1995:209.
18. Connidis I. Life transitions and the sibling tie: A qualitative study. *Journal of Marriage and Family*. 1992;54(4):972.
19. Cicirelli VG. *Sibling Relationships Across the Lifespan*. New York, NY: Plenum Press; 1995:61.
20. Walker A, Allen KR, Connidis I, eds. Theorizing and studying sibling ties in adulthood. In: *Sourcebook of Family Theory and Research*. Thousand Oaks, CA: Sage; 2005:168.
21. Campbell LD, Connidis IA, Davies L. Sibling ties in later life: A social network analysis. *Journal of Family Issues*. 1999;116. 114DOI:10.1177/01925139902001006.
22. Walker A, Allen KR, Connidis I, eds. Theorizing and studying sibling ties in adulthood. In: *Sourcebook of Family Theory and Research*. Thousand Oaks, CA: Sage; 2005:177.
23. Bank SP, Kahn MD. *Sibling Bond*. New York, NY: Basic Books; 1982:28.
24. Connidis IA. *Family Ties and Aging*. Thousand Oaks, CA: Sage; 2001:214–215.
25. Cicirelli VG. *Sibling Relationships Across the Lifespan*. New York, NY: Plenum Press; 1995:57.
26. Cicirelli VG. *Sibling Relationships Across the Lifespan*. New York, NY: Plenum Press; 1995:63.
27. Cicirelli V. *Sibling Relationships Across the Lifespan*. New York, NY: Plenum Press; 1995:56–57.
28. Connidis I. Life transitions and the sibling tie: A qualitative study. *Journal of Marriage and Family*. 1992;54(4):972.
29. Cicirelli V. *Sibling Relationships Across the Lifespan*. New York, NY: Plenum Press; 1995:2.

30. Cicirelli V. *Sibling Relationships Across the Lifespan*. New York, NY: Plenum Press; 1995:55.

31. Cicirelli V. *Sibling Relationships Across the Lifespan*. New York, NY: Plenum Press; 1995:57.

32. Connidis IA. *Family Ties and Aging*. Thousand Oaks, CA: Sage; 2001:223.

33. Cicirelli V. *Sibling Relationships Across the Lifespan*. New York, NY: Plenum Press; 1995:64.

34. Scott JP. Sibling interaction in later life. In: Brubaker TH, ed. *Family Relationships in Later Life*. Thousand Oaks, CA: Sage Publications; 1990:99.

35. Ramey C, Cress CJ. Integrating late life relocation: The role of the GCM. In: Cress C, ed. *Handbook of Geriatric Care Management*. 2nd ed. Sudbury, MA: Jones and Bartlett; 2007:283.

36. Schulman G. Siblings revisited: Old conflicts and new opportunities in later life. *Journal of Marital and Family Therapy*. 1999;October.

37. Scott JP. Sibling interaction in later life. In: Brubaker TH, ed. *Family Relationships in Later Life*. Thousand Oaks, CA: Sage Publications; 1990:87.

38. Blieszner R, Bedford VH, eds. *Handbook of the Aging Family*. Westport, CT: Greenwood Press; 1995:211–212.

39. Floyd K, Morman MT. *Widening the Family Circle, New Research on Family Communication*. Thousand Oaks, CA: Sage; 2006:23.

40. Cicirelli VG. *Sibling Relationships Across the Lifespan*. New York, NY: Plenum Press; 1995:3.

41. Connidis IA. *Family Ties and Aging*. Thousand Oaks, CA: Sage; 2001:196.

42. http://wwwstepfamilies.info/faqs/factsheet.php

43. Rosenberg E. Siblings in therapy. In: Kahn MD, Lewis KG, eds. *Siblings in Therapy*. New York, NY: Norton; 1988.

44. Greer J. *Adult Sibling Rivalry, Understanding the Legacy of Childhood*. Fawcett Crest;1992:25.

45. Cicirelli VG. *Sibling Relationships Across the Lifespan*. New York, NY: Plenum Press; 1995:161.

46. Suitor JJ, Pillemer K. *Mother's Favoritism in Later Life: The Role of Children's Birth*. Sage:44. DOI:10.1177/0164027506291750.

47. Riggo H. Measuring adult sibling relationships: The Lifespan Sibling Scale. *Journal of Social and Personal Relationships*. 2000;17:710, 723–724. 707DOI;10.1177/0265407500176001.

48. Leder JM. *Adult Sibling Rivalry: Sibling rivalry often lingers through adulthood*. Available at http://psychologytoday.com/articles/index.php?term=19930101-000023&page=1. Accessed on July 11, 2008.

49. Cicirelli VG. *Sibling Relationships Across the Lifespan*. New York, NY: Plenum Press; 1995:56.

50. Leder JM. Adult sibling rivalry. *Psychology Today*. 1993, Jan–Feb.

51. Walker A, Allen KR, Connidis I. Theorizing and studying sibling ties in adulthood. In: *Sourcebook of Family Theory and Research*. Thousand Oaks, CA: Sage; 2005:172.

52. Lustbader W, Hooeyman NR. *Taking Care of Aging Family Members, A Practical Guide*. New York, NY: Macmillan; 1994:70.

53. Lustbader W, Hooeyman NR. *Taking Care of Aging Family Members, a Practical Guide*. New York, NY: Macmillan; 1994:68.

54. Lustbader W, Hooeyman NR. *Taking Care of Aging Family Members, a Practical Guide*. New York, NY: Macmillan; 1994:70.

55. Riggo H. Measuring adult sibling relationships: The Lifespan Sibling Scale. *Journal of Social and Personal Relationships*. 2000;17:724. 707DOI;10.1177/0265407500176001.

56. Merril DM. *Caring for Elderly Parents, Juggling Work, Family, and Caregiving in Middle and Working Class Families*. Westport, CT: Auburn House; 1997:51.

57. Keith C. Family caregiving systems: Models, resources and values. *Journal of Marriage and the Family*. 1995;57:180.

58. Matthews S, Rosner TT. Shared filial responsibility: The family as the primary caregiver. *Journal of Marriage and the Family*. 1988;50:188.

59. Cicirelli VG. *Sibling Relationships Across the Lifespan*. New York, NY: Plenum Press; 1995:123.

60. Coward RT, Dwyer JW. The association of gender, sibling network composition, and patterns of parent care by adult children. *Research on Aging*. 1990;12(2):173–174.

61. Blieszner R, Bedford VH, eds. *Handbook of the Aging Family*. Westport, CT: Greenwood Press; 1995:215.

62. Cicirelli VG. *Sibling Relationships Across the Lifespan*. New York, NY: Plenum Press; 1995:125.

63. Cicirelli VG. *Sibling Relationships Across the Lifespan*. New York, NY: Plenum Press; 1995:125.

64. Lustbader W, Hooeyman NR. *Taking Care of Aging Family Members, a Practical Guide*. New York, NY: Macmillan; 1994:67.

65. Matthews S, Heidorn J. Meeting filial responsibilities in brothers-only sibling groups. *Journal of Gerontology: Social Sciences*. 1998;53B(5): S278–S286.

66. Tonti M. Relationships among adult siblings who care for their aged parents. In: Kahn MD, Lewis KG, eds. *Siblings in Therapy*. New York, NY: Norton; 1988:425–426.

67. Cicirelli VG. *Sibling Relationships Across the Lifespan*. New York, NY: Plenum Press; 1995:129.

68. Lustbader W, Hooeyman NR. *Taking Care of Aging Family Members, a Practical Guide*. New York, NY: Macmillan; 1994:81.

69. Cicirelli VG. *Sibling Relationships Across the Lifespan*. New York, NY: Plenum Press; 1995:129.

70. Cicirelli VG. *Sibling Relationships Across the Lifespan*. New York, NY: Plenum Press; 1995:129.

71. Cress C. Understanding the causes of elder abuse. *Care Management*. 2004;10(4):33.

72. Cicirelli VG. *Sibling Relationships Across the Lifespan*. New York, NY: Plenum Press; 1995:136.

73. Cicirelli VG. *Sibling Relationships Across the Lifespan*. New York, NY: Plenum Press; 1995:132.

74. Matthews SH, Rosner TT. Shared responsibility: The family as the primary caregiver. *Journal of Marriage and the Family*. 1988;February:191.

75. Cicirelli VG. *Sibling Relationships Across the Lifespan*. New York, NY: Plenum Press; 1995:132.

76. Lustbader W, Hooeyman NR. *Taking Care of Aging Family Members, a Practical Guide*. New York, NY: Macmillan; 1994:65–79.

77. Morano B, Morano C. *Psychosocial Assesment: Handbook of Geriatric Care Management*. Sudbury, MA: Jones and Bartlett; 2007;2;25.

78. Lustbader W, Hooeyman NR. *Taking Care of Aging Family Members, a Practical Guide*. New York, NY: Macmillan; 1994:83–86.

79. Herndon NP, Thorpe V. Supporting quality of life: Drawing on community, informal networks, and care manager creativity. In: Cress C, ed. *Handbook of Geriatric Care Management*. Sudbury, MA: Jones and Bartlett; 2007:357.

CHAPTER 9

Dying, Grief, and Burial in the Aging Family

Diane M. LeVan and Gwen Lazo Harris

Families of the dying are faced with the challenge of coping with the impending loss of a loved one and yet are still very involved in providing care for their dying family member. For care managers, working with families at this time presents a unique challenge, because death exacerbates rifts in the family, unresolved interpersonal conflicts, and other unfinished business. Helping family members cope with these stresses requires that a supportive environment be established where they can openly discuss death, grief, and loss. A care manager becomes the supportive presence that helps family members know what to expect, calms their fears, helps them make difficult decisions that are in the best interest of their loved one, and helps them deal with their grief. *Certainly the road toward dying is a difficult one.* But a road map of the stages and a list of the tasks can be reassuring for both care manager and family and lead the family to opportunities for healing and transformation.[1]

THE ROLES OF FAMILIES IN END-OF-LIFE CARE

End-of-life (EOL) care management involves working with both the dying and their family members. This is because of the critical role that family members assume in the care of terminally ill patients. In a national survey by the Agency for Healthcare Research and Quality (AHRQ), it was determined that most terminally ill patients relied totally on family members and friends for assistance. Ninety-six percent of the caregivers were family members, and 72% of the caregivers were women. The services these caregivers provide to the dying include the following:

- Domestic care (housekeeping, laundry, meal preparation, shopping)
- Personal care (bathing and dressing)
- Transportation
- Nursing care (administering medication, collecting and giving information about functional and psychological capacities and needs)[2]
- Social care (emotional comfort and support)
- Planning care (obtain and coordinate care from health and social service providers)
- Medical care decision making (if acute hospitalization becomes necessary)[3]

It should be noted that the care provided by family members is unpaid and often provided around the clock. Without their assistance the health and well-being of the terminally ill patient is much poorer.

THE NEEDS OF FAMILIES IN END-OF-LIFE CARE

Given that family members provide so much of the care terminally ill elderly patients receive, care managers must be concerned about their needs. The concerns of families facing terminal illness are similar in many ways to those of the dying. They include:

- The need for information and clarification to be able to make healthcare decisions
- Preparation for death
- Help to achieve closure[4]

However, for family members, the following needs and concerns are more important:

- Support for their emotional well-being
- Assistance advocating for the best care of their loved one
- Help find ways to enhance self-efficacy

In the context of EOL care, self-efficacy refers to the need that family caregivers have to be more confident about their abilities to care for their loved one.[5]

In addition, the responsibilities of the caregiving role can have a tremendous impact on the life of the caregiver. Caring for a loved one has a physical, emotional, and financial cost. Caregiver burden, which is the strain or load borne by a person giving care, becomes an issue care managers need to monitor.

The AHRQ report examined the types of interventions that will improve the outcomes for the dying person and their family. The desired outcomes include reducing caregiver burden (depression, tension, anger, burden, negative affect), stress, and anxiety. The desired outcomes also include increasing decision-making confidence, coping, life satisfaction, and morale.[6]

Both palliative care and care management have been found to lessen the negative impact of caregiving. The interventions found to help lessen the impact of caregiving were palliative care, education, counseling, and support groups. The use of respite care and home care services were also helpful.[7]

FAMILY-CENTERED CARE

The foundation of EOL geriatric care management is family-centered care. This approach during palliative care and bereavement provides a method of enhancing family functioning and improving the overall outcome. Family-centered care is a way that care managers arrange and coordinate care services. It involves collaboration between the patient, family, and other healthcare professionals. Family-centered care can be thought of as an extension of patient-centered care, whose underlying premise is that patients should be active participants in their own care and that the services they receive should be centered on their needs and preferences. Patient-centered care contrasts with a more traditional disease-centered model where physicians have all the control and make almost all treatment decisions based largely on their clinical experience and data from various medical tests.[8]

The family in family-centered care is defined broadly. The dying individual decides who they mean when they say they want family support.[9] This family network may extend beyond biological or legal relations and includes people with whom the patient has close emotional ties. This may include siblings, same sex partners, or close neighbors and friends.

In this model, care is not solely focused on the needs of the dying individual. Family-centered care organizes treatment plans around both the patient and their family. Because family caregivers play a vital role in assisting dying elders, care plans are developed to include interventions that address caregiver burden.

Family-centered care also incorporates the beliefs and cultural values of the client and his or her family.[10] To make informed healthcare decisions, information needs to be presented in the native language of the patient and their family. Likewise, cultural and religious beliefs about causes of illness or how illness is treated should be taken into consideration. For example, Asian cultures use acupuncture and herbs to cure illness and are often skeptical of Western medicine. Many times the care manager needs to explain to the client the value and benefit of the medical treatment that is recommended to them.

The communication process is key to EOL family support and intervention. The dying and their families need to know what medical options are available as well as what the ramifications of these options are. They cannot make informed healthcare decisions without adequate information. They need to be fully aware of the invasive nature of a procedure and any potential side effects as well what possible outcomes and quality of life to expect.

For the care manager, communication and information sharing are excellent tools for enhancing family well-being. A diagnosis of a terminal illness creates feelings of powerlessness and lack of control. Families need timely, accurate, complete, and unbiased information to be able to understand their loved one's situation and participate in end-of-life decision making. Care managers obtain their research information from a variety of sources including hospitals and national health organizations such as the American Cancer Society or the Alzheimer's Association. They also get information from family support organizations like the Family Caregiver Alliance. The Internet is also a vast resource of information. For families with access to the Internet, information and tools to help them manage a chronic disease or condition are available at such Web sites as mayoclinic.com, webmd.com, and webhealth.com.

Supporting dying clients and their families as they navigate through their reactions to terminal illness is also a part of family-centered care. The Kubler-Ross grief model (denial, anger, bargaining, depression, acceptance) is commonly used to understand these reactions and to help one come to terms with terminal illness.

- Denial functions as a temporary buffer to bad news. It is a way to try to avoid the inevitable and allows patients and their families time to collect themselves until they can begin to deal with a painful and uncomfortable situation.
- As denial dissipates, anger associated with losses in the present and future sets in.
- Bargaining is when people are looking for ways to avoid having the inevitable happen. Pleas to God may be made: "If you will only spare her life, I'll devote the rest of my life to helping others." They are trying to negotiate their way out of hurt and pain.
- Depression is when the person finally understands the inevitability of what is going to happen. They often turn inward and have feelings of deep sadness.
- Often the final stage, acceptance, is when the person comes to peace with the situation and begins to live with the threat of loss.

Sadness may not entirely go away, but it diminishes. It is important to note that these stages are not always sequential as Kubler-Ross originally thought. People's responses vary, and coping with them, like the grief process itself, involves many ups and downs with gradual improvement over time.[11]

PALLIATIVE AND HOSPICE CARE

Family-centered care is the underlying framework of palliative and hospice care. Palliative and hospice care address both the client's needs and the family's needs and offers them support as well. Palliative and hospice care are team-oriented approaches. These teams are interdisciplinary, meaning they include professionals with several different skill sets and specialties. The care manager is part of this team. The services provided by the team include expert medical care and pain management as well as emotional and spiritual care tailored to each client's needs and wishes.

The focus of hospice is care, not cure. Hospice care pays for and orders medication and durable equipment and provides medical oversight from doctors, nurses, and a social worker. The emphasis is on pain and symptom management. Hospice clients have been diagnosed with a life expectancy of 6 months or less, and all curative treatments have stopped. Because most clients and their families hold on to the hope that a cure may be found, they are unwilling to stop curative medical treatments. This prevents them from starting hospice care. Most clients wait until the very end of their lives; often, it's too late to gain benefit from hospice care at this point. This is where care managers play an important role. They can assist clients and their families to determine when hospice care is the most appropriate and beneficial type of care.

Palliative care, on the other hand, extends itself to a broader population. Palliative care also focuses on pain and symptom management but is not just for the dying. The client does not have to be terminally ill and may still pursue aggressive medical treatment. No specific medical therapy is excluded from consideration. Since palliative care may be obtained during any part of the disease continuum, clients are more likely to access this type of care. Palliative care may segue into hospice care as the illness progresses. Palliative care helps clients transition from hospital care to other healthcare settings.

Because emotional, psychosocial, physical, and spiritual aspects of advanced illness are addressed, clients report higher levels of satisfaction with their end-of-life care.

Care Manager's Role

Care managers usually become involved at one of two points in the client's living–dying interval. For some clients, the care manager has been caring for them through the chronic illness phase and their disease has progressed to the terminal phase. The second way care managers become involved is with clients who have a terminal illness and need care management services. In both cases the care manager's role is to manage medical treatments and to treat the needs of the client and family members. Care managers research information about the specific terminal disease, treatment options, and perform ongoing assessments of the client's medical status and care needs.

Once hospice is in place, care managers work together with the hospice team, acting as a liaison and overseer of:

- Medical treatments
- Communication with medical staff and families
- Making sure durable equipment is on site and that caregivers know how to use equipment

The care manager will:

- Provide support for client and families.
- Arrange transportation to treatments or doctor visits.
- Manage caregivers and practical service providers.
- Explain procedures to family members.
- Collaborate with client and social worker to see that all the needs are met.

The care manager needs to know when to call in hospice nursing or medical staff.

Social workers are often part of the hospice team. When that is so, their role often overlaps the care manager's role and thus responsibilities are shared. It's important for the care manager to develop a good working relationship with the hospice social worker.

FIVE PHASES OF TERMINAL ILLNESS

People usually learn that they have a terminal illness from a doctor who gives them a diagnosis. To work with terminally ill patients and their families, the care manager must understand both the physical and emotional aspects of the dying trajectory. Due to recent advances in medical technology, the period between diagnosis and death has lengthened. This period is termed the *living–dying interval*.[12(p5)]

During this time, the progression of most terminal illnesses will be similar to that of a chronic illness. There may be intensive medical treatments involving drug regimens, surgeries, and dietary modifications that improve the quality of life or extend the time left to live. However, the client never fully regains their former level of functioning. Progress fighting the disease is followed by relapse. The disease progresses and mental and physical symptoms slowly get worse over time. As an individual progresses to the final stages of terminal illness, problems such as infections gradually become more difficult to treat and the ability to speak, eat, dress, and toilet oneself deteriorates. With the help of an interdisciplinary team of healthcare professionals, the care manager monitors these changes and decides what they mean in terms of ongoing care. These changes will be reflected in updated care plans.

After the diagnosis, coping and accepting one's own death or the impending death of a loved one can take some time. It begins with an intellectual realization followed by an exploration of feelings. As the dying and their family members begin to accept what is happening they begin to make adjustments to accommodate the changes that come as the disease progresses.

This process of acceptance and adjustment to terminal illness has five phases:

• Before the diagnosis
• The acute phase
• The chronic phase
• The recovery phase
• The terminal phase[13]

Interventions vary according to the phase. As a care manager may be brought in when the family is negotiating through any one of these phases, the care manager's work begins with making a determination of what phase the client is in during the initial assessment. These phases do not mark specific points in the progression of the disease itself.

The Phase Before Diagnosis

The phase before diagnosis of a life-threatening illness begins with the time directly before an official diagnosis of an illness is made. This phase is characterized as

the period of time when a person begins to recognize symptoms and realizes that he or she may have contracted an illness. This phase is not a single instant of recognition, but instead is more of a period of time when the person undergoes physical examinations, various tests, and ultimately ends when the person is told they are suffering from a terminal illness.[14]

Care manager tasks (these are ongoing throughout the continuum of illness) include:

- Schedule medical appointments.
- Assist the family in having questions answered by healthcare professionals.
- Before visiting the client, maintain an up-to-date medication list and list of any drug allergies.
- Assist the family to organize documents.
- Arrange for someone to go to medical appointments with the patient to take notes and ask questions. This is important because people often don't understand or remember important parts of conversations with their doctors.
- Ask caregivers to use a calendar to keep a log of important medical information, questions, and things out of the ordinary that happen to the ill person.
- Create a notebook to store information.[15]

The Acute Phase

The acute phase begins at the time of diagnosis. The person has heard their terminal diagnosis from a doctor or other medical staff person and is then forced to understand their situation. Many people can't absorb or understand their diagnosis the first time they hear it.

Shock is often the first reaction. People are immobilized and temporarily shut down. This makes concentration and listening next to impossible. They may also want to avoid acknowledging the illness. People need time to process such news. The care manager can help clients cope by encouraging them to talk things out. Unless a decision needs to be made immediately, decision making should be postponed until there has been some time to talk things through.[16] If the caregiver's performance of family tasks interferes with timely medical treatment, then the care manager needs to intervene.

Ultimately decisions must be made regarding the patient's medical care and available treatment options. Once treatment begins, the reality of the illness becomes a part of the family's life, and adjustments and accommodations need to be made. At this point, the family is hopeful that a cure can be found.[17]

Care manager tasks include:

- Arrange in-home support.
- Arrange for durable medical equipment, if needed.
- Coordinate and facilitate family meetings.
- Assist compiling and organizing documents needed for advance care planning.

The Chronic Phase

The chronic phase is the period of time between the diagnosis and the result from the treatments. During this phase, the dying person tries to cope with the demands of daily life while also going through necessary medical treatment, "often having to struggle with the unpleasant side effects of their treatment."[18] Chronic illness may also involve repeated episodes of deterioration in which the patient confronts and adjusts to these losses. Examples of these losses include cognitive function, sexuality, toileting, and the ability to ambulate, eat, and dress. The focus of life for both the family and the patient needs to be redefined, shifting from hope for a cure to coping with the illness.[19]

Care manager tasks include:

- Assist the family to determine the type of long-term care that may be safest and healthiest for the loved one (hospital chronic care, nursing home care, in-home nursing care, or family care) and make arrangements.
- Coordinate help from community organizations.

- Assist the client and family to connect with support groups.
- Assist learning management of disease skills from healthcare staff, videos, manuals, or brochures.
- Monitor anticipatory grief needs.
- Learn about disease in order to help the patient make good decisions about his or her care and to help family members monitor their expectations.[20]
- Monitor caregiver burden by ensuring caregivers take time for themselves, take breaks, get rest, get to medical appointments. Monitor for grief needs.

The Recovery Phase

The recovery phase occurs when people finally are able to cope with the mental, social, physical, religious, and financial effects of their disease.[21] In the disease process, this is the period of time after a medical procedure such as chemotherapy, radiation, or surgery. The client's response to treatment is being monitored. "Recovery does not always mean remission, but instead it is the ability to accept and deal with the struggles of their illness."[22]

CASE STUDY:
CLIENT TAKING CARE OF FAMILY

Edgar Enlightened was diagnosed with pancreatic cancer. Because his prognosis was so grim, he was undergoing trial cancer treatments in the hope of finding a cure. He had just finished one such treatment. He was feeling good and hopeful that this time he would be cured.

Edgar now thought that this was the best time to address concerns about his family. Edgar's parents lived in another country, and each time they visited they stayed in bed and breakfast accommodations to reduce the costs. But Edgar knew that the travel and lodging costs were eating up their retirement money. He also worried

about other family members. He knew that his prognosis was not good and wanted them all to seek some group counseling.

Edgar sought the help of a care manager to find affordable housing for his parents and appropriate therapy assistance for the family. The care manager was able to find housing that was subsidized by a local charity that supports families facing life-threatening illness. The care manager was also able to find therapists trained to talk to groups about facing life-threatening illnesses. Edgar's family members were able to express their fears, and Edgar was able to express his appreciation for their support and love. Having this period of recovery allowed time for Edgar and his family to heal and prepare for the eventual advancement of his illness.

The Terminal Phase

The terminal phase of any life-threatening illness is the time between diagnosis and the final decline when no cure or extension of life is in the offing. The individual confronts progressive decline and deterioration. Death is imminent. The focus of doctors and patients now changes from attempting to cure the illness or prolong life to trying to provide relief from pain and to comfort the sufferer. Religious concerns such as what happens after someone passes away or how to handle the suffering at the end of life or how to give comfort to family members are the focus during this time as well as tying up any loose ends.

Care manager tasks include:

- Monitor and continue tasks from previous phases.
- Monitor anticipatory grief needs.
- Communicate that this is the end (and time to say good-bye).
- Assess spiritual needs, and contact the appropriate religious spiritual counselors to provide comfort and healing.

- Encourage family members to say the four things that matter most: "Please forgive me," "I forgive you," "Thank you," and "I love you."[23(p3)]

ADVANCE CARE PLANNING

Once the diagnosis is known, the care manager is often the one who will initiate and guide advance care planning discussions. As difficult as these discussions may be, the burden on the family is significantly lessened if decisions about advance care planning are made before the client's condition worsens. Communication between clients and their loved ones greatly improves the quality of care received as an advanced illness progresses. Conversations about quality versus quantity of life enables care managers to better coordinate services for continuity of care and plan for or stay away from various medical treatments.

The client's decisions about these issues relieve the family from stress and the burden of having to make these decisions. In one study, when family members participated in EOL discussions about their dying loved one's healthcare preferences, 63% said the burden of making treatment decisions was lessened. Although 48% of family members singled out their attending physician as the preferred source of information and reassurance,[24] studies on EOL care highlight intense communication and the role of the interdisciplinary team in reducing family burden, avoiding futile life-sustaining therapies, and providing effective comfort care.

Advance Directives

Advance directives are legal documents that allow clients to make decisions about their health care and finances in advance of when they are not mentally or physically able to do so. These documents must be signed, dated, and witnessed, and name another person to make decisions for you.

Durable Power of Attorney for Health Care

A durable power of attorney (DPOA) for health care is a type of advance directive that names another person to make medical decisions for you. Clients appoint a person who is entrusted to learn what their healthcare wishes are and make medical decisions on their behalf should they be incapacitated. This person is called a healthcare agent. A primary agent is chosen, as well as an alternate agent in case the primary agent is not available. The agent must be willing and able to speak for the client. The most important aspect of choosing an agent and alternate agent is to have conversations with both of them, making sure they know what issues are important to the client and how he or she would like to live and die. Clients may choose their spouse, partner, or family member. However the best choice for an agent may be somebody else. The agent and alternate agent will act as the voice and mind of the client. They must be willing to follow the healthcare instructions exactly and be able to be assertive in an aggressive medical environment. A family member who is too emotionally upset to make these difficult but necessary decisions should not be chosen.

Once the client chooses the agents, decisions are then made about the various types of healthcare options, including:

- Life-support equipment
- Artificial feeding and hydration
- Pain management and antibiotics
- Do not resuscitate (DNR) and cardiopulmonary resuscitation (CPR)

Withdrawal of Life Support

Research indicates that it is very likely that it will be a family member and a physician discussing withdrawal of life support due to the fact that less than 5% of patients in the ICU are able to communicate or have decision-making capacity at the time decisions are made.[25] Discussions about the withdrawal of life-sustaining treatments are the most difficult conversations physicians can have with family members. "Beyond mastery of medical facts, they require the ability to really talk with (not just report to) family members about powerfully emotional subjects."[26(p70)] ICU conferences are typically lead by a physician who becomes the spokesperson for the healthcare team. The decisions often revolve around honoring the patient's wishes or honoring the family's wishes, which can be difficult to determine when no healthcare agent has been selected and contradictory versions of the patient's wishes exist. Family members often have opposing opinions on withdrawing or withholding life support; it may be seen as allowing the patient to die, or it may be viewed as killing the patient.[27]

The care manager's role will be to help facilitate the understanding of the medical decisions that were made at the conference. This may involve providing further information or setting up a meeting with the doctor so that further questions can be asked. Knowing the facts helps families feel that they've made the right decision. The care manager's job involves reassuring them that the best choice possible was made given the circumstances. Knowing that the care manager's assurances are backed by years of experience lends them support and helps them to feel confident and comfortable with the decisions they've made.

Artificial Feeding and Hydrating

A natural part of the dying process is the withdrawal from food and liquids. The discussion of whether or not to use a feeding tube and IV comes up as part of the family's desire to keep their loved one comfortable. Often family members are afraid that the patient is dying of starvation and thirst. Denys Cope, a hospice nurse and EOL educator, states that withdrawal from food and fluids is a natural process that actually supports the dying person's comfort and does not create suffering. It naturally puts the body into a fasting mode that serves two purposes: cleansing and the enhancement of spiritual experiences.

> Therefore, what the dying person is doing is entering an altered state that makes disconnection from the body and the connection with the spiritual realm much easier. Fasting actually creates *comfort* for the person at this stage; it has a sedative effect. If you give someone an IV at this point, it will bring them right back into their body and out of the altered state. As a result, they come back into an awareness of any discomfort their body may be in, and meanwhile the body cannot effectively use the fluid from the IV. They have withdrawn from eating and drinking for a reason. The body has its own wisdom, and when we override that with our human "wisdom" in an effort to provide comfort, we can actually create the opposite effect. The body is unable to use the fluid because it is in the process of shutting down. If a person is given fluids at this stage it can result in swelling, or edema, and eventually the lungs can fill with fluid. In this care [the] loved one will be in great respiration distress as a result of something we were doing to try and create comfort.[28(p13)]

The care manager relays this information to the family so that they can make a decision that is in the best interest of the client.

Pain Management

Another decision families may be confronted with is how to best handle pain.

While they don't to want see their loved one suffer, very often their fears about the use of narcotics for alleviating pain result in patients getting inadequate pain control. Uncontrolled physical discomfort and pain become the life focus, greatly diminishing the dying person's quality of life. Families need to know that pain is related to advancing illness, not to dying. According to Denys Cope, the dying process, which is when the body's functions close down, is not painful. The same can be true for many of the diseases that may be causing the death:

> In many people's minds, dying and pain are always interconnected. They think the more pain someone is in, the closer to death that person must be. Advancing pain is related to advancing illness, and there are many excellent ways available to control pain and discomfort. Death on the other hand, comes in its own timing, regardless of the presence or absence of pain.[29(p4–5)]

Narcotic medications are appropriately given for this purpose. Morphine is the most commonly used medication for managing a terminally ill patient's pain. Families often are afraid its use will cause addiction or hasten the death of their loved one. As a result, morphine does not get used often or soon enough. When prescribed properly, morphine has been found to be a safe and effective drug, often considered to be the gold standard against which other pain drugs are compared.[30]

When used to alleviate pain, morphine is not being used in an addictive way. Drug addiction involves the use of drugs in order to alter consciousness, often as a way of coping with emotional difficulties. It may be helpful for families to know that the dose of morphine may have to be gradually increased, and that this is not due to addiction:

> Rather, it is because the condition creating the discomfort is advancing, with in-

creasing pain. There is also a gradual tolerance to the medication that develops over time that requires a gradual increase in dosage.[31(p18)]

Physicians providing pain management and symptom control adjust drugs and doses to individual patients so that they can be comfortable and are able to live with an improved quality of life until they die.

Explaining these distinctions to the family members can reduce the family's anxiety and facilitate their understanding of the use of pain medication. Most families want there to be enough pain management for their loved one to be comfortable but not so much that they cannot communicate or that death is hastened.

CASE STUDY: WHEN HEALTHCARE AGENTS DO "HEAR" WHAT THE CLIENT EXPRESSES

Clara Clarity survived breast cancer 10 years earlier and was now diagnosed with liver cancer. After 6 months of chemotherapy, Clara had surgery to remove small cancerous tumors from her liver. During her stay at the hospital, Clara suffered from an infection and was in excruciating pain. Because her liver was compromised, her physician was reluctant to give her pain medication. Her healthcare agent heard her say over and over again "Please give me all the pain medication available—I do not care whether or not it is life threatening." Her healthcare agent knew what she heard but could not face taking a chance with Clara's life. "I keep seeing her walking and talking—I couldn't take the chance that she might die." When the crucial moment came for her healthcare agent to follow Clara's decision, she followed her own idea for what she thought was best for Clara. Clara eventually healed from the infection but decided to change her healthcare agent.

Durable Power of Attorney for Finances

A durable power of attorney (DPOA) for finances is a type of advance directive that names another person (an agent) to act on a patient's behalf regarding financial decisions should incapacitation occur. Durable power of attorney allows the agent to pay bills, manage assets, sell property, and so forth.

Personal and Financial Records

Personal and financial documents must be gathered for the purposes of preparing instructions regarding financial matters and for the purposes of writing a will to bequeath money and property. Assembling these personal and financial records is helpful to families who will need them at a later date. Personal records consisting of facts, dates, names, and documents should be collected and documented on a personal information sheet like the one shown in Exhibit 9-1.

Financial records should include sources of income and assets (pension funds, IRAs, 401Ks, interest income, etc.). You may need to involve the family attorney, accountant, or family services advisor to accomplish some of these tasks. Always verify the costs of these services before using them. Free legal and financial services are often available to families:

- Social Security and Medicare information
- Investment income (stocks, bonds, property, and any brokers' names and addresses)
- Insurance information (life, health, and property) with policy numbers and agents' names
- Bank account numbers (checking, savings, and credit union)
- Liabilities—what is owed to whom and when are payments due?
- Mortgages and debts—how and when paid
- Credit card and charge account names and numbers

- Property taxes
- Location of all personal items such as jewelry or family treasures

---

CASE STUDY: CLIENT PUTS FINANCIAL AFFAIRS IN ORDER

When Clyde Compassion and his wife Sarah grew up, they were taught that men take care of the family's finances. Sarah did not know how to write a check or balance a checkbook. She also did not know where their money was invested. When Clyde was diagnosed with lymphoma at the age of 83, he knew that he had to teach Sarah as much as he could about their family finances.

The problem was that every time Clyde tried to teach Sarah, she would break down and cry. She felt that she could not handle the finances and that taking this task "away from Clyde" would make him leave her sooner. Since they did not have any children to take on this responsibility Clyde contacted a care manager to help them solve this dilemma. The care manager set the Compassion family up with a financial management system through their investment company. This type of financial conservatorship for Sarah took care of all the bill paying, income deposits, and investment decisions. Sarah was free to spend the available time with Clyde and not worry about learning a new financial system she felt unable to handle. After Clyde's death, Sarah felt that she was somehow still being cared for by Clyde in his choice of financial management.

STRATEGIES TO HELP FAMILIES MAKE DECISIONS

A prevailing theme of end-of-life care is the right of a terminally ill person to make decisions about what type of medical treatment will be received and how their last days will be spent. Making these decisions can help the dying and their family have a sense

Exhibit 9-1 Personal Records Information Sheet

My Personal Information

Name _____   U.S. Citizen   YES   NO
Social Security Number _____   Naturalization Number _____
Street Address _____   Marital Status _____
City of Residence _____   Spouse (maiden name) _____
County of Residence _____   Ancestry _____
State/Province _____   Race _____
Country of Residence _____   Father's Full Name _____
Zip _____   Father's
Sex   M   F   Birth Place _____
Age Last Birthday _____   Mother's Full Name _____
Date of Birth _____   Mother's
Birth Place _____   Birth Place _____
City _____   Education Highest Level _____
State _____   College _____
Country _____

Military Info

                                      Place where Entered _____
                                      Separation Place _____
Military Service Branch _____   Grade or Rank _____
Date Entered _____   Grade Rank/Rating _____
Separation Date _____   Service Serial Number _____

My Documents Location

Birth Certificate _____   Income Tax Returns _____
Marriage License _____   Military Discharge Papers _____
Mortgage _____   Automobile Titles _____
Other Mortgage 1(?) _____   Other Title 1(?) _____
Other Mortgage 2(?) _____   Other Title 2(?) _____
Deed or Notes 1(?) _____   Other Title 3(?) _____
Deed or Notes 2(?) _____   Safety Deposit Box _____

Medical History

Personal Physician _____   Have Had Treatment for
Address _____   Cancer   Kidney Disease
City _____   Circulatory   Tuberculosis
State _____   Diabetes   Other
Zip _____   Heart   Other
Phone _____
Additional Important Medical Information/History:

Allergic Reactions To:

My Children [Address & Phone Numbers]

Organizations I Want Notified [Phone No.]   **People To Notify** [Address & Phone No.]

Source: With permission from the Final Arrangements Network (http://www.finalarrangementsnetwork.com).

of control and enhances their ability to cope with other stressful aspects of their illness. Care managers fill a crucial role in educating both the patient and family. They also foster communication between all of the interested parties, enabling the family and patient to be aware of the available care options and to make these decisions with confidence.

Supportive Communication

Supportive communication requires being aware that how information is relayed can promote either a "positive attitude" with faith in the ultimate outcome, or a "negative attitude" with corresponding feelings of "despondence and despair."[32(p127)] Supportive communication relays to the family and patient care, concern, or comfort and allows people to feel understood and less alone. Some examples of supportive communication include simple acts such as going into the patient's room, sitting by their bed, spending some time with them, and being willing to listen. This goes a long way toward "creating a climate that encourages and supports sharing feelings."[33] Open-ended questions such as "What happened to make you feel that way?" encourage discussion. Paying attention to a patient's verbalized concerns and responding to their needs and the needs of their family promotes trust and communication. Implementing these techniques does not necessarily make their diagnosis easier to accept, but it does help create a safe environment where the possibility exists for the patient to begin to express a desire to talk about uncomfortable issues such as death or understanding the diagnosis.[34]

For the care manager, communication and information sharing are excellent tools for enhancing family well-being. A diagnosis of a terminal illness creates great feelings of powerlessness and lack of control. Families need timely, accurate, complete, and unbiased information to be able to understand their loved one's situation and participate in end-of-life decision making. Supportive communication helps create a caring environment where the dying and his or her family may express and articulate their physical, emotional, and spiritual needs. Communication and information sharing are empowerment strategies. They help patients and their families achieve a sense of control over their lives and thereby reduce the anxiety and depression produced by the uncertainty of the situation.[35]

Family Conferences

Life-threatening illness produces considerable distress for family members caring for their dying loved one. Family conferences can be used to establish a safe environment where plans, decisions, conflicts, and grief issues can be discussed honestly and openly. The aforementioned elements of family-centered care are an integral part of family meetings. The overall goal of family conferences in end-of-life care is to enhance supportive communication and family functioning. The dimensions of family functioning that are targeted include the following:

- Promotion of cohesiveness
- Reduction of conflict
- Encouragement to share thoughts and feelings with each other
- Promotion of "cooperation and communication among family members in decision making"[36]

Integral to this process is the sharing together of family grief. When this happens, "The family's strengths and successful ways of coping together are affirmed."[37]

It's important to realize that discussions involving EOL decisions can be quite lengthy and often involve numerous family members in a series of meetings spaced over time.[38] Family conference process steps (Exhibit 9-2) offer a detailed outline of how to conduct a family conference. Setting an agenda for the meeting and letting all parties know ahead of time what you plan to discuss is an important

---

Exhibit 9-2 Conducting a Family Conference

At some point during the course of a terminal illness, a meeting between healthcare professionals and the patient and family is usually necessary to review the disease course and develop end-of-life goals of care. Learning the process steps of a family conference is an important skill for physicians, nurses, and others who are in a position to help patients and families reach consensus on end-of-life planning.

1. **Why are you meeting?** Clarify conference goals in your own mind. What do you hope to accomplish?
2. **Where:** A room with comfort, privacy, and circular seating
3. **Who:** Patient (if capable of participating), legal decision maker/healthcare power of attorney, family members, social support, key healthcare professionals
4. **Introduction and relationship building:**
   - Introduce self and others; review meeting goals; clarify if specific decisions need to be made.
   - Establish ground rules: Each person will have a chance to ask questions and express views. No interruptions. Identify legal decision maker, and describe importance of supportive decision making.
   - If you are new to the patient and family, spend time seeking to know the "person"—ask about hobbies, family, and so on.
5. **Determine what the patient and family already knows:** "Tell me your understanding of the current medical condition." Ask everyone in the room to speak. Also ask about the past 1–6 months—what has changed in terms of functional decline, weight loss, and so on?
6. **Review medical status:**
   - Review current status, prognosis, and treatment options.
   - Ask each family member in turn if they have any questions about current status, plan, and prognosis.
   - Defer discussion of decision making until the next step.
   - Respond to emotional reactions.
7. **Family discussion with decisional patient:**
   - Ask the patient, "What decision(s) are you considering?"
   - Ask each family member, "Do you have questions or concerns about the treatment plan? How can you support the patient?"
8. **Family discussion with nondecisional patient:**
   - Ask each family member in turn, "What do you believe the patient would choose if he could speak for himself?"
   - Ask each family member, "What do you think should be done?"
   - Ask if the family would like you to leave room to let them discuss alone.
   - If there is consensus, go to Step 10; if no consensus, go to Step 9.
9. **When there is no consensus:**
   - Restate goal: What would the patient say if he or she could speak?
   - Use time as ally: Schedule a follow-up conference the next day.
   - Try further discussion: "What values is your decision based upon? How will the decision affect you and other family members?"
   - Identify other resources: Minister or priest, other physicians, ethics committee
10. **Wrap-up:**
    - Summarize consensus, disagreements, decisions, and plan.
    - Caution against unexpected outcomes.
    - Identify family spokesperson for ongoing communication.
    - Document in the chart who was present, what decisions were made, and follow-up plan.
    - Don't turf discontinuation of treatment to nursing.
    - Continuity: Maintain contact with family and medical team. Schedule follow-up meetings as needed.

Source: Courtesy of Weissman D. Fast fact and concepts #16: Conducting a family conference. End-of-Life Physician Education Resource Center. www.eperc.mew.edu. June 2000.

part of the process. Research on improving care planning with older people and their families shows that a family meeting is unsatisfactory when they go into it with an unclear agenda. The patient, the staff, and the family members must all be clear on the meeting's purpose. "This requires conveying and gathering information with the patient, adjusting expectations of all parties, and resolving any differences."[39(p579)] Information from meetings with other professionals or results from medical tests are two examples of the type of information that may be needed. When the meeting begins, it is good for the care manager to review the meeting goals and to clarify if specific decisions need to be made. Before the meeting ends the team checks back with the participants and each other to debrief and identify any unmet needs.[40]

Who Should Attend

The patient, family members, the care manager, and other healthcare professionals whose expertise is needed for the matter at hand should be present. Whenever possible or practical, the meetings should include the sick person. If he or she is unable to attend, let him or her know who has been invited and exactly what you plan to discuss. If he or she is unable to attend, report back to him or her immediately about the meeting. This keeps the locus of control with the patient, where it belongs. It is after all their life being discussed. If the sick person is unable to attend, then the person most familiar with the needs of the dying person should attend. An appointed spokesperson (a legal decision maker or person with the healthcare power of attorney) should attend if the patient is unable to speak for him- or herself.[41] There may be some cases where because of dementia or some other condition it might be appropriate to hold a meeting without the patient present. Depending on the condition, a follow-up with

the sick person may be appropriate. Another situation where the ill person should not be present is if the family members need to share with each other thoughts or feelings about family grief or other issues that would be too painful for the ill person to hear. In this case it would be appropriate to hold one meeting to focus on these matters only.[42]

Care Manager's Role

The care manager's role is to facilitate meetings, communicate information, explain, negotiate care, and have empathy and understanding.

CULTURAL DIVERSITY

Each member of the family will have a mental framework for understanding death, dying, end-of-life decision making, grief, and bereavement. Beliefs and practices that influence attitudes about EOL care preferences also vary from family to family. They also vary according to the country of origin and religious beliefs. An individual's beliefs will also vary by degree of acculturation into the mainstream society. The overall effectiveness of the EOL services provided requires knowledge about the culture and languages of the families served.

Culture shapes this mental framework, tempered by the level of acculturation. Although attitudes change unevenly, first generations are more likely to hold on to traditional beliefs. Interventions for a traditional person who knows little English and practices the "old ways" would need to be different than for a person who is assimilated and has adopted dominant cultural values and abandoned the "old ways."[43]

Therefore, care managers need to develop some familiarity with cultural variations regarding healthcare preferences and communication styles. Keep in mind that variations exist within each group. Stereotyping and generalization can be avoided by a comprehensive assessment process. Along with other specifics of individual or family needs, establishing the level of acculturation should be part of the assessment process. If available, use an assessment tool to measure acculturation. For Latinos, use the Marín and Marín Acculturation Scale found at http://chipts.ucla.edu/assessment/Assessment_Instruments/Assessment_files_new/assess_si.htm. For Asians, either modify the Marín and Marín scale or use the Suinn-Lew Asian Self-Identity Acculturation Scale. The Suinn-Lew scale can be found along with other psychosocial assessment tools for Asian-American populations at http://www.columbia.edu/cu/ssw/projects/pmap/ethnicities.htm.

If no assessment tool is available, a simple approach is to ask the client and family members about their preferences and rituals using the interview questions listed in Exhibit 9-3 or others like them. This approach avoids assumptions of the patient's ethnic heritage and level of acculturation. It also acknowledges that there may be differences from mainstream culture.

Three basic dimensions of end-of-life care may vary culturally. These are the communication of bad news, the communication of needs about pain, and the locus of decision making. Some cultures view directly informing patients of bad news as harmful to health. Talking about death or terminal illness is thought to bring on depression or to cause the dying person to lose hope. "Some cultures believe that speaking aloud about a condition, even in a hypothetic sense, makes death or terminal illness real because of the power of the spoken word."[44(p517)]

Pain management is one of the most important aspects of care for terminally ill patients. If pain is left untreated, a patient may stop participating in life, feel anxious, experience depression, and give up hope. Some ethnic patients don't get pain treatment because they value emotional self-control and wish to appear stoic in relation to pain. With ethnic clients, instead of asking about how much pain they are experiencing, ask: "May I get you something for pain?"[45]

In the United States, the dying individual is thought to be the autonomous decision maker, and so the family's opinion is secondary to the client's. Healthcare professionals communicate the diagnosis and other options directly to him or her. In contrast, in many ethnic communities, "Authority shifts for the elderly, and the family may take the responsibility of decision making for the older family member."[46]

Exhibit 9-3 Semistructured Interview Questions

Grand tour question: What is it like in your culture when a family member dies?

Probes:
- What does the immediate family do when a family member dies?
- What do friends and other relatives do when a family member dies?
- What expectations do people in your culture have for the immediate family and for other relatives?
- How long is bereavement expected to last?
- What is different if it is a child or an adult who dies?
- What meaning is attached to the death of an infant or child?
- How does religious affiliation affect what family members do and what is expected of them?

Source: With permission from Jannetti Publications.

Care manager tasks include:

- Assess degree of acculturation.
- Assess language preferences; if you do not speak the language, use a trained interpreter.
- Assess religious preferences.
- Assess food preferences and restrictions.
- Establish use of traditional medicines.
- Establish who is to be told healthcare status.
- Establish client preferences for disclosure or nondisclosure of medical information.
- Request educational materials in preferred language from hospitals and family disease support networks such as the American Cancer Society.
- Inform other providers of culturally specific requirements.
- Assess if special arrangements are required for after-death care of the body.

FAMILY PROBLEMS AND ISSUES

Caregiver Burden and Stress

Caregiving at the end of life

has a dramatic impact on the health and well-being of family caregivers. Between 40% and 70% of caregivers have been found to have clinically significant levels of depressive symptoms, and as many as 50% may meet criteria for a diagnosable depressive disorder at some point in their caregiving careers. Caregivers have been found to have an elevated risk of death compared with age- and sex-matched control subjects who are not providing care.[47]

Family conferences can be used by the care manager to meet the need for support and to reduce caregiver burden. In contrast to other types of family meetings, support meetings can be used by a care manager as a tool to combat caregiver stress, which is often the

result of providing constant care to a terminally ill family member.

Balancing the caregiving needs of the patient against their own needs, the level of responsibility, and guilt that some caregivers feel when they can't do everything being required of them are some of the primary stressors.[48] A support type of family meeting does the following:

- Fosters emotional support
- Provides information from professionals about illness and coping techniques
- Focuses on emotional support
- Clarifies misperceptions
- Provides information and education

The role of the care manager includes:

- Listening empathetically and responding to the concerns, thoughts, and feelings of the family member(s)
- Monitoring caregiver expectations about their ability to give care
- Providing information and mobilizing resources and other types of support
- Looking for ways to help family members take time for themselves and take breaks[49]

Not all family members are physically or emotionally able to provide hands-on care for their dying loved one. This meeting can also be used to redefine the concept of caring by letting them know that there are other tangible ways to provide care. Some examples of other types of caregiving tasks are bill paying, running errands, or keeping friends and families updated on the health status via e-mail or phone.

Conflict Resolution

Family disputes have the potential to be very destructive and can cause a breakdown in a family's ability to provide needed care and support for elder members.[50] Conflict resolution is one of the five most frequent interventions social workers from home healthcare agencies make. Sources of conflict around elder care decisions include:

> feelings of guilt, grief connected with the loss of the elder member's health, disparate investments and interests in the caregiving arrangements of elders, scarce resources for elder caregiving that demand commitment and substantial sacrifice from family members, limited experience with joint decision making, and the rejuvenation of old conflictual family dynamics.[51(p122)]

The care manager can facilitate this process by planning a family conference to address the conflicts that come up. In more extreme cases, family-oriented mediation with the help of a professional counselor or an attorney may be necessary to resolve disputes before progress on decision making can be made.

Anger

Not dealing effectively with anger can impede the decision-making process, adversely impacting the health of the elder family member and his or her ability to cope with the illness. Anger and emotional outbursts are common reactions of families of the dying. They are dealing with the illness and impending death of someone they love. They are faced with losses in the present and in the future. One source of anger stems from the failure of the dying person to fulfill their customary family roles and responsibilities—both now and in the future. Family members must also

> struggle with their anger over the [subsequent] emotional, physical, economic, and

social drains that impact both their lifestyle and standard of living. This becomes increasingly problematic as the resource drains escalate and, despite the sacrifices, the patient declines anyway.[52(p109)]

Often as a patient's condition deteriorates, old unresolved family conflicts emerge and dysfunctional families frequently become more dysfunctional. These conflicts may present as inappropriate anger, which can be very stressful for the care manager. Realize that the anger about the situation may be directed at the care manager as part of a psychological defense against what is too painful to contain within themselves: grief, sadness, and anxiety.

Care Manager Tasks

Empathetic listening tends to resolve anger. Through conversation and empathetic listening you are building trust, reducing anxiety, and creating a healing relationship.[53] This relationship has emotional components that require clear emotional boundaries. One technique is called "engaging but not enmeshing":

> A non-enmeshed statement supports the patient's capacity to process their own emotions and protects the professional's well being. A non-enmeshed statement would be: If I were in your situation I would certainly feel upset.[54(p5)]

Normalizing can help move a person through the anger stage of grief. It is perfectly reasonable that a family is angry. They are about to lose someone they love who may be faced with dealing with a great deal of pain.[55]

Give permission to ventilate feelings, and encourage appropriate expressions of anger during a family conference.

Clarifying or asking the person to provide more information, to elaborate upon their statement, or answer specific questions deflects the anger and helps you explore what the real cause of the anger is.

Explore what scares or troubles them the most about their present and future. Just asking the question, "Tell me what frightens you," will help them to focus on circumstances they may not have considered. [56]

Knowledge and positive action "can help mitigate fears and reduce anger. How are they handling the dying—are they making concrete plans about their finances, their things, their family? Have they thought about formal counseling to help deal with the depression and the anger?"[57]

CASE STUDY: EMPATHETIC LISTENING

After Andy Anger's colon cancer prognosis and chemo treatments, which made him very weak and dizzy, he had to give up his driver's license. Andy continually expressed anger about having to give up his driver's license and complained that no one gave him a ride when "he really needed one." So the care manager wanted to set up a transportation schedule to make sure that Andy had a ride every time he needed one. She normalized his feelings of anger about the unfairness of not being able to drive and gave him permission to express his anger at his doctor, who signed the discontinuance of license forms, and the family members, who were unable to drive him to places he wanted to go. She clarified with him the reasons why his dizziness and weakness made it unsafe for him to drive, and they explored possible transportation alternatives. After Andy talked about it they discovered the knowledge behind his anger about not being able to drive was his fear of being helpless and abandoned given his colon cancer prognosis. The care manager was then able to set up a transportation schedule based on Andy's most impor-

tant destinations and appointments. This positive action resulted in Andy being able to express his fear and his grief during subsequent care manager monitoring visits.

STRATEGIES TO HELP FAMILIES COPE AND GRIEVE

Anticipatory Grief

Anticipatory grief is any grief that occurs prior to a loss, as opposed to grief that occurs after a death.[58] When a family learns that a loved one is going to die, they begin to anticipate what that loss is going to mean to them personally. This sets in motion the bereavement process of which anticipatory grief is a facet.[59] Usually grief and bereavement intervention focuses on assisting the survivor to cope with a death that has already happened.

> It is in the area of anticipatory grief that the care manager has the opportunity to use primary prevention strategies and to make therapeutic interventions that may facilitate [grief work resulting in] a more positive bereavement experience for the survivor-to-be. It is well known that the experience of terminal illness—that period of time in which anticipatory grief occurs—has a profound influence on post death bereavement. To the extent that healthy behavior, interaction, and process can be promoted during this time, the individual's post death mourning can be made relatively better than it would be if the experience lacked the therapeutic benefits of appropriate anticipatory grief.[60(p4–5)]

Typically grief and loss issues are examined within the context of how individuals cope and experience loss. But what we need to do is to understand that the family is a separate functioning unit that has its own grieving process. According to research anticipatory grief work diminishes the impact of the actual death and the intensity of the grief that follows. For the family this "lead time" can be an opportunity to prepare for the impending death through accomplishing the grief work and preparing for the necessary adaptations that may be required because of it.[61]

Grief and loss issues may be dealt with by means of supportive counseling. This fundamentally involves employing active, empathetic listening techniques in response to the feelings of sadness, helplessness, anxiety, anger, and fear.

Talking to your client and their loved ones about anticipatory grief is the primary prevention strategy. According to Rando, the process of anticipatory grief involves six adaptational tasks for the dying patient's family.[62] Adaptation has to do with "active coping, struggling well, and forging the strengths to meet the many challenges that unfold over time."[63(p9)]

Remain Involved with the Patient

The goal of the care manager is to facilitate communication so that family members can maintain their relationship with the dying loved one. Family members need to continue to respond to what the dying family member is going through and to include him or her in family events. It is a natural reaction for some to want to withdraw themselves emotionally and distance themselves physically from the dying person. The care manager must monitor for premature withdrawal and help family members focus on continuing to experience the pleasure and joy of the dying person's company. Often, much of the contact that family members have with the dying patient involves assisting with the tasks of daily living or attending to their medical needs. A task of the care manager is to help arrange caregiving tasks so family members can spend time alone with their loved one.

Remain Separate from the Patient

Each family member must recognize that they will continue to live once the patient has died. Therefore, they must begin to recognize their own needs and begin to plan for life in the future. The care manager's role is to be a supportive presence.

Adapt to Their New Role in the Family

The family must start to reorganize itself to maintain its stability following the imbalance created by the dying patient. The other family members must survive, and they must grieve for the death of the family unit as it has been known to them. A new role may involve something as simple as reassigning who will host holiday parties to helping a surviving spouse assume all the responsibilities of the household. The care manager's role is to be a facilitator who will encourage and delegate tasks that were previously performed by the client or to hire the necessary support services such as housekeeping, yard work, or financial management.

Tolerate the Effects of Grief

The care manager tasks are to provide supportive counseling encouraging the family members to express their emotions. Point out to family members that it is normal to experience intense feelings and that these feelings need to be expressed. Depending on the client, it may be appropriate to make a referral to other counseling professionals such as clergy or a marriage and family therapist with a specialty in aging.

An additional care management task is to continue to monitor for quality of life. It is not uncommon to hear that family members are not eating or sleeping well, not going to their doctor appointments, not taking breaks, nor engaging in other activities that nurture or give them pleasure. They often feel guilty or feel they cannot take time away from the dying loved one. However, most people cannot tolerate an unrelenting confrontation with loss. Taking breaks and "the healthy use of minimization or selective focus on the positive, as well as timely doses of humor" are part of healthy coping and need to be encouraged.[64(p233)] Care managers need to encourage family caregivers to take good care of themselves so they can effectively take care of their loved one. This includes encouraging them to continue to exercise, meditate, and participate in other stress-relieving activities.

Come to Terms with the Reality of the Impending Loss

The family passes through the stages of grief and begins to accept the impending loss. They need to start to "anticipate a future without the loved one and to tolerate some thoughts of and planning for themselves in that future."[65(p341)] The care manager tasks include education so the family can understand what is happening medically, advance care planning, and pre- and postdeath planning on such things as funeral plans.

Get Closure

As family members confront the death of their loved one, they often feel the need to have a sense of closure. Closure is a sense of completion, of tying up loose ends, and completing unfinished business. Getting closure may involve attending to practical matters, but just as often it involves the need to feel complete in relationships. In his book, *The Four Things That Matter Most*, Byock states that "We are complete in our relationships when we feel reconciled, whole, and at peace."[66(p18)] There are no regrets about something left unsaid. For families who have

had difficulties in their relationships, helping them to achieve reconciliation may be an important part of this process. Completing relationships is both a need for the family as well as for the dying.

Say Good-Bye

The care manager's job at this time is to let the family members know that the end is near and that good-byes need to be said. It is hoped they will be able to take advantage of opportunities to talk to the dying person while they are awake and communicative. But this is not always the case. If the person dying is not able to speak, let the family members know that hearing is the last sense to leave. They should assume everything they say can be heard and understood, even if the person is not responsive.[67] Others may want to simply hold the hand of their dying loved one.

Some people want to be with their loved one at the time of death. Other family members may not be comfortable with being in the room when their loved one dies. Letting family members know that it is all right to be present or not is helpful to them. It is possible for someone who has been keeping a vigil to miss the actual moment of death. So whether it is their wish to be present at death or not, you can suggest that they simply say, "I'm going to leave the room for awhile. I love you."[68(p18)]

Give Permission to Die

As the patient nears death the family must give him or her permission to die. A soft touch or your quiet presence may be the reassurance and good-bye someone needs to be able to let go.

This does not mean that the family is unmoved that the patient is dying; far from it. It signifies that, despite their wishes to the contrary, they love the patient enough to recognize that his or her death is natural and inevitable, and do not act in ways that will meet their needs at the expense of the dying patient's need to let go.[69(p348)]

Care Manager Tasks

- Offer supportive counseling, and encourage expressions of grief.
- Monitor for quality of life and caregiver burden.
- Refer to professionals.
- Mobilize support.
- Help family to spend quality time with dying.
- Facilitate closure.
- Help the family to say the four things: "Please forgive me," "I forgive you," "Thank you," and "I love you."[70]
- Say good-bye.

Spirituality

One of the ways that care managers can alleviate the suffering of the dying and their families coping with terminal illness is to help them to find hope and meaning through spirituality.

> Spirituality is integral to who we all are as human beings. It is very relevant to the healthcare setting, because it is the way people understand who they are and is a lens through which people understand the world. It is a way people may cope with suffering, and also a way people come to understand what their illness and their dying mean.[71]

Spirituality may involve connecting or reconnecting with an individual's religion. Spiritual beliefs and practices are often interwoven with religious identity. Religion provides standards for family relationships, offers community, and most importantly offers ways of properly dealing with death as well as providing support for the bereaved.[72]

Research findings on older adults and religion show that "while other sources of well-being decline, religion becomes more important over time. [It also shows that] when religious support is most needed, older persons are less able to access it (due to failing health, immobility, or lack of transportation)."[73]

Spirituality also refers to something that can be experienced outside religious structures. It is a broader concept than religion, although religion is one form of spirituality as is meditation or prayer. "A broad, inclusive definition of spirituality is that which gives meaning to one's life and draws one to transcend oneself."[74]

The concept of spirituality is found in all cultures and societies. Philosophies and practices of spirituality may differ, but similar positive outcomes are derived.[75]

Keep in mind it is not our role as care managers to impose our own template of values on our clients. In the patient–family-centered approach the role of the care manager is to assess and respond to the diverse spiritual and religious practices and beliefs of their clients.

Care Manager Tasks

- Perform a spiritual assessment.
- Elicit information by asking such open-ended questions as: "Do you have spiritual beliefs that help you cope with difficult situations, or do you belong to a religious community?"
- Listen to the response, trying to discern how important these beliefs are to the patient, whether they give meaning to his or her life, and how they influence his or her healthcare decisions.
- Encourage the family to continue to participate in regular rituals derived from their religious belief system, such as family nights, prayer times, creating simple altars, and readings and stories from holy books.

- Suggest the use of meditation, music, or other types of artistic expression.

The care manager can make a referral upon the request of the family to a trained spiritual care provider, such as a chaplain, spiritual director, or pastoral counselor.

STRATEGIES TO HELP THE DYING COPE AND GRIEVE

Although the experience of dying varies from person to person there are common issues that confront them. Dr. Byock reframes the idea that dying is an "end to a meaningful life" by saying "dying is a part of living." He proposes that human development is a lifelong process that continues while someone is dying. He created a developmental model of landmarks and tasks for the end-of-life experience (Exhibit 9-4). The successful completion of these tasks is meaningful both to the person dying and to the family.

In his article "The Nature of Suffering and the Nature of Opportunity at the End of Life," Byock states:

> Encountering a patient who is suffering in the midst of terminal illness is an all too common occurrence for clinicians who care for the elderly. [...Yet] Clinical observation documents that some persons experience a subjectively heightened sense of well-being as they die. The concept of personhood and the model of life-long human development are applied to the explication of this apparent paradox, enabling an understanding of the nature of opportunity at the end of life.

To Have a Sense of Meaning and Purpose

Life review, the process of thinking back on one's life and communicating about one's life to another person, is one task in Byock's model for bringing one's life to a close. As life ends, one wants to know that one has truly been seen by someone in this world, that one's life has had value and meaning. It is a way of putting one's emotional life in order by reexamining it and finding purpose in the life one has lived.

Completion of Worldly Affairs

Having a sense of completion by getting one's worldly affairs in order is a task in this model. Advance care planning is one step in completing this task. Personal and financial documents are gathered for the purposes of writing a will to bequeath money and property and to help the decision makers have the information needed to act on the client's behalf.

Beyond transferring one's material assets, we also want to pass on information, wisdom, and skills. A care manager can suggest that the client create an ethical will as a vehicle for accomplishing this task. "Ethical wills are a way for people to leave their loved ones with 'values' instead of just 'valuables.'"[76] The origins of the term *ethical will* are unknown, but the practice began as an oral tradition. It has long been in use in Jewish history to bequeath a "spiritual legacy, a heritage of values."[77(p518)] An ethical will transmits the lessons life has taught you, personal values, beliefs, and family stories that you hope to pass on to the next generation. Unlike a last will and trust, ethical wills are not legally binding documents. But they can be used to explain the will and preserve family harmony. Traditionally ethical wills are a written document. But they can come in a variety of forms such as a short letter, an autobiographical statement, an audio-recorded message, or a memory book. Whichever format your client chooses, the process helps him or her to come to terms with their mortality. Creating an

Exhibit 9-4 Developmental Landmarks and Task Work for the End of Life

Landmarks	Task Work
Sense of completion with worldly affairs	Transfer of fiscal, legal, and formal social responsibilities
Sense of completion in relationships with community	Closure of multiple social relationships (employment, commerce, organizational, congregational)
	Components include expressions of regret, expressions of forgiveness, and acceptance of gratitude and appreciation
	Leave taking—the saying of goodbye
Sense of meaning about one's individual life	Life review
	The telling of one's stories
	Transmission of knowledge and wisdom
Experienced love of self	Self-acknowledgment
	Self-forgiveness
Experienced love of others	Acceptance of worthiness
Sense of completion in relationships with family and friends	Reconciliation, fullness of communication, and closure in each of one's important relationships
	Component tasks include expressions of regret, expressions of forgiveness and acceptance, expressions of gratitude and appreciation, acceptance of gratitude and appreciation, and expressions of affection
	Leave-taking—the saying of goodbye
Acceptance of the finality of life—of one's existence as an individual	Acknowledgment of the totality of personal loss represented by one's dying and experience of personal pain of existential loss
	Expression of the depth of personal tragedy that dying represents
	Decathexis (emotional withdrawal) from worldly affairs and cathexis (emotional connection) with an enduring construct
	Acceptance of dependency
Sense of a new self (personhood) beyond personal loss	Developing self-awareness in the present
Sense of meaning about life in general	Achieving a sense of awe
	Recognition of a transcendent realm
	Developing or achieving a sense of comfort with chaos
Surrender to the transcendent, to the unknown—"letting go"	In pursuit of this landmark, the doer and task work are one. Here, little remains of the ego except the volition to surrender.

Source: With permission from Dr. Ira Byock.

ethical will is meaningful and gives a sense of importance, belonging, power, and peace.

Completion of Relationships

Beyond the need to put their worldly affairs in order, the dying need to deeply connect with the people they love and to feel at peace with their relationships before they die. Like the members of their family, they need to have a sense of closure. They may wish to resolve guilt about harm done to another. They may want to say something that should have been said, to apologize, or to reconcile with someone in their life. In the time they have left they want to reach out to those closest to them to let them know they are loved and appreciated. Helping the dying talk about these things with their loved ones is one of the most important tasks of a care manager.

Completing relationships involves four components: asking and accepting forgiveness, expressing gratitude, expressing love, and saying a final good-bye. Engaging in these steps of completion is beneficial and healing both for the dying person and for their family members. Relationships can be healed; emotional burdens can be lightened. Memories of these last conversations are carried into the future. From his work with hundreds of dying patients, Byock distilled this process into four simple phrases: "Please forgive me. I forgive you. Thank you, and I love you."[78] The use of these four simple statements is a powerful healing tool that the care manager can teach to their dying clients and family members to help them let go of negative feelings and to bring wholeness and closure to their relationships.

Forgiveness is multifaceted. There is self-forgiveness, which has to do with accepting oneself as a human who has faults and makes mistakes. Forgiveness by others allows a person to let go of guilt for past failures, errors, and mistakes. And finally, forgiving others is about giving up anger and resentment against them. It is important to help dying patients understand that forgiveness of others does not mean condoning unkind actions that were hurtful. Forgiveness is more about freeing the self from the feelings attached to those acts:

> Whether or not the person who abused [or hurt] you benefits from your forgiveness is not the issue. The issue is the quality of your life. Forgiveness is an act of affirmation on your part. It is a way of letting go of old wounds that weigh you down.[79(p76)]

Another step in this search for emotional peace is gratitude. Gratitude is a feeling of being appreciative for benefits received. Research indicates that gratitude enhances well-being,[80] and it may assist individuals in reframing their dying experience. Helping a dying person express gratitude helps them heal emotionally in the face of terminal illness by looking at what is meaningful in their lives.

In the face of death, many clients experience an intensification of life and have a profound connection to life and to those around them. So it is natural that expressing love would be something the dying need to do. To express love is to connect to something that is positive—a reflection of a deep kind of happiness and peace. Love is something that is beyond one's suffering.

And finally there is saying good-bye. Although the authors cannot point to any evidence as to why or how this occurs, we've seen people seemingly delay their death until a loved one arrives at their death bed. It indicates to us how important it is to the dying to be able to have this sense of closure, which can be simple words such as, "I've always loved you," or it can be a nonverbal way such as a look or a handshake. This is not an easy thing to do, but the peace it brings to the dying and their loved ones makes it worth our efforts.

We have previously discussed the five stages of grief an individual goes through when coming to terms with a terminal illness. Suffering of another kind arises after the awareness sinks in that death is approaching and that medical problems have been addressed. Emotional, social, and psychological issues come to the forefront.

Acceptance of the Finality of Life: The Body

Helping a dying person accept the finality of life so that they can begin to move through the experience of leaving the physical body is part of the care manager's role. "How can we honor the physical body, which has been the host of the person for a lifetime, and yet at the same time prepare to discard it?"[81(p131)] There is a great need to pay attention to the physical body in order for the dying person to be able to let go of it in a peaceful way.[82]

Most of the focus of attention given to the body at the end of life revolves around medical treatments. The body may have been through surgery resulting in scars, open wounds, bruises, and require treatments involving tubes inserted into it or injections. For family members touching a person in this state may be off-putting; yet, touch for relief and comfort may be what's most wanted and needed.[83] However, each dying person's situation is unique and must be respected. Touch may be painful in some cases, or there may be cultural prohibitions against touching.

In her book, *Sacred Dying*, Megary Anderson writes that there are some things that are universally appropriate: "Keeping the physical body clean and purified, keeping the person comfortable and at ease, and offering some kind of physical contact for assurance or as a sign of love and affection."[84(p134)] The dying are not excluded from having a sense of self-esteem or from feeling refreshed once they have bathed. Some other healing ways to deal non-medically with the person include massage, washing hands and feet, the use of scented oils, incense, reciting family prayers, and playing favorite music or sacred or ethnic songs. Family members can participate in these activities or simply be present. These healing acts are loving, meaningful, and healing for both the dying and the family.

Care of the Body

At a certain point a person knows that their body is dying and may be receptive to the care manager introducing the question of how they might want to honor the physical body once death has occurred. Specifically one wants to ascertain if they want to be buried or cremated and if there are any specific instructions or rituals that must be followed for the physical care of the body after death. Some religious traditions have very specific customs that "involve respectful washing and purification, sometimes anointing, and the wrapping and clothing of the body to ready it for after the funeral. The body is physically purified for this death-to-afterlife transition."[85(p132)]

Often the dying want to be involved in planning what will happen to their remains and what type of funeral service will be held. Many times the family will also want to be involved in the funeral planning process. The final arrangements include whether the body will be buried or cremated, where the remains will go, and the details of the service. At the Web site for the Final Arrangements Network (www.finalarrangementsnetwork.com) you can find a planning guide and forms that will help you in this process.[86]

Funeral Arrangements

A funeral is a ceremony commemorating the life and death of an individual. This ritual often helps surviving families and friends acknowledge death. It can be held at home or at a funeral home. Home funerals, for some, offer an alternative to handing a body over to a mortician for embalming and display before cremation or burial.

Home funerals are legal in most states. In California, the Department of Consumer Affairs regulates the funeral industry. They publish a consumer guide to funeral and cemetery purchases that has this to say about home funerals:

> The law allows consumers to prepare their own dead for disposition. If you choose to do this, you must provide a casket or suitable container and make arrangements directly

with the cemetery or crematory. A properly completed certificate of death, signed by the attending physician or coroner, must be filed with the local registrar and a permit for disposition obtained before any disposition can occur."[87]

Although the most common method of disposition in the United States is embalming and casket burial, recent alternatives include cremation, home funerals, and green burial.

Cremation

Some cultures and spiritual traditions such as Hinduism choose to have the body cremated. As with the home funeral and green burial, cremation has become a popular option for environmentally sensitive people, and it is a low-cost alternative to ground burial of the body. The body is essentially reduced to ashes (cremains) by burning. The ashes are then placed in some sort of urn. The urn can be buried at a cemetery in a permanent or biodegradable urn marked by a grave stone. Alternatively, the urn can be placed above ground in a mausoleum marked by a plaque. Many people prefer to keep the urn.

Rather than keeping the ashes, some people prefer to scatter them in a place special to the deceased such as over water or on public or private land. Some places such as parks may require permits, so check before deciding where to dispose of ashes.

For the environmentally conscious and those who love the sea, memorial reefs are another option. Memorial reefs are reefs made of environmentally safe cast concrete that includes the cremains. After they are cast, they are placed at sea and create new marine habitats for fish and other forms of sea life.[88]

Green Burial

As the baby boomers age and look at what is next, natural burial grounds address their desire for environmentally conscious solutions. Green burial grounds are environmentally sustainable alternatives to conventional cemeteries. They are located at nature preserves throughout the United States.

Green burial has also been called natural burial because the body is returned to the earth to decompose naturally. The site itself remains as natural as possible. The body is prepared without chemical preservatives such as embalming fluids, and it is placed in a biodegradable casket or a simple shroud. The grave markers are natural elements from the environment such as shrubs, trees, or indigenous stones that may or may not be engraved. As in all cemeteries, careful records are kept of the exact location of each burial.

This less institutionalized approach to death helps people accept death as part of the natural order of life and promotes healing and closure. The participation in the preparation of the body, the familiar family environment, and the sharing of the planning and participation in the funeral celebration help all participants acknowledge the death and provides a creative and healing outlet for their feelings of grief.[89]

BEREAVEMENT

Bereavement is the period of grief that takes place after a death. The family's process of mourning the deceased is similar to that of an individual's process. Individually, each family member must allow mourning to occur, accept the reality of the loss, and work through the pain of grief while caring for themselves physically, emotionally, socially, and spiritually.[90]

But there must also be a shared acknowledgment of the reality of death, worked through as a family. This can be difficult because the grief of the individual family members may inhibit their ability to care for each other. As a result, their loss can be compounded by their grieving for the family unit that may no longer be meeting their needs.[91]

Consequently, a significant part of the grief process for the family involves directing its emotional energy toward reestablishing equilibrium in the family unit. Death of a family member always requires some change in family roles. Someone will need to fill the role that has been left vacant, and spouses and other family members will need to perform new functions and adjust to their new identities.[92] As this is being worked out, conflict may arise. Rules for behavior and new expectations must be discussed and negotiated:

> It is also important to note that family members are not equal players in the family system. Some family members will occupy more central positions in the system than others (in terms of communication with other family members, knowledge of family members and family events, influence over family members, and perceived responsibility for meeting the needs of other family members). Also, some family members may be linked to others in coalitions, either in specific situations or in general. Understanding these structures is important in understanding the impact of a loss on family relationships and on individual family members. For example, if the deceased was a communication link for other family members, that loss may complicate efforts to communicate about matters relating to grief and the shared loss. Similarly, a person who has lost a coalition partner may feel comparatively alone or powerless.[93(p107)]

Individually and collectively it takes time to grieve. It is a process. Grief has no time line, and there is no right way to do it. Expressions of grief vary and arise and recede at different times for each person. Often these expressions, which include anger and other hostile feelings, get directed at other family members. The family and the care manager need to learn to tolerate the differences in other's grief styles and accommodate and respect them.[94]

As family members move through grief they begin to accept the reality of the loss and adjust to life without the deceased. The focus is on trying to move on without forgetting the old. Holidays and anniversaries are symbolic of this process. These are times when the absence of that person is especially noticeable. These events begin to redefine the family. Family members consider how they can share this time together. They try to integrate cherished memories of the deceased. Old traditions are reinvigorated, or new ones are started. As their grief lessens, the individual family members begin to reinvest in other relationships and life pursuits.

WELL-BEING IN WIDOWHOOD

Thus far we have discussed the role of families in end-of-life care and their various roles in the dying trajectory as well as the grief process itself. This section addresses the death of a client's spouse. Factors that correlate to a successful bereavement outcome are identified so that care managers can develop appropriate interventions. The death of a spouse is rated as one of the most stressful life events that a human can experience. In addition to the loss of the loved one, widowhood causes "a loss of social, emotional, and physical support and frequently entails a notable reduction in income."[95(p197)] The average duration of widowed life is approximately 14 years for women and 7 years for men.

Research indicates that survivors report poorer physical health than before the loss and that the odds of new or worsened illness increase, as does medication usage.[96] Widows and widowers are more likely to be institutionalized than married persons.[97] Higher mortality rates are reported for both sexes; men have higher rates of mortality shortly after their loss (during the first 6 months) in contrast to women who are at higher risk 2 or 3 years later.[98]

Widowhood has a negative impact on mental health as well. The death of a spouse or significant other is associated with higher depressive symptoms, and suicide rates are high among the recently widowed, with men being at particularly high risk. Bereavement is a cause of acute stress. Unlike other stressful events, rather than there being a single event, there are ongoing stresses such as adapting to a new social role, coping with serious economic problems, and assuming the household tasks of the deceased spouse. The inability to perform these tasks is a great source of difficulty. Research indicates that learning new skills needed to perform even some of these tasks enhances self-esteem, self-efficacy, the ability to get along with others, and coping with grief.[99]

The transition to widowhood brings many challenges. Widowed men have a greater difficulty than women adapting to the emotional demands of being alone, whereas older widowed women frequently have the greatest difficulty with practical concerns such as home or car maintenance.[100] But the single greatest source of suffering and difficulty for bereaved spouses is loneliness.[101] As people age, their primary networks of friends and relatives diminish. Older widows and widowers have lower levels of social support, which normally can buffer the effects of bereavement. Because of the uniqueness of each individual, it is difficult to measure which interventions are helpful for everyone. In general, the literature indicates that initial family support is helpful, but single friends and other widowed friends proved to be the most important support over time.[102] A crucial task of the care manager is augmenting social support by initiating contact with self-help support groups, counseling, or helping the individual get access to his or her existing social network.

Ultimately, the great majority of men and women demonstrate considerable resiliency and resourcefulness in adapting to major life change and to the secondary changes associated with loss.[103] In spite of bereavement and the subsequent burden of widowhood, older widows and widowers adjust psychologically and believe themselves to be as healthy and as able to perform daily activities as older married individuals. This does not mean that the loved one has been forgotten or that some sense of loss does not remain, but rather it means that individuals learn to cope with their losses and that "widowhood ultimately ceases to have much effect on day-to-day mood and functioning."[104(p206)]

Care Management Strategies

That the majority of men and women show psychological recovery after widowhood does not mean that bereavement is not a major trauma or that there aren't things that can be done to speed and improve recovery. From a care management perspective there are three domains that correlate to a successful bereavement: depression status, use of general coping strategies, and social supports:

> There is evidence that a majority of widows have some warning of the impending death, and that using that time to prepare, or rehearse, for widowhood is associated positively with long-term adjustments. . . . Rehearsal activities include social comparison with other individuals in similar situations, beginning to plan and make decisions, and actually beginning to try to do things on their own, such as making new friends, becoming involved in the community, taking over family finances [and] learning to get around on their own.[105(p373)]

Depression early on in bereavement negatively affects the subsequent adjustment.[106] Focusing on early treatment of depression is recommended both to reduce its effects and to make way for "fuller engagement in the bereavement process."[107(p238)]

For the recently widowed, interventions aimed at ameliorating psychological distress and psychosocial impairment are best.[108] These include encouraging the coping strategies of expressing sadness, seeking to find a purpose, and positive self-talk.[109]

Given the higher rates of suicide among men, providing network enrichment for older males in the early stages of bereavement is critical. Suicidal people often feel isolated and feel there is no one they can turn to. If you suspect that a client is not coping, you should ask him if he's thinking about hurting himself.

Care Manager Tasks

- Help with funeral planning if not completed in advance care planning.
- Address such practical issues as collecting documents, filing for benefits, and dealing with money and legal matters.
  - Final details: A checklist www.aarp.org/families/grief_loss/a2004-11-15-final checklist.html
  - Final details: Necessary papers http://www.aarp.org/families/grief_loss/a2004-11-15-necessarypapers.html
  - Final details: Steps to take http://www.aarp.org/families/grief_loss/a2004-11-15-finaldetails.html
- Final details: Claiming benefits http://www.aarp.org/families/grief_loss/a2004-11-15-claiming.html
- Use a family conference to go over the list of final details and assign tasks.
- Perform assessments: psychosocial, functional, home environment, and depression.
- Monitor for suicide warning signs.
- Identify tasks formerly performed by the deceased spouse that need to be adopted by survivor or performed by someone else.
- Connect with support groups and self-help groups such as Widows and Widowers.
- Connect survivor with grief counseling.

CONCLUSION

The death of a family member can easily be the most profound experience of a person's life. Emotions run high. The hours are long, unpredictable, and disruptive to one's normal life. Every decision is fraught with importance and peril.

Care managers create a foundation on which family members can make difficult decisions and assess what they want to do with the time they have left together. We can give clients the opportunity to answer the big questions: Did my life have meaning? Are people going to remember me when I'm gone? Will my family be all right? By creating a less chaotic space for the participants, care managers have the opportunity to change what can be a profoundly horrible experience into a meaningful resolution of a life.

REFERENCES

1. Byock I. *Dying Well: The Prospect of Growth at the End of Life.* New York, NY: Putnam/Riverhead; 1997.
2. Lorenz K, Dy S, Lynn J, et al. *End-of-life care and outcomes.* Evidence Report/Technology Assessment No. 110 [Electronic version]. Rockville, MD: Agency for Healthcare Research and Quality. December 2004. AHRQ Publication No. 05-E004-2.
3. Blaylock B, Johnson B. *Advancing the Practice of Patient- and Family-Centered Geriatric Care.* Bethesda, MD: Institute for Family-Centered Care; 2001.

4. Steinhauser KE, Clipp EC, McNeilly M, et al. In search of a good death: Observations of patients, families, and providers. *Annals of Internal Medicine*. 2000;132(10):825–832.

5. Teno JM, Carey V, Okun S, Rochon T, Welch L. Putting the patient and family voice back into measuring the quality of care for the dying: Toolkit of instruments to measure end-of-life care (TIME) [slide presentation]. Available at: http://www.chcr.brown.edu/pcoc/toolkitconcepts.pdf. Accessed August 20, 2007.

6. Lorenz K, Dy S, Lynn J, et al. *End-of-life care and outcomes*. Evidence Report/Technology Assessment No. 110 [Electronic version]. Rockville, MD: Agency for Healthcare Research and Quality. December 2004. AHRQ Publication No. 05-E004-2.

7. Lorenz K, Dy S, Lynn J, et al. *End-of-life care and outcomes*. Evidence Report/Technology Assessment No. 110 [Electronic version]. Rockville, MD: Agency for Healthcare Research and Quality. December 2004. AHRQ Publication No. 05-E004-2.

8. Stanton M. Expanding patient-centered care to empower patients and assist providers. *Research in Action*. 2002;5. AHRQ Publication No. 02-0024.

9. Blaylock B, Johnson B. *Advancing the Practice of Patient- and Family-Centered Geriatric Care*. Bethesda, MD: Institute for Family-Centered Care; 2001.

10. Blaylock B, Johnson B. *Advancing the Practice of Patient- and Family-Centered Geriatric Care*. Bethesda, MD: Institute for Family-Centered Care; 2001.

11. Andrist L, Nicholas PK, Wolf K. *A History of Nursing Ideas*. Sudbury, MA: Jones and Bartlett; 2005:205.

12. Rando TA. *Loss & Anticipatory Grief*. New York, NY: Lexington Books; 1986.

13. National Cancer Institute. *Phases of a life threatening illness*. 2006. Available at: http://www.cancer.gov/cancertopics/pdq/supportivecare/bereavement/Patient/page3. Retrieved July 15, 2007.

14. Asbestos Resource Center. *Dealing with grief terminal illness phases*. Available at: http://www.asbestosresource.com/grief/phases.html. Accessed July15, 2007.

15. Center for Caregiver Training. *Caregiving 101. How to be prepared for a ten-minute doctor's visit* (mod. 2: Lesson 3). Available at: http://www.caregiving101.org/LessonContent/m2/m2l3.asp. Accessed July 18, 2007.

16. Matzo M, Sherman D. *Palliative Care Nursing: Quality Care to the End of Life*. New York, NY: Springer; 2001.

17. National Cancer Institute. *Phases of a life threatening illness*. Available at: http://www.cancer.gov/cancertopics/pdq/supportivecare/bereavement/Patient/page3. Accessed July 15, 2007.

18. National Cancer Institute. *Phases of a life threatening illness*. Available at: http://www.cancer.gov/cancertopics/pdq/supportivecare/bereavement/Patient/page3. Accessed July 15, 2007.

19. Waters C, Crary W. *Learning to cope with chronic illness*. Available at: http://seniors-site.com/coping/chronic.html. Accessed July 20, 2007.

20. Waters C, Crary W. *Learning to cope with chronic illness*. Available at: http://seniors-site.com/coping/chronic.html. Accessed July 20, 2007.

21. National Cancer Institute. *Phases of a life threatening illness*. Available at: http://www.cancer.gov/cancertopics/pdq/supportive care/bereavement/Patient/page3. Accessed July 15, 2007.

22. Asbestos Resource Center. *Dealing with grief terminal illness phases*. Available at: http://www.asbestosresource.com/grief/phases.html. Accessed July15, 2007.

23. Byock I. *The Four Things That Matter Most: A Book About Living*. New York, NY: Free Press; 2004.

24. Abbot KH, Abernaty AP, Breen CM, Sago JG, Tulsky JA. (2001). *Families looking back: one year after discussion of withdrawal or withholding of life-sustaining in support*. Available at: http://www.ncbi.nlm.nih.gov/sites/entrez?cmd=Retrieve& db=PubMed&list_uids=11176185. Retrieved July 20, 2007.

25. Hsiu-Fang H, Curtis J, Shannon S. Contradictions and strategic communication during end-of-life decision making in the intensive care unit. *Journal of Critical Care*. 2006;21:294–304.

26. Chipman JG, Beilman GJ, Schmitz CC, Seatter SC. Development and pilot testing of an OSCE for difficult conversations in surgical intensive care. *Journal of Surgical Education*. 2007;64(2):79–87.

27. Hsiu-Fang H, Curtis J, Shannon S. Contradictions and strategic communication during end-of-life decision making in the intensive care unit. *Journal of Critical Care*. 2006;21:294–304.

28. Cope D. *Dying: A Natural Process*. Santa Fe, NM: Beyond Coping; 2004.

29. Cope D. *Dying: A Natural Process*. Santa Fe, NM: Beyond Coping; 2004.

30. Dunn G, Johnson GP. *Surgical Palliative Care*. New York, NY: Oxford University Press; 2004.

31. Cope D. *Dying: A Natural Process.* Santa Fe, NM: Beyond Coping; 2004.

32. DeSpelder LA, Strickland AL. *The Last Dance: Encountering Death and Dying.* (6th ed.). Boston, MA: McGraw-Hill Higher Education; 2002.

33. Hospice Net. *What you can do to be a supportive caregiver.* Available at: http://www.hospicenet.org/html/supportive_how.html. Accessed July 20, 2007.

34. DeSpelder LA, Strickland AL. *The Last Dance: Encountering Death and Dying.* (6th ed.). Boston, MA: McGraw-Hill Higher Education; 2002.

35. Azoulay E. The end-of-life family conference: Communication empowers. *American Journal of Critical Care Medicine.* 2005;171:803–805.

36. Kissane DW. *Importance of family-centered care to palliative medicine.* Available at: http://jjco.oxfordjournals.org/cgi/content/full/29/8/371. Accessed August 1, 2007.

37. Kissane DW. *Importance of family-centered care to palliative medicine.* Available at: http://jjco.oxfordjournals.org/cgi/content/full/29/8/371. Accessed August 1, 2007.

38. Chipman JG, Beilman GJ, Schmitz CC, Seatter SC. Development and pilot testing of an OSCE for difficult conversations in surgical intensive care. *Journal of Surgical Education.* 2007;64(2): 79–87.

39. Griffith J, Brosnan M, Keeling S, Lacey K, Wilkinson T. Family meetings—A qualitative exploration of improving care planning with older people and their families. *Age and Ageing.* 2004; 33(6):577–581.

40. Griffith J, Brosnan M, Keeling S, Lacey K, Wilkinson T. Family meetings—A qualitative exploration of improving care planning with older people and their families. *Age and Ageing.* 2004;33(6):577–581.

41. McFarlane R, Bashe P. *The Complete Bedside Companion: A No-Nonsense Guide to Caring for the Seriously Ill.* New York, NY: Fireside; 1998.

42. Family Caregiver Alliance. *Holding a family meeting.* Available at: http://www.strengthforcaring.com/manual/balancing-work-and-family-family/holding-a-family-meeting. Accessed July 20, 2007.

43. Iyer R, Cheng B, Kwong-Wirth S. *The end of life: Coping with death and dying in the Asian family.* Available at: http://www.cacf.org/wwwboard/messages/205.html. Accessed July 20, 2007.

44. Family Caregiver Alliance. *Holding a family meeting.* Available at: http://www.strengthforcaring.com/manual/balancing-work-and-family-family/holding-a-family-meeting. Accessed July 20, 2007.

45. University of Washington Medical Center. *Culture clues: Communicating with your Chinese patient.* Available at: http://depts.washington.edu/pfes/pdf/ChineseCultureClue4_07.pdf. Accessed October 26, 2007.

46. Iyer R, Cheng B, Kwong-Wirth S. *The end of life: Coping with death and dying in the Asian family.* Available at: http://www.cacf.org/wwwboard/messages/205.html. Accessed July 20, 2007.

47. Zarit SH. *Family care and burden at the end of life.* Available at: http://www.cmaj.ca/cgi/content/full/170/12/1811. Accessed August 20, 2007.

48. Brodie K, Gadling-Cole C. The use of family decision meetings when addressing caregiver stress. *Journal of Gerontological Social Work.* 2003; 42(1):89–100.

49. Winefield HR, Harvey EJ. Tertiary prevention in mental health care: Effects of group meetings for family caregivers. *Australian and New Zealand Journal of Psychiatry.* 1995;29:139–145.

50. Parsons R, Cox E. Family mediation in elder caregiving decisions: An empowerment intervention. *Social Work.* 1989;34(2):122–126.

51. Parsons R, Cox E. Family mediation in elder caregiving decisions: An empowerment intervention. *Social Work.* 1989;34(2):122–126.

52. Rando TA. *How to Go on Living When Someone You Love Dies.* Lexington, MA: Lexington Books; 1998.

53. Feil N. *V/F Validation: The Feil Method, How to Help Disoriented Old-Old.* Cleveland, OH: Edward Feil Productions; 2003.

54. Houston R. The angry dying patient. *Journal of Clinical Psychiatry.* 1999;1(1):5–8.

55. Houston R. The angry dying patient. *Journal of Clinical Psychiatry.* 1999;1(1):5–8.

56. Wang-Cheng B. *Fast fact and concept #059: Dealing with the angry dying patient.* Available at: http://www.mywhatever.com/cifwriter/library/eperc/fastfact/ff16.html. Accessed July 20, 2007.

57. Wang-Cheng B. *Fast fact and concept #059: Dealing with the angry dying patient.* Available at: http://www.mywhatever.com/cifwriter/library/eperc/fastfact/ff16.html. Accessed July 20, 2007.

58. Caroff P, Dobrof R. Social work: Its institutional role. In: Schoenberg B, Carr A, Kuitscher A, Peretz D, Goldberg I, eds. *Anticipatory Grief.* New York, NY: Columbia University Press; 1974:251–263.

59. Rando TA. *How to Go on Living When Someone You Love Dies.* Lexington, MA: Lexington Books; 1998.

60. Rando TA. *Loss & Anticipatory Grief*. New York, NY: Lexington Books; 1986.

61. Caroff P, Dobrof R. Social work: Its institutional role. In: Schoenberg B, Carr A, Kuitscher A, Peretz D, Goldberg I, eds. *Anticipatory Grief*. New York, NY: Columbia University Press; 1974: 251–263.

62. Humphrey MA. Effects of anticipatory grief for the patient, family member, and caregiver. In: Rando TA, ed. *Loss & Anticipatory Grief*. New York, NY: Lexington Books; 1986:68.

63. Walsh F, McGoldrick M. *Living Beyond Loss: Death in the Family* (2nd ed.). New York, NY: W.W. Norton & Company; 2004.

64. Rolland JS. Helping families with anticipatory loss and terminal illness. In: Walsh F, McGoldrick M, eds. *Living Beyond Loss: Death in the Family* (2nd ed.). New York, NY: W.W. Norton & Company; 2004:213–236.

65. Rando TA. *Grief, Dying, and Death: Clinical Interventions for Caregivers*. Lexington, MA: Lexington Books; 1993.

66. Byock I. *The Four Things That Matter Most: A Book About Living*. New York, NY: Free Press; 2004.

67. Center on Aging, University of Hawaii. *Preparing to say good-bye: Care for the dying*. Available at: http://www.hawaii.edu/aging/ECHO3.pdf. Accessed October 26, 2007.

68. Center for Caregiver Training. *Caregiving 101. How to be prepared for a ten-minute doctor's visit* (mod. 2: Lesson 3). Available at: http://www.caregiving101.org/LessonContent/m2/m2l3.asp. Accessed July 18, 2007.

69. Rando TA. *Grief, Dying, and Death: Clinical Interventions for Caregivers*. Lexington, MA: Lexington Books; 1993.

70. Byock I. *The Four Things That Matter Most: A Book About Living*. New York, NY: Free Press; 2004.

71. Puchalski C. *Listening to stories of pain and joy: Physicians and other caregivers can help patients find comfort and meaning at the end of life*. Available at: http://www.chausa.org/Pub/Main Nav/News/HP/Archive/2004/07julyaugust/articles/SpecialSection/hp0407h.htm. Accessed July 20, 2007.

72. Walsh F, McGoldrick M. *Living Beyond Loss: Death in the Family*. (2nd ed.). New York, NY: W.W. Norton & Company; 2004.

73. Center on Aging Studies at the University of Missouri-Kansas City. *Spirituality and aging*. Available at: http://cas.umkc.edu/casww/sa/Spirituality. htm. Accessed October 26, 2007.

74. Teno JM, Carey V, Okun S, Rochon T, Welch L. *Putting the patient and family voice back into measuring the quality of care for the dying: Toolkit of instruments to measure end-of-life care (TIME)* [slide presentation]. Available at: http://www.chcr.brown.edu/pcoc/toolkitconcepts.pdf. Accessed August 20, 2007.

75. Center on Aging Studies at the University of Missouri-Kansas City. *Spirituality and aging*. Available at: http://cas.umkc.edu/casww/sa/Spirituality.htm. Accessed October 26, 2007.

76. ACFNewsource. *Ethical wills*. Available at: http://www.acfnewsource.org/religion/ethical_wills.html. Accessed October 23, 2007.

77. Gessert C, Baines B, Clark C, Haller I, Kuross S. Ethical wills and suffering in patients with cancer: A pilot study. *Journal of Palliative Medicine*. 2004;7(4):517–526.

78. Byock I. *The Four Things That Matter Most: A Book About Living*. New York, NY: Free Press; 2004.

79. Byock I. *The Four Things That Matter Most: A Book About Living*. New York, NY: Free Press; 2004.

80. Watkins P, Grimm D, Kolts R. Counting your blessings: Positive memories among grateful persons. *Current Psychology*. 2004;23(1):52–67.

81. Anderson M. *Sacred Dying: Creating Rituals for Embracing the End of Life*. New York, NY: Marlowe & Company; 2003.

82. Anderson M. *Sacred Dying: Creating Rituals for Embracing the End of Life*. New York, NY: Marlowe & Company; 2003.

83. Anderson M. *Sacred Dying: Creating Rituals for Embracing the End of Life*. New York, NY: Marlowe & Company; 2003.

84. Anderson M. *Sacred Dying: Creating Rituals for Embracing the End of Life*. New York, NY: Marlowe & Company; 2003.

85. Anderson M. *Sacred Dying: Creating Rituals for Embracing the End of Life*. New York, NY: Marlowe & Company; 2003.

86. Family Caregiver Alliance. *Making funeral arrangements*. Available at: http://www.strengthforcaring.com/money-insurance/end-of-life-planning-choosing-a-funeral-home/making-funeral-arrangements/. Accessed July 20, 2007.

87. Centre for Natural Burial. *Natural burial*. Available at: http://www.naturalburial.coop/about-natural-burial. Accessed October 26, 2007.

88. Eternal Reefs. *Memorial reefs*. Available at: http://www.eternalreefs.com/reefs/reefs.html. Accessed October 26, 2007.

89. Final Passages. *Legalities.* Available at: http://www.finalpassages.org. Accessed October 26, 2007.

90. Worden W. *William Wordens four tasks of mourning.* Available at: http://www.vitas.com/bereavement/providers1.asp. Accessed May 26, 2008.

91. Rosenblatt PC, Grief: The social context of private feelings. In: Stroebe MS, Stroebe W, Hansson RO, eds. *Handbook of Bereavement Research: Consequences, Coping, and Care.* New York, NY: Cambridge University Press; 1993:102–111.

92. Rando TA. *Grief, Dying, and Death: Clinical Interventions for Caregivers.* Lexington, MA: Lexington Books; 1993.

93. Rosenblatt PC, Grief: The social context of private feelings. In: Stroebe MS, Stroebe W, Hansson RO, eds. *Handbook of Bereavement Research: Consequences, Coping, and Care.* New York, NY: Cambridge University Press; 1993:102–111.

94. Rando TA. *Grief, Dying, and Death: Clinical Interventions for Caregivers.* Lexington, MA: Lexington Books; 1993.

95. McCrae RR, Costa PT. Psychological resilience among widowed men and women: A 10-year follow-up of a national sample. In: Stroebe MS, Stroebe W, Hansson RO, eds. *Handbook of Bereavement Research: Consequences, Coping, and Care.* New York, NY: Cambridge University Press; 1993:196–207.

96. Gallagher-Thompson D, Futterman A, Farberow, N, et al. The impact of spousal bereavement on older widows and widowers. In: Stroebe MS, Stroebe W, Hansson RO, eds. *Handbook of Bereavement Research: Consequences, Coping, and Care.* New York, NY: Cambridge University Press; 1993:227–239.

97. McCrae RR, Costa PT. Psychological resilience among widowed men and women: A 10-year follow-up of a national sample. In: Stroebe MS, Stroebe W, Hansson RO, eds. *Handbook of Bereavement Research: Consequences, Coping, and Care.* New York, NY: Cambridge University Press; 1993:196–207.

98. Rando TA. *Grief, Dying, and Death: Clinical Interventions for Caregivers.* Lexington, MA: Lexington Books; 1993.

99. Lund DA, Caserta MS, Dimond MF. The course of spousal bereavement in later life. In: Stroebe MS, Stroebe W, Hansson RO, eds. *Handbook of Bereavement Research: Consequences, Coping, and Care.* New York, NY: Cambridge University Press; 1993:240–254.

100. Gallagher-Thompson D, Futterman A, Farberow, N, et al. The impact of spousal bereavement on older widows and widowers. In: Stroebe MS, Stroebe W, Hansson RO, eds. *Handbook of Bereavement Research: Consequences, Coping, and Care.* New York, NY: Cambridge University Press; 1993:227–239.

101. Lund DA, Caserta MS, Dimond MF, The course of spousal bereavement in later life. In: Stroebe MS, Stroebe W, Hansson RO, eds. *Handbook of Bereavement Research: Consequences, Coping, and Care.* New York, NY: Cambridge University Press; 1993:240–254.

102. Stylianos SK, Vachon ML. The role of social support in bereavement. In: Stroebe MS, Stroebe W, Hansson RO, eds. *Handbook of Bereavement Research: Consequences, Coping, and Care.* New York, NY: Cambridge University Press; 1993:397–410.

103. Lund DA, Caserta MS, Dimond MF, The course of spousal bereavement in later life. In: Stroebe MS, Stroebe W, Hansson RO, eds. *Handbook of Bereavement Research: Consequences, Coping, and Care.* New York, NY: Cambridge University Press; 1993:240–254.

104. McCrae RR, Costa PT. Psychological resilience among widowed men and women: A 10-year follow-up of a national sample. In: Stroebe MS, Stroebe W, Hansson RO, eds. *Handbook of Bereavement Research: Consequences, Coping, and Care.* New York, NY: Cambridge University Press; 1993:196–207.

105. Hansson RO, Remondet JH, Galusha M. Old age and widowhood: Issues of personal control and independence. In: Stroebe MS, Stroebe W, Hansson RO, eds. *Handbook of Bereavement Research: Consequences, Coping, and Care.* New York, NY: Cambridge University Press; 1993:367–380.

106. Gallagher-Thompson D, Futterman A, Farberow, N, et al. The impact of spousal bereavement on older widows and widowers. In: Stroebe MS, Stroebe W, Hansson RO, eds. *Handbook of Bereavement Research: Consequences, Coping, and Care.* New York, NY: Cambridge University Press; 1993:227–239.

107. Gallagher-Thompson D, Futterman A, Farberow, N, et al. The impact of spousal bereavement on older widows and widowers. In: Stroebe MS, Stroebe W, Hansson RO, eds. *Handbook of Bereavement Research: Consequences, Coping, and Care.* New York, NY: Cambridge University Press; 1993:227–239.

108. McCrae RR, Costa PT. Psychological resilience among widowed men and women: A 10-year follow-up of a national sample. In: Stroebe MS, Stroebe W, Hansson RO, eds. *Handbook of Bereavement Research: Consequences, Coping, and Care*. New York, NY: Cambridge University Press; 1993: 196–207.

109. Gallagher-Thompson D, Futterman A, Farberow N, et al. The impact of spousal bereavement on older widows and widowers. In: Stroebe MS, Stroebe W, Hansson RO, eds. *Handbook of Bereavement Research: Consequences, Coping, and Care*. New York, NY: Cambridge University Press; 1993:227–239.

Care Managers Working with the Clinical Aging Family Issues

CHAPTER 10

Loss, Dependence, Filial Maturity, and Homeostasis in the Aging Family

Cathy Jo Cress and Leonie Nowitz

THE MYTH OF AMERICAN AUTONOMY AND CULTURE OF INDEPENDENCE AMONG TODAY'S ELDERS

As John Wayne blazed across the silver screen of the 1940s and '50s, he heralded in celluloid form what the 1800s had falsely taught Americans. Wayne, as the perennial Wild West cowboy, embodied the myth of the American Adam, a heroic figure who came to the United States to start a new history. American literature from 1820–1840 ripened this myth through Melville, Hawthorne, and Henry James. The fable told us all New World settlers used the traits of rugged individualism—doing it yourself, pulling yourself up by your bootstraps—to conquer the new land, and push westward across the continent. They believed they had the right to do this and that it was their manifest destiny.

After World War II, Wayne atop his Hollywood horse brought the myth to the masses in movie theaters and then as reruns on television. Returning World War II soldiers and their wives already knew from their Depression-era history books the glorious vanquishing of the Red Man, along with the uncharted territory of the West. This matched their own recent victory in the Old World, where Hitler and the Japanese were poised to destroy them in World War II. When these soldier-heroes took their wives to the movies,

they made babies afterward, and lots of them. The now-famous baby boom was launched out of the flourishing Eisenhower economy.

The falsehood of the American Adam let Americans believe when immigrants left the Old World of Europe behind, they were reborn in the new American Eden. This fostered the myth of American independence and a do-it-by-yourself mentality. These baby boomers, born in 1940s and '50s, are now facing aging parents whose health is declining yet who still are attempting to live out the myth of rugged individualism. These elderly parents resist their adult children's attempt at care. The baby boomer's challenge is to help their aging parents accept depending on their adult children.

The Results of the Myth of American Autonomy and Culture of Independence on Today's Old-Old

Many aging couples and individuals live in isolation. Their baby boomer children moved away from their parents for jobs, forging their own destiny from coast to coast. Adult children have left their mothers and fathers in their original communities where family members who might provide the basket weave of support no longer live.

Now the isolated parents are aging and need help. These present day old-old (85 years and above) think they should remain independent as long as possible. So, they are stricken when accidents and illness manifest in broken hips, stroke, arthritis, cancer, and dementia and make them dependent on assistance from their adult baby boomer children.

Thus, dependence and loss, forced on older Americans through the natural progression of aging and illness, collides with the spirit of John Wayne and Teddy Roosevelt in the old-old of the 21st century. They were immersed in the Adamic myth of independence that was bound to devastate them as they aged.

Baby Boomer Caregiver Stressors When Old-Old Parents Are Dependent on Them

The baby boomer children conceived in the Eisenhower era of American world dominance and tutored in 1950s schoolrooms in American independence, have their own conflicting feeling about their aging parents' reliance of them. During their childhood, when the 1950s Russian *Sputnik* challenged the United States, the American response of sending Neil Armstrong to walk on the moon led some baby boomers to believe the American Adamic myth as well. As their seemingly indominatable parents become dependent and suffer the losses of old age, these boomers are at times as befuddled as their aging parents as to how to get their parents to accept help. The adult children are caught up in the dilemma of the impact on their own lives by the increasing needs and dependence of their parents.

After a lifetime of seeing their parents as the resolute force in their lives, baby boomer children are shocked and baffled when their now aging parents are no longer that John Wayne father figure who can root out every bad guy with his gun and horse. When their mother or father need help following diminished health in old age, their adult children are often thrown into crisis.

THE FILIAL CRISIS—THE PARENT NEEDS CARE

The crisis that adult children are thrown into when their parent needs care has been labeled a "filial crisis" by pioneering social worker Margaret Blenkner. A breaker of new ground in the social sciences, Blenkner was the first director of the Benjamin Rose Institute in Cleveland and introduced the concept of the filial crisis.[1]

This crisis, she theorized, happened when the adult child realized that their parents were not invulnerable. Like the Twin Towers crumbling after America's 9-11, these adult children in midlife saw their invulnerable parents start to disintegrate and, with them, the hope of continued financial, economic, and emotional support. This filial crisis is in essence a new developmental phase in life, the loss of one's parents' independence and their now dependence on their grown children.

Prior Life Transitions Do Not Prepare Adult Children or Aging Parents for This Filial Crisis

Blenkner's research and ideas are little known outside the field of aging or even within it. Unlike other major developmental phases, such as becoming a mother or father, parenting a teenager, or marrying, the developmental phase of beginning to take responsibility for your parent is not part of the wider popular culture that is written about. Compared to popular books available for young parents, such as the Dr. Spock books, there are few definitive how-to books for the filial crisis. Baby boomer children and their old-old parents are unprepared for this new developmental phase.

They do not expect this parental care emergency like they did the nights of the crying newborn or the rebellious teen; thus, most are thrown off balance by the sometime sudden and usually unexpected losses of the aging parents. Indeed what must happen in this new developmental phase is that the adult child must evolve beyond expecting his or her parents to care for him or her through providing fiscal, emotional, and social support. The baby boomer must transition to what Blenkner calls filial maturity or a new mature state where they as midlife adults can give up their former dependence on their parents and move toward providing care to their old-old parents.[2]

Resulting Family Dysfunction and Crisis with Increase in Dependence and Loss in Aging Family Members

In the normal healthy family system this filial crisis can usually be overcome, and the adult children can let go of their former dependent roles and confront their parents' loss by organizing and providing care. In the dysfunctional aging family this filial crisis is incredibly hard to surmount from both the parent's and the adult child's point of view. With both the normal and the abnormal aging family, the culture of "pull yourself up by your bootstraps" and the accepted autonomous point of view of "do your own thing" filtered through the media in literature, film, and television contribute to baby boomers and their aging parents refusing to accept the losses of aging. This is exacerbated by the continuing American Adamic myth and these adult children's own cultural stereotype of themselves as perennial free spirits from the 1960s whose needs will always be met by their parents.

Dennis Hopper, director and writer of the explosive antiestablishment 1969 film *Easy Rider*, which propelled many baby boomers toward their own self-absorption and self-examination, now plays on that theme on 2007 television. Talking to boomers in a commercial about retirement planning, Hopper says, in that craggy easy rider voice, "You can still have it all." So, the myth that these adult children can remain free of responsibility is still touted by the media, making it even more difficult for baby boomer adult children to confront the losses of their once invulnerable parents.

LOSSES EXPERIENCED BY AGING PARENTS AND THE CONFLICTS IN BELIEFS OF THE CULTURE OF INDEPENDENCE

Constant Losses in Old Age

The old-old parent is confronted with constant loss as she or he passes through their last stage of life. Loss has been present in every stage of the elder's life, but he or she has clung to the American myth of self-reliance and self-determination and believed that no matter what the loss, he or she could regain control through sheer will. These survivors of the Great Depression and World War II have matured and aged on the idea that they could turn any deficit around. Old age and the vicissitudes of the body do change all this in spite of the stratospheric leaps of American medicine.

Loss of Mental Functioning in Old Age

Old-old individuals in the family may confront the unconquered universe of diminishing cognition. In spite of years of research in dementia, American medicine has yet to defeat the gradual breakdown of the brain in the old-old. In fact 50% of people 85 and older suffer with dementia.

Because their families and adult children often do not live nearby, many older people are able to hide this slow loss of metal functioning until a crisis occurs, like getting lost while driving or an unexpected hospitalization during which the medical staff detect the progress of dementia. At this point the filial crisis usually explodes as the adult children are called in, and the aging adult must confront the loss of independence that he or she has always considered sacrosanct.

Loss of Physical Abilities in Old Age

The loss of physical abilities is another characteristic of aging and can also cause a filial crisis. As people grow older and face functional loss through all the common disease processes of the body, they are confronted by the gradual inability to control their own lives through the basic activities of daily living. To remain independent without the help of others the aging parents must be able to bathe, groom, dress, eat, transfer themselves, and be able to go to the toilet without assistance. These functions are considered the basic activities of daily living, which when lacking will be provided by a personal or professional caregiver. After age 85, when parents are considered in the older echelons, they will be dependent on assistance from others in many activities of daily living. Again, in our isolated American society, where family members do not live next door to each other, older parents may have retired some years ago to "snowbird communities" where they can golf and remain independent. In this state of isolation the older adult may be able to cope with these gradual losses in function for many years until a health crisis, like a fall from poor ambulation, initiates an emergency call to an adult child. At this point the older adult is forced into confronting the loss of their independence and either anticipating or denying needing to depend on the younger family members.

Loss of Social Networks in Old Age

Social networks are further diminished as older adults move toward 85 years and the old-old stage. Many older adults experience friends and family moving away or becoming ill and unable to visit, and many of these friends or family members die.

These older adults may themselves reduce their social interaction with others because of their own physical decrements or functional losses. The ties that bind through attending church, synagogues, mosques, clubs, recreational activities, and travel all become more difficult with age and eventually have to be curtailed when mental or physical losses become overwhelming. This increases the isolation that older people often experience.

Financial Losses in Old Age

Finally, as we age we often experience financial losses. The old-old in our society grew up during the worldwide bankruptcy of the Great Depression and in their adulthood valued financial security much more than their baby boomer children. But in retirement the loss of steady income and the sheer length of life, because seniors are now retired for sometimes 40 plus years, diminish all but the largest nest egg. As the functional deficits of old age occur, care must be brought in to assist the elder, and the costs can diminish and eradicate savings. Elders are frequently faced with fiscal loss as they age, which for low- or middle-class elders can make them face dependence on their children and the federal government through Medicaid.

LOSSES TO ADULT CHILD AS PARENT AGES

Adult children have great difficulty facing the needs of their aging parents. As the old-old and, to a lesser degree, the young-old lose their mental, functional, social, or fiscal abilities to be independent, the adult child is many times in shock about what to do. Part of this alarm comes from the adult child having to relinquish their own needs, both basic and perceived. The parents of baby boomers, raised in the deprivation of the worldwide depression of the 1930s, wanted to give their children much more than they themselves received as children. With the booming post–World War II economy in the United States, their newly affluent parents were able to provide for them materially. These boomers' lives filled with Davy Crocket raccoon hats, poodle skirts, and the affluent toys of a secure middle-class America. These were things the Depression-raised adult parents never received as children. Baby boomers were raised in the era of "It's all about me"—first taught to them by their devoted mothers and fathers. This was reinforced by the turbulent 1960s when Americans and the world began to radically question authority. From the free speech movement at UC Berkeley through the Vietnam War, these baby boomers and then the national media questioned why they should march lockstep into another foreign war and their own deaths. The Vietnam War, unlike the World War II of their parents, had no clear threatening enemy. In addition, these boomers were happily and warmly tucked into their college life, unlike their post-Depression parents, who hardly had enough money to go to college.

Many youths of the 1960s did not see anything positive about the Vietnam War, and they participated in nationwide protests and draft card burnings. They got married or received deferments to escape the draft. The nation's most recent two presidents escaped being sent to Vietnam, reflecting this generation's rejection of authority and belief in individual choice as opposed to meeting the

perceived collective need. So, when the collective need of the family calls, baby boomers have conflicting feelings over meeting their own perceived needs and the needs of their parents.

Conflict of Adult Children with Feeling of Loss of Their Parent in Their Lives and Resulting Ambivalence

Today, adult children of aging parents not only confront the postponement of their own needs when their parents' dependence calls them to the family table, they also confront their own future and the much more impending loss of the central figures in their lives—their own parents. When functional and mental decrements of old age begin to show in parents, adult children are forced to face their parents' mortality. This brings about the new idea that these adult children will have to step forward and be the new caregivers. In the normal family, where aging parents and their adult children are emotionally supportive and healthy interdependence among members has guided the family norms, accepting the shift in care can be considered appropriate by the family members. Adult children may have already been assisting in family festivities, by making the turkey at Thanksgiving or overseeing the Seder during the holidays. So, moving to taking care of parents may be a big step for the adult children, but one that is consistent with the interdependent style of their family.

Adult Children's Confrontation of Mortality Through Parents Nearing Death

When older parents need assistance in their care, their adult children may experience a range of emotions including fear, denial, and anger. This is because our present culture reinforces the denial of death and its impact on everyone in the family, including the older person who will be leaving this world and the adult children who will be assuming roles as heads of the family.

Death used to be a routine part of life. Children and adults died at home with the family around them. Family members understood death in a visceral way—the smells, the heartbreak, and keening, and the passing on of the head of family responsibilities when the family elder died.

In our culture death and birth are hidden in the halls of hospitals where we are unable to experience it fully. Baby boomers have a more difficult time than previous generations facing the loss of their parents. They may live far away and may be unable to spend long periods of time with their parent who is hospitalized or is on hospice care at home. Boomers may not have seen the gradual losses leading to the end of their parent's life. When this comes about, adult children are often shocked and totally unprepared.

Adult Children Facing Their Own Mortality

The filial crisis of a parent's care needs not only makes the adult child face their parent's death but brings them face to face with their own mortality. Adult children of aging parents, brought up in the 1950s and 1960s youth culture, often cling to the feeling of adolescent invulnerability. This compounds their own denial of death pushed by the American culture of cloaked mortality, away from the reality of death in past generations. The adult child is often unprepared for the spectral reminder of their own mortality brought about by their parent's imminent death. These fears can move boomers away from the responsibility of caring for their parents and prevent them from being fully en-

gaged in the dependence and eventual dying of their parent.

Baby Boomers' Conflict with Their Own Aging

The adult child, by being brought face to face with the dependence of their parents, is forced to come to grips with their own aging. Being raised in a world that venerated youth culture, delayed responsibility by going off to college (as opposed to their parents who many times had to either go fight a war or take any job to support their family), today's baby boomers have not been prepared for the culture of aging. They watched their own grandparents age from a distance. In the 1950s and 1960s when the largest growth in the aging population started to explode, the societal ethic was not community care or serving the older person at home but institutional care in the form of nursing home placement. So, these baby boomers' grandparents were routinely placed in a nursing home, many times inappropriately, where the present young-old, who were then their grandchildren, rarely saw them and most importantly never saw them age. By the 1970s, the federal government confronted the huge expense of nursing home care by establishing community care for the elderly. This was much less costly to the federal budget, and through the Older American's Act we now have a broad community care system in place that allows the now old-old to age in place. This has had the result of allowing these baby boomers to see their parents age at home. The raw power of now watching their own parents go through the losses of aging—even from a distance—has forced these adult children to not only confront their parents' mortality but their own.

Finally, baby boomers face their own aging when the filial crisis occurs, and their parents need care. These adult children see their mother and father suffering the decrements of age and understand they are not too far behind. Today, adult children of aging parents are usually in their fifties and sixties and their parents are in their seventies, eighties, or nineties. With the life span increasing in the United States and people living longer, these adult children see their lives following the course of decrements and loss experienced by their parents. They see in their future the possibility of having Alzheimer's disease, experiencing a loss of function, and loss of control of their lives. Brought up in the youth culture of the late 20th century, these baby boomers are afraid of getting old. They are the Dorian Grays of our society, and they consider easy access to face lifts and tummy tucks and erectile dysfunction pills to be their fountain of youth. When they are stopped in their tracks by their parents aging, the adult children look away for fear they will see themselves.

THE EFFECTS OF STRESS AND LOSS IN THE NORMAL FAMILY

When an Aging Parent Is Unable to Parent

The family is an emotional unit. It is a living, breathing system and the emotional workhorse of our society. It is the system that keeps us moving toward the future while nurturing us in the present. Most families are nearly normal. This means that they are not always the *Leave It to Beaver* family, and they have their flaws. However, the nearly normal family can generally be characterized as being healthy with mostly unstrained relationships. The family usually has the ability to resolve conflicts and can move forward emotionally. It has generally dealt with former life transitions in the family, such as

birth, adolescence, and marriage in a healthy way. It is characterized by intact parental figures, whether they are the nuclear mother and father, just the mother or father, two mothers or two fathers, or a relative or friend acting as parent figure.

These parents and parent figures nurture their children and generally establish clear rules. There are obvious roles for everyone in the family with the chief role being the parent. The family members are also grounded in the feeling that the parent figure is there for them and nurtures and guides them. When the parent figure in a family ages and begins to suffer the losses that come with getting old and the filial crisis occurs, a healthy family is also thrown off balance. The person who has the lead role on the family stage will not be able to fulfill this role and his/her cognition may limit his/her ability to make decisions regarding health and care. At this giant pause in the family play, the normal family will face a change in roles in their family system

What has happened is that the role of parent has shifted, and the family must reorganize to find a new way of responding to the change in roles and functioning. In the nearly normal family, the parent was generally nurturing and financially or emotionally supported the younger family members, who are now young-old themselves. Over time, the role shifts may have occurred gradually, but when the parent has diminished functioning, he or she may not be physically or mentally able to continue in the activities that nurtured their families. They can continue to be loving and caring and supportive of their younger family member, but they will begin to depend on their adult children who in turn will assume new responsibilities. When family members have many other responsibilities or live far away from their parents, the reorganization of roles and finding assistance for their parents can be turbulent. As older parents need their money to care for themselves, panic can set in among the adult children who depended on their parents' financial support.

Anger and Ambivalence Over the Loss by Adult Children

Adult children can suffer ambivalence and anger at the parent who is unable to continue supporting the adult child because of illness or age. The adult child can feel torn between his or her need to nurture his or her parent and also feel resentful that he or she must take on duties, roles, and responsibilities that were assumed by the parent before. With baby boomers, this can manifest in the delaying of care for a parent when he or she clearly needs it. Their conflicts in providing necessary assistance can put the parent in harm's way.

Another symptom of anger or ambivalence is when adult children have difficulty in moving into the role of making decisions with and for their parents. Without someone to lead the family through the family traditions and holiday rituals that help bind the family together, the family can be thrown off balance. The balance in the family or in any system is called homeostasis. Every system must achieve balance to survive, whether it be a big corporation, your body, or the family. A system is characterized by multiple parts that work together for the system to function well. If one part of the system changes, the rest of the parts need to change.

Shifting Balance in Homeostasis

Change is difficult for most systems. The filial crisis of the parent needing care is an especially significant change in the normal and abnormal family. When the aging parent relinquishes his or her role because of the losses of old age, then the adult children and their siblings must provide care for that parent plus take over some of the roles the parent formerly assumed. This transition is gut wrenching to the system even in the normal family, because care of the parent is such a new life transition, particularly in our youth-focused society. The young-old children may not have anticipated a health crisis of a parent, and neither has the parent, so both the aging parent and their adult children may experience this period as a titanic crisis.

THE EFFECTS OF STRESS AND LOSS IN THE DYSFUNCTIONAL FAMILY

The filial crisis in a normal family is just a hand grenade compared to the nuclear bomb of the filial crisis in a dysfunctional family. Dysfunctional families lack the ability to resolve conflicts and have frequent psychosocial blockages that prevent the family from growing emotionally. Most life transitions in the family, such as birth, adolescence, and marriage may have been very difficult, marked by a lack of support from the parents. The parental figures are usually not in charge and are unable to nurture or establish clear rules. There are murky roles for everyone in the family. The chief role of the parent is characterized, at times, by a lack of leadership of the family and ability to nurture the children. The family members generally do not believe the parent is there for them or that the parent can be depended on. The dysfunctional family is typified by strained relationships and unresolved conflicts.

It is also the inspiration for great literature. O'Neil's wrenching play *A Long Day's Journey into Night* portrays the most miserable of dysfunctional families. The use of alcohol and the presence of family secrets that have been kept for generations color every scene of this great drama. A novel, *Prince of Tides*, by Pat Conroy is a more recent tale of a southern dysfunctional family; it gives us a more timely glimpse of a family whose center can never hold together and whose emotionalism affects everyone from one generation to the next.

Common Themes Care Managers Find in Aging Dysfunctional Families

When working with the dysfunctional family care managers face common themes identified by Emily Saltz.[3] Saltz says there are recurring characteristics that dysfunctional families demonstrate when they face a filial crisis and their parent needs care. These families come to the care managers projecting a sense of urgency. They call the care manager in a crisis and expect instant service. These dysfunctional families may call many care managers to help them. They may do unproductive research and may be unable to make a decision to hire a care manager after all the investigation to engage a care manager. They have conflictual relationships with the care manager they finally hire and often argue and find fault with the professional's opinions. They may exhibit a sense of entitlement. They feel that their family's problem should get priority with the care manager, and they balk at limits and want the care manager to bend the rules. They feel personally criticized by the care manager's recommendations and are frustrated if the care manager's suggestions do not give them instant gratification. They have extreme emotional reactions to the care manager's perspective and to opinions of other family members.

Most of the family lacks the ability to agree with each other about the elder's problems. They may blame each other when things go wrong, and some family members are unable to take responsibility for their own actions. They can blame the care manager, the staff, and the service providers. Family members can have poor listening skills when professionals try to explain, talk about, or resolve a problem. The adult children tend to be unrealistic about the elderly parent's diminished capacities and can deny the older person's functional and emotional limitations. They also can have little tolerance for the initial and possibly ongoing difficulty the older person has in accepting either their cognitive or physical challenges. These families are characterized by contentiousness, and many times old fights erupt over "Mom loved you best." There is usually little love to go around in these families. These adult children are forever fighting over the inadequate love and support in the family. Anger is a characteristic of these families and has lingered with them all of their emotional lives. They have experienced emotional abuse and at times physical abuse and anger from the parent and among themselves. Dysfunctional families are very practiced at distancing and cutting each other off. Their members often pull away, and patterns of isolation among family members are often present.

Fusion and Triangulation in the Aging Dysfunctional Family

The care manager may note that some family members take on the personality of another family member; this is referred to as fusion. This describes the process in which a person is unable to differentiate his feelings and reactions from that of another family member—for instance, the eldest daughter might respond exactly in the manner as her older parent does. The care manager's challenge would be to help the daughter differentiate from her parent and find her own voice, which is often a difficult and long process.

Family members will often, when stressed, form alliances, such as two family members joining sides against another family member. This process, triangulation, is described by Murray Bowen as a way people cope under intense stress.[4] Engaging family members in focusing on changes they need to make is difficult when they are fixed in their different viewpoints regarding their parent's care.

Abuse and Addiction in the Aging Dysfunctional Family

In the dysfunctional family, as in O'Neil's family and in Conroy's family, there are often symptoms of problems such as alcohol abuse, child abuse, or other negative behaviors throughout the generations. These dysfunctions usually create a barrier to nurturing, and this affects everyone in the family. The system is also marked by ambivalence, and all adults and children live in a love–hate relationship with other family members.

Adult Children in the Dysfunctional Family Asked to Care for a Parent Who Did Not Care for Them

Family systems resist change, so it is even more difficult for members of the dysfunctional family to make changes when their parent needs care. The nearly normal system is shaken to its core by the parent becoming dependent. However a care manager can guide the family members into reorganizing their family roles when the parents can no longer care for themselves, while acknowledging the shift and changes they need to make both emotionally and practically.

The members of the dysfunctional family, who may have experienced a lack of nurturing by their parent and have no role model of positive caring, may be angry and resentful at being asked to care for the parent and thus will find it difficult to provide the practical and emotional care their parent needs.

One way to view the difficulty of the adult child from the dysfunctional family is the lack of integration of the parent of the past and the parent in the present, who is old, dependent, and in need of care. The parent of the past (the internalized parent), who is perceived as not loving and possibly harmful, could evoke angry responses from the adult child who may have been abused either emotionally or physically.

The challenge to the adult child of the dysfunctional family is how to meet the dependency needs of the here-and-now old-old parent when the parent did not meet their dependency needs as a child. The challenge to the care manager is to bring the adult child of the dysfunctional family into the here-and-now and see their parents for who they are— an aging older person, flawed and imperfect, but a human being nonetheless, who needs their love, support, and nurturing.[5] The parent is not a child, and there is no role reversal, as Margaret Blenkner points out.

Adult Child Responding to Two Parents—Internalized and Real

Strikingly, the adult child experiences the internalized and real parents from the point of view of two people. One of her selves is her internal self, who may be 12 years old and who was mistreated by the internalized bad parent. Neither this 12-year-old child nor the 40-year-old parent exists except in the mind of the adult child. The adult child is also herself in the here-and-now—probably 55 years old with an 80-year-old father. These two people do exist. The adult child in both the dysfunctional and nearly normal family clings to that internal parent. They were the parent who either nurtured them or did not take care of them. To achieve filial maturity, the adult child needs to move into the here-and-now, grieve for the needy child, have compassion for him or her, and then gradually begin to relinquish the earlier perception of the parent. He/she needs to change her role in the family from the past angry/backed-off role and assume the role of his/her present self in the here-and-now, someone who is ready to have a mature relationship with his/her here-and-now 80-year-old parent. This means abandoning that internal 40-year-old parent as well. This is done by forgiving past wrongs and beginning to understand the circumstances of the parent in terms of their history and relationships with their own family of origin. These steps, with the assistance of a supportive care manager, can create the possibility of providing care for a parent who was not there for the adult child.[4]

Both adult child and their parent(s) have the opportunity to create a new here-and-now based on mutual dependence. Both adult child and older parent have the opportunity to reframe dependency in terms of interdependence on each other for both the emotional and concrete aspects of care. The role of the care manager is to help adult children and their aging parents heal old wounds and accept the limitations of each other, while forging a new reality that can heal the relationship between them. By being available to the family members and understanding and supporting them, the care manager can facilitate the adult children reaching out to their parent and providing care for them, as well as working with the aging parent to help them accept care.

THE CARE MANAGER'S ROLE IN DEPENDENCY AND LOSS WITH ADULT CHILDREN

The care manager's role with the aging family around dependency, loss, and filial maturity is to work with the adult children, the older client, and the aging family. This requires extensive intervention especially with the dysfunctional aging family.

The care manager must have good psychosocial and clinical skills and years of experience in the field. This work is not for the novice. Care managers are encouraged to work with the adult child who they feel is most receptive and to work on a one-to-one basis. The care manager can help the adult child shift their experience of their parent to a more productive one. This is achieved by building a good relationship with the adult child and to be empathetic to their experience, while helping them see their parents' lives over the long spectrum of time to get the overall picture of their parents' lives. Many adult children carry the hurts experienced in childhood. They may be able to camouflage their feelings in adulthood. When facing a health crisis of their parents, adult children are often conflicted by past hurts and a sense of obligation to care for their parents. This situation offers the opportunity to work on the earlier feelings about their parents, by helping them broaden their perspective about their parents' behavior and the message of their parents' lives to themselves and others. Working with the care manager can help the adult children see the broader picture of their parent's life and enable them to be able to experience their love and connection with their parents in the last part of their lives.

CASE EXAMPLE: MRS. SHREBERG, MRS. TAISON, AND MR. TAISON, JR.

Mrs. Shreberg called the care manager to help her manage her mother's care. Her mother, an 89-year-old widow who had cognitive deficits, lived alone in her apartment.

Mrs. Taison, the mother, had difficulty walking and was unstable at times. She was visually impaired and smoked incessantly. Mrs. Taison, whose father had been persecuted and killed in Europe during WWII, was writing a memoir about her father. Mrs. Shreberg's older brother, Mr. T, Jr., had left home after school and lived on the West Coast. He was an alcoholic and seldom called or visited his mother. Mrs. Shreberg said that her mother had always been emotionally distant from her and her brother. When asked about her mother's background, the daughter shared a history of her mother's courageous behavior during World War II: After her grandfather was killed, her mother found a way to save her grandmother and other members of the family and brought them to America. Her husband died before they emigrated.

The adult daughter was currently married, and she lived with her family, a few hours away from her mother. She had a full-time job. She had found unique resources for her mother, such as researchers who volunteered to assist her mother translate the memoir she was writing. Mrs. Taison didn't want any home health aide in her home even though she couldn't cook or clean for herself. The daughter engaged the care manager to meet her mother and develop a relationship with her. Gradually over time, the mother accepted caregivers that the care manager brought for her to select to work for her for a few hours, several days a week. The daughter respected her mother's wish for autonomy and spoke with the care manager about increasing hours of care when safety issues arose for her mother.

The care manager met with the mother on a regular basis to review her life, her accomplishments, and the challenges of diminished health. The care manager spent time getting to know Mrs. T and understand her values about her life, both past and present. When the mother needed more care, the care manager reviewed her care needs with her, and the mother reluctantly, over time, increased the number of hours of service that was needed. This success may have been caused by any of the following factors: improved communication between Mrs. Taison and her

daughter, Mrs. Taison's increased comfort with the caregivers, and her trust in her relationship with the care manager, as well as her gradual acceptance of her need for care. The care manager also listened to the daughter's sadness about her mother's unavailability to her as a child, but was able to get a full picture of the mother, in light of her life and circumstances, and recognized that her mother's emotional unavailibility to her were not a reflection of lack of care or love, but was one of the ways her mother coped in difficult times, having been responsible for bringing her family to the United States and also assuming the role of breadwinner.

Over time, the daughter began to recall the virtues of her mother: physically saving and providing for her family, being an advocate for the rights of workers in the United States and being an advocate and leader on their behalf, and her friendships with people at work as well as other friends who had since died.

The care manager asked both Mrs. Shreberg and Mrs. Taison if she could contact their brother and son. Mrs. Shreberg thought there would be no point; he didn't have a relationship with her or her mother. Mrs. Taison gave the care manager permission to call him, though she hadn't spoken to him in a long while. The care manager called Mr. T, Jr., to let him know her role in Mrs. Taison's life and invite him to share his perspective. Mr. T called back and said he wasn't interested in talking with the care manager—his relationship with his mother was a private matter. The care manager mentioned that his mother was ill and was receiving care. Mr. T said he'd check with his mother and ended the conversation. When Mrs. Taison's illness progressed further, the care manager called the son again, and spoke with him. He thanked the care manager for the call, and said he'd be in touch with his mother.

A few months later, in a meeting with Mrs. T, she said her son called. He couldn't visit her, but said he'd call again. She seemed pleased with his concern. She shared how difficult he'd been as a child, and that she didn't have time to discipline him. Her daughter was an easier person. She admitted to feeling bad that she didn't have more time to devote to him, but she was busy working long hours. The care manager acknowledged her for all she did do for him, and suggested she might share some of her thoughts with her son. She said she'd think about it.

The daughter encouraged her mother to visit her over the holidays when this was possible for the mother (despite the difficulties in caring for her mother in the daughter's home). As her mother's health declined, the daughter was able to increase the hours of the caregivers at home, and she herself spent time at her mother's home, caring for her.

When Mrs. Taison had a stroke, her daughter respected her mother's prior wishes not to be hospitalized, and Mrs. Shreberg spent the last week of her mother's life caring for her by herself. She was able to tell her mother how much she loved her and acknowledge that she knew her mother loved her. She helped her mother die a peaceful death by her physical and emotional presence.

The care manager witnessed the caring the adult daughter and mother shared for each other and the increased comfort between them over the 2-year period of her work with them.

After listening actively to the adult child's story and pain, the care manager needs to encourage the adult child toward seeing the bigger picture. The care manager should attempt to get the adult child to see the overall family story, not just their own version, which is the family drama from their point of view, scripted with what they recall happened between themselves and their parent in the past. If the adult child has perceived a parent as neglectful or unloving, the care manager can attempt to reframe that perceived lack of love by reviewing the parent's life with the adult child in order to see the larger picture.

In this case, the care manager listened to the daughter's sadness and her mother's unavailaibity to her as a child. But with the care manager's guidance the daughter was able to gain a full picture of her mother, in light of her life and circumstances. The care manager had facilitated the shift in the daughter's perspective through encouraging her to grieve and then encouraged her viewpoint and perception of her mother's journey in her life—which demonstrated the larger picture of her mother saving their family and advocating for others all her life.

The care manager reframed the mother's caring to the larger picture—her family and the people she worked to help. Over time, the adult child focused less on her mother's emotional unavailability to her as she recognized how supportive her mother was to their entire family and the world. This allowed the adult child to forgive her mother, see the parent for who she was by reviewing her life—an older person who had done many brave and caring things in her life. She and her mother had moved to a filially mature relationship.

The care manager was able to move the adult child away from her painful past into the present by listening to her grieve and share her sadness at her mother's emotional unavailability over a long period of time. This helped the adult child begin to be open to seeing the larger picture of who her mother really was and the values that motivated her in her courage and ability to save and fight for others including family and coworkers. She could see her mother now as an older person moving toward death, who had done some great things in her life and some hurtful things, including being distant to the daughter. In addition, by guiding the daughter away from only focusing on the smaller picture (her relationship with her mother many years ago) to the bigger picture (her mother's overall life from the point of view of the old woman she was now) the care manager was able to help her reframe her mother in a filially mature way. In this manner the care manager could bring the daughter to the present, as an adult in the here-and-now who saw her mother for who she was, a flawed older person who had done great things in her life but also had not been as loving as the daughter wished she had been.

The care manager was able to intervene in the mother–son relationship in a limited way. Mr. Taison, Jr., had been alienated from the family since he left home. However, he did maintain a relationship with his mother, however infrequent his contacts with her were. The care manager created an opening for him to engage in discussing his response to his mother's situation, particularly as she approached the end of her life. She was respectful of his wishes to not engage with the care manager, but he seemed appreciative when the care manager called informing him that his mother's health was declining. Mrs. Taison was able to share her sadness and regret at not being able to provide more emotional nurturance and availability to her son. By encouraging Mrs. Taison to share her feelings with her son, the care manager hoped Mrs. Taison could engage more openly with her son and share her regrets, which could bring them closer.

It is hard to know at the outset which adult child is able to move from a position of anger, to recognize their hurt at their parent, and to know whether they are open to engage with the care manager. Many adult children who are wounded prefer not to share their negative experiences beyond naming them; they often direct the care manager to provide the care the parent needs. Their unresolved feelings can be reflected in intrafamilial struggles and anger at the care manager, their parent, their siblings, and professional caregivers.

It is important to begin by checking each family member's availability by listening to their concerns and being supportive of them. Family members can display a range of responses from being open to sharing their thoughts and feelings, to remaining stuck in their hurt, anger, and unavailability. The care manager should not view the situation as static and should reach out from time to time to the unavailable family members during their work with the parent because there may be opportunities of engaging more openly over time.

The care manager can offer family members who are available ways to collaborate with each other on issues that require attention in their response to the care of their parents. This work takes great psychodynamic skill on the part of care managers, including expert listening and reframing skills and experience. The care manager can offer consultation that may include therapy to these families and encourage members to listen to each other's experience. Because of the intensity of family members' reactions to their parents and each other, the care manager should have a great deal of expertise in order to take the "psychodynamic pulse" of the family (see Chapter 11). It is helpful to have a background in family therapy with extensive experience in working with aging families in crisis. The care manager needs to have a good theoretical framework of the tasks the family needs to achieve and an assessment on how to move toward accomplishing that plan. The care manager may have to engage family members both individually or in family meetings to discuss the parent's needs, the family's resources, and each family member's point of view on how to accomplish this plan. This is difficult work and should not be attempted by care managers new to the field. If the care manager does not have these skills, then he or she should refer the client to a private therapist with a background in family therapy with extensive experience in families in later life and an educational background in aging. Another possibility is to work with an experienced professional in order to learn the skills needed. This could be facilitated by both care manager and professional participating in the meetings with the family, as well as being supervised by the experienced professional regarding ongoing work with the family.

COACH ADULT CHILDREN TO DEAL WITH THEIR OWN FEARS OF AGING AND DEATH

Blenkner tells us that the adult child's ability to resolve the filial crisis and deal with his or her parents' care sets the stage for the adult child's capacity to face his or her own mortality. The care manager's role includes helping the adult child face their fears of their own mortality. Many times adult children are resistant to fully engage with their parent's care because it may get them in touch with their parent's approaching death and their own fear of dying. A terminal diagnosis or one that inevitability leads to death (like Alzheimer's disease) brings the adult child's attention to the irrefutable truth of his or her own demise. This sometimes creates a feeling of powerlessness and lack of control in the adult child. If the care manager believes this is an issue, he or she may want to acknowledge the adult child's feelings and fears by using listening skills, giving complete attention both mentally and empathetically to the adult child's reactions to their situation. An adult child may be ambivalent about providing care when he or she is angry at the parent.

The care manager should create a climate of acceptance of the adult child and one that gives the adult child permission to share feelings. This supportive climate is set up by use of self (body language, tone, and setting). In this sympathetic environment the care manager might ask open-ended questions such as, "What are you most upset about?"

Allowing the adult child to share their difficulties with the care manager can create the beginning of a relationship to help the adult child move forward in relationship with their parent. Questions such as "What does your parent's illness bring to mind?" can acknowledge the fears and unresolved issues that the adult child is experiencing. Having a trusted professional to listen to their point of view is important in this work (see Chapter 9, "Dying, Grief, and Burial in the Aging Family").

CARE MANAGER HELPING BREAK ADULT CHILDREN'S PATTERN OF GENERALIZATION

The care manager needs to find a way to help wounded adult children see what is positive or good in the parent. This at times is challenging to their model of reality. Often adult children may describe their experience with their family members by expressing generalizations, such as the parent "never cared." *Can't*, *won't*, and *always* are words that describe a model of a world that cannot change. Bandler and Grinder, family therapists who drew heavily on Virginia Satir and Fritz Perls, suggested that in creating a model of experience, people use these generalizations and generate an impoverished model of reality that loses the detail and richness of the original experience.[6] The care manager may need to listen to the adult child's recounting of negative experiences, to help him or her feel understood and heard, before the move to make a shift. Through active listening, the care manager can gently challenge the adult child's model, a model that had deleted many experiences that could be viewed differently. The care manager can use such questions as "Can you recall one time when your mother was loving to you?" Or "Can you think of something your mother did (that you thought was bad—for example, punishment for bad grades) that resulted in a positive outcome for you?" Questions like these can reconnect the adult child's model with his or her actual experience. Other possibilities are to have family members share their viewpoints in a meeting with the care manager.

It is unlikely that all experiences were bad experiences with the parent, so some positive aspects may emerge. The care manager can also encourage the adult children to speak to contemporaries of their parents— aunts, uncles, and friends of their parents to ask questions about their parents and how they lived their lives. This is a way to gain additional information about the parent and a different perspective other than their own, thus creating the possibility of broadening their view of the parent.

Murray Bowen named this process *coaching*.[7] Here the care manager can reduce some of the obstacles that decrease the earlier vision of the parent by the adult child and help the adult child view their parent in a more realistic light. The adult children have the opportunity to add detail and richness to their parent's life that they never before considered.

Although this period is frightening for many adult children, in seeing their distant future move forward they have the opportunity to review their own lives, accomplishments, and think how they would want to live the final chapter of their own story.

Their parent's own journey can inspire them to follow in their parent's footsteps or perhaps do things differently for themselves and their families. If they can make a shift in resolving some of their earlier issues with their parents and are able to show and provide care for their parents, they will provide a positive model to their children and improve their relationships within their own families.

CARE MANAGER WORKING WITH THE OLDER CLIENT TO ACCEPT LOSS

The care manager's role with the older client is to help him or her acknowledge his or her need for care and be willing to accept it. This is a very difficult task given the older person's feelings about dependency in this culture and denial in recognizing his or her need for care. It is also difficult to give up one's image of how one has experienced oneself most of one's adult life—as an independent and self-sufficient person. Many times the first complaint a care manager hears from an adult child at intake is, "How do I get my mother to accept care?" This is usually said in complete frustration.

According to Saltz, the aging parent must go through their own process to be open to accepting care from their adult children. This takes the elder entering into a reciprocal caring relationship and at the same time being able retain their own self-esteem, dignity, and integrity. Saltz refers to this new task as "mutuality" in older families. By the parent allowing the adult child to render or arrange care, the adult child can move to a new phase of adulthood. This results in mutuality by both sides of the parent–child relationship.[8]

The care manager can use active listening with the older client to identify values that the adult child and the aging parent have in common that can move them toward mutuality. When family members have shared values, the care manager is much more likely to achieve a productive care planning process. Care managers need to identify the values that the older person has in common with their adult child and use these to strengthen the care plan. With a focus on the shared values and common goals, the care manager can help adult children and their parents move toward mutuality.

The care manager for Mrs. Kauffman, the client mentioned in the case described in Chapter 5, was able to show Mrs. Kauffman, who was not agreeing to home care, that she and her daughter shared the same value, which was aging in place. The care manager identified this through careful listening to both the older client and the daughter during the assessment process. Once she showed Mrs. Kauffman that she and her daughter had a mutual value, the care manager was also able to assuage Mrs. Kauffman's fear that if she accepted care, her daughter would not be involved with her mother. By hearing the older client's fears and getting the daughter to agree to a schedule of visits during each week, the care manager was able to bolster her case for the needed care for Mrs. Kauffman and get Mrs. Kauffman to accept care. Mrs. Kauffman was finally able to receive care at home, instigated by her overwhelmed daughter and resisted before the care manager intervened. So, care management skills of active listening and encouraging clients to identify and communicate mutual values help older people to accept dependence on others for care.

LIFE REVIEW OR REMINISCENCE WITH THE OLDER CLIENT AROUND LOSS AND DEPENDENCE

The care manager can offer life review or reminiscence to the older person to help them both verbalize and mourn the extreme losses that they experience and accept their new dependent role. Old age is a time of profound loss for the elderly. Many times the searing loss of their spouse or their friends occurs, and it seems like death is taking every loved one and confidante one by one. Older people lose many of their roles in life, like the role of a crackerjack businessperson or a capable parent or a talented writer or artist. They retire and lose their jobs and many times their incomes. They slowly and sometimes rapidly lose their physical capabilities. Many times they lose their homes because they have to downsize or move near relatives because of diminished activities of daily living, such as the ability to climb stairs. With their homes go the markers of their lives, the furniture they collected over a lifetime and treasured family heirlooms. These aging clients then are left with facing the ultimate loss—that of their own life. This process of multiple loss requires a period of mourning and is often an intense process. Freud said that mourning is the working through of personal loss. Mourning is intense as the losses are manifold at this time of life. Older people focus on a lost role, person, or changes in their health and functioning. Mourning is different from melancholia because it is a healthy letting go of what is lost as we age rather than a loss of personal esteem.[9]

Life review can offer the opportunity to help the client make meaning of his or her life as he or she approaches the end of the life span. If the care manager has a background in counseling or training in life review, the care manager could guide the older person through reminiscence. The goal could be to mourn the losses in the person's life in a healthy way and view more positively their need for help. The older person is letting go of the lost object, lost role, or lost person in a manner that keeps self-esteem intact rather than as a form of melancholy.

Life review has been posited as being a way of reviewing one's life and making meaning of it. When the older person loses significant roles and objects they begin to turn inward. The self-observation that can occur when one is reminiscing can help to replace in part the self-gratification formerly experienced with objects, people, and roles.[10]

Reminiscence can also identify unresolved conflicts, move the older person toward forgiveness, and also be a way to review accomplishments. If the point of the life review is to create an oral history and pass down family stories and the life of the older person, the care manager can involve the family. The care manager can suggest to the family members some guidelines for the life-review process. They could review their older relative's life with him or her on occasions of family gatherings spurred by ritual holidays or general family get-togethers. In fact, life review is often stimulated by ritual holidays and often happens naturally as a part of anniversary dinners and rites of passage, like bar mitzvahs and retirement dinners for younger members of the family. Life review can increase an older person's self-esteem and pride when reviewing accomplishments of the past and can be a gift to the family in cataloging for themselves their family history.

Care managers can also use care providers to work with the client in doing a life review. If an older person is open to sharing stories about his or her life with the care providers, the care manager can encourage the care providers to be interested in the stories the older person's shares. This is an excellent opportunity to connect the care providers with interests of the older person and to validate them in the process. It is a good addition to a care plan for care staff. If the older person suffers from dementia or cannot be easily understood, having the care providers tell the older person stories about their life, which the client has related in the past, can be a soothing practice under the guidance of the care manager. Encouraging the older person

or care provider to do this can be an educational function of the care manager.

Even if the older person is experiencing memory loss, care managers can involve the older person in reminiscence groups, women's or men's groups at senior centers, or adult day centers where they can share their life and losses in a group. This process has been demonstrated in research studies to improve both mental and physical health and functioning.

Older people sometimes feel belittled by younger family members for frequently repeating their stories. Or they may be made to feel that their life events are not significant. Thus, the care manager should educate both the client and the family about the importance of reminiscence in creating meaning for the older person and in transmitting history to the family members. It is a good use of a care manager's skills.

The care manager can refer the older person to therapists in the community who specialize in working with older people who might need a more positive identity in their aging process or who seek to derive meaning from their life. For example, an older man who experiences the loss of himself as virile and handsome and sees himself now as wrinkled and sexually impotent might benefit from individual therapy.

Care managers can use reminiscence to review the difficulties that the older parent had in caring for their own parent. In touching on this nerve there is a possibility of the aging mother or father empathizing with their own adult child's frustration in getting them to accept care and dependence and move toward mutuality.

Care managers should be especially cautious in working with someone who is clinically depressed or has a history of a serious mental illness. Reminiscence with older people with this diagnosis should be attempted by only a very seasoned care manager with a clinical background. Otherwise, the older person should be referred a mental health professional.

Late-Life Siblings and Reminiscence

The major avenue of communication with elderly siblings comes through reminiscence. Life review or reminiscence appears to be both a way to better adjust to old age and to also heal the wounds of early childhood. See Chapter 8.

Reminiscence gives old-old brothers and sisters comfort. Sharing recollections about childhood can provide a font of warm feelings, and speaking about early life with the people who know it best, siblings, allows people to have a second feeling of that warmth that the family either really had or had only in the older person's imagination. Doing this work with a highly skilled care manager or therapist with an aging backgound might be necessary, particularly if there are tensions between siblings that need to be resolved.

CARE MANAGERS WORKING WITH THE FAMILY AROUND LOSS AND DEPENDENCE AND FILIAL MATURITY

To help functional and dysfunctional families change and work toward filial maturity the care manager must move on all fronts. We have reviewed how the care manager can work with the adult children and the older client individually around dependency, loss, and filial maturity. Added to this repertoire is the care manager working with the whole family. A family meeting is one of the best tools a care manager can use to interact with the whole family (see Chapter 6, "Family Meetings and the Aging Family). Family

meetings succeed if adequate preparation in made. Part of this preparation can be individually meeting with family members as outlined in earlier sections.

Getting the family to come together as a whole to solve or begin to tackle issues with dependency, loss, and filial maturity can sometimes be better solved in a family meeting. Cicirelli studied decision-making beliefs and caregiving decisions among siblings. He found that siblings constructing care decisions as a group make decisions that better respect their parents' autonomy than a single sibling making decisions alone. He feels that a group offers checks and balances together to ensure that the parent's view is respected. Although this research reflects siblings, it is probably true for all family members.[11] By including the family, whoever they may be (partners, siblings, friends, spouses, or ex-spouses) as a group, the care manager can monitor the family's advocating for the older client because those group checks and balances are present.

When a decision that is critical needs to be made about a parent who has undergone losses that will involve changes in care, a family meeting is a choice that a care manager should consider. Decisions that might need to be made include moving a client to a higher level of care such as providing more care at home or transfer of the parent from their home to a facility. This will involve preferences of the older person, availability of family members to assist in care, and government entitlements and financial resources to provide for such care.

Family meeting are generally beneficial to plan interventions and set goals. Achieving either of these is supremely difficult with the dysfunctional family. In general, family meetings are scheduled to create a plan that provides for the safety, health, and psychosocial well-being of an older adult.

With dysfunctional families these family meetings can be extremely challenging. Only a psychodynamically or systems-oriented trained care manager should approach these families, especially in a family meeting. Some of the family members may suffer from mental health diagnoses in a dysfunctional family. In a family meeting, when they are all together, the interaction of those mental health problems is greater than all of the parts, and the care manager has to have a high level of education and training to manage these families. The care manager who works with these families must feel comfortable in working with difficult-to-serve families and should be able to withstand emotional drama and intense family communication. The care manager should also be able to work with aggressive family members who at times will totally devalue him or her. The care manager who uses the tools of a family meeting must also know how to come up with procedures and goals and critically move the family toward those goals during the meeting. Keeping on track with the dysfunctional family is challenging, so rock-solid planning and mediating skills are needed.

It is important to have a skilled elder mediator at family meetings who is either a care manager or a mental health professional who works with dysfunctional families. It is also important to have a specific tight agenda that is action oriented.

At the end of the family meeting the care manager should have an action-oriented plan. That plan should be a summary of all the issues covered, each issue raised, actions to take, each decision made, and who is responsible for each action agreed on at the meeting. If this is too much to accomplish, the care manager can arrange shorter meetings, with only a few items on the agenda to discuss. This could help the family members feel a sense of accomplishment in reaching goals and action plans. Follow-up meetings can reinforce success achieved and discover next steps to take when problems arise.

FAMILY MEETINGS WHEN THE CASE MANAGER MUST USE TECHNOLOGY BECAUSE FAMILY CANNOT ATTEND

Family meetings that take place when one or even several of the family members live out of the area are covered in Chapter 3. The care manager can hold a family meeting and include long-distance care providers through the telephone or more advanced technology. Face-to-face meetings are always best, but as families are far flung today, especially baby boomer children, a family meeting using technology may be the next best thing. The meeting can be held over the telephone if one or even all parties are out of the area, using the teleconferencing feature of the care manager's telephone service. The care manager can also use a teleconference or videoconferencing service. (See Chapter 3 on long-distance care for more specific information.) The care manager can also use a digital voice recorder to record office meetings and conference phone calls via speakerphone. If requested or helpful to the caregivers and client, the care manager can e-mail or save the files to a CD and give it to any persons who were unable to attend. This guarantees that everyone is privy to the same issues addressed in the meeting. This is an excellent tool for working with dysfunctional families because they present with such denial and conflict over events. This can give them the text of exactly what was said and agreed upon. Before the telephonic meeting, the care manager can work with all of the participants, either in person, by telephone, or by e-mail, fax, or regular mail, to develop an agenda. In advance of the meeting the care manager can work individually with the participants on main issues they want covered even if the work must be done on the telephone.

The care manager can attend to each participant's point of view and "hot button" topics that might come up. It is important to cover each participant's feelings in advance because dysfunctional families may have intense emotional reactions and respond in an angry or contentious manner. It is important that the telephone call meeting not break down.

Using an E-Mail Newsletter to Work with Families

Another tool a care manager can use with dysfunctional families is an e-mail newsletter, weekly report, or monthly report. Dysfunctional family members live mainly in their past memories, which to them seem as nightmares.[11] These anchors to the past usually center over the lack of love in their childhood, with each family member focusing on what piece of that nurturing they did not get. Although the very skilled care manager can work individually with family members on these past pieces, the main job of the care manage is to ensure that the aging parent, facing their losses in aging, has the best level of care. So, it is important for the care manager to focus the family on the present, which is the proper level of care their parent is receiving and their parent's health and safety.

For very fractured and dysfunctional families, with the hallmarks of quarreling over past events, denial, and triangulation, it is good for the care manager to keep reframing reality back to the present and the care of the parent. One way to do this is for the care manager to frame the reality him- or herself by supplying a narrative of each week or month, from the care manager's point of view. In spite of these dysfunctional family's penchant to undervalue the care manager's point of view, an e-mail newsletter or weekly or monthly report sent via e-mail or hard copy will define the reality of the client in the care manager's narrative, in the present. This moves the family toward playing with the same deck of cards and the care manager being the dealer.

In each e-mail newsletter the care manager should cover what happened during the period since the last newsletter, any new problems that developed, any old problems that occurred, and most important, the status of the present problems taken directly from the care manager's updated care plan. It is important to make the report sound personal and authoritative at the same time. These dysfunctional families "only want the best," so the care manager must come off as an authority. Yet, the families will respond better to authority that also reaches out to them personally because dysfunctional families tend to be narcissistic in nature.

The care manager will pick up the overview of issues in the family when he or she does the initial psychosocial assessment. This assessment should give the care manager the name and locations of all members of the family. The relationship that each family member has to each other and to the older client can be arrived at by constructing a genogram, which can graphically allow the care manager to see the family system. The genogram can tell the care manager basic client information about all family members but also each family member's relationship to the older parent.[12] This is a valuable tool but should be done at the beginning of the work at the assessment and perhaps updated throughout the work with the family. It is not a tool to be constructed in a crisis.

USING THE CONTINUUM OF CARE WITH THE WHOLE FAMILY

The last thing that the care manager can use with the whole family regarding dependence, loss, and filial maturity is a core tool of the care manager—the continuum of care in the care manager's community. The continuum of care is all the services in the community that serve the older population and their families. The care manager needs to not only know what services are useful to aging families in the area in which they live, but where to find them. This information needs to be in the care manager's knowledge base. Care managers should have access to or create their own database of community resources and the continuum of care.

A major part of the care manager's job, then, becomes referral. Family caregivers seek out care managers for education on resources. They seek information on what resources are available that solve the problems they have and are suitable to their specific needs. They also want to know how to access these resources. Information on specific resources to support family caregivers and the aging family must be at the care manager's fingertips. This also means knowing where to go on the Web to find resources in the community. A care manager cannot possibly have everything in their own continuum of care database, so adding other databases such as the Area Agency on Aging's Senior Information and Referral Web site is essential to help care managers serve aging families.

Helping family members access these resources is an important part of the work. The care manager's relationship with day care facilities, volunteers who can visit, and other needed services can improve their accessibility to the client. The care manager can assist the older person and their family members in visiting programs to choose which they prefer and can be present when they make these visits.

CONCLUSION

Working with dependence, loss, and filial maturity with the aging family requires sophisticated skills of the care manager. It takes a clinical background, years of care management experience, and a willingness to serve the hardest-to-serve clients. A care manager without this background needs to have an understanding of these issues and know where to get help for these problems in the community they serve. In larger agencies care managers can work under the supervision of more skilled care managers who have a background in these issues. If they are in private practice, care managers need to find good clinical supervision in working with these families.

So, the losses of the aging family can be mitigated when the family engages a care manager to help them solve these issues. Care managers can truly be one of the lights at the end of the aging family tunnel, and the care manager can gain skills and knowledge through working with these complex and all-too-human passages.

REFERENCES

1. Blenkner M. Social work and family relationships in later life with some thoughts on filial maturity. In Shanas E, Sttreib G, eds. *Social Structure and the Family: Generational Relations.* Englewood Cliffs, NJ: Prentice Hall;1965:46–59.
2. Saltz E. Difficult families: Conflict, dependence, and mutuality. In: Cress C, ed. *Handbook of Geriatric Care Management* (2nd ed.). Sudbury, MA: Jones and Bartlctt; 2007.
3. Saltz E. Difficult families: Conflict, dependence, and mutuality. In: Cress C, ed. *Handbook of Geriatric Care Management* (2nd ed.). Sudbury, MA: Jones and Bartlett; 2007.
4. Hoffman L. *Foundations of Family Therapy: A Conceptual Framework for Change.* New York, NY: Basic Books; 1981:28–32.
5. Cress C. Geriatric fiblits, necessary white lies or bad therapeutic techniques: How to do an ethical

query in your practice. *Geriatric Care Management Journal.* Spring 2006; 6(2):10.

6. Bandler R, Grinder J. *The Structure of Magic.* Palo Alto, CA: Science and Behavior Books; 1975: 40–56.

7. Bowen M. *Family Therapy in Clinical Practice.* New York, NY: Jason Aronson; 1978.

8. Saltz E. Difficult families: Conflict, dependence, and mutuality. In: Cress C, ed. *Handbook of Geriatric Care Management* (2nd ed.). Sudbury, MA: Jones and Bartlett; 2007.

9. Wrye H, Churill J. Looking inward, looking backward, reminiscence and life review. *Frontiers, A Journal of Women Studies*; 1977:2(2):98.

10. Wrye H, Churill J. Looking inward, looking backward, reminiscence and life review. *Frontiers, A Journal of Women Studies*; 1977:2(2):100.

11. Cicirelli VG. *Sibling Relationships Across the Life Span.* New York, NY: Plenum Press; 1995:64.

12. Morano C, Morano B. Psychosocial assessment. In Cress C, ed. *Handbook of Geriatric Care Management* (2nd ed.). Sudbury, MA: Jones and Bartlett; 2007:26.

CHAPTER 11

Entitlement in the Dysfunctional Family

Claudia Fine and Nick Newcombe
(Edited by Joseph Canarelli)

INTRODUCTION

Dysfunction in the family, as in the individual, is defined by the utilization of less than optimal defense mechanisms, thus promoting inadequate biopsychosocial coping and adaptation. These weakened defenses give rise to constellations of symptoms and behaviors that result in poor judgment and decision making, as well as unsuccessful social and professional relationships. They lead families to isolation, chaos, and, finally, crisis. Within families, these methods of coping and adaptation are established psychodynamically and are passed on from parents to children. If care managers are to intervene effectively with dysfunctional families, they must actually enter the family system and address the needs, symptoms, defenses, and behaviors of the client, adult children, and, in fact, the entire care network. Most importantly, care managers must be aware of their own familiarly transmitted dysfunctions.

Assessment and diagnosis must occur prior to intervening with the client and family. This process entails labeling and categorizing defenses and constellations of symptoms and psychiatric entities that will help the care manager to differentiate one family from another, much as psychiatric labels such as schizophrenia, major depression, bipolar disorder, and borderline personality disorder differentiate one person's emotional position and biopsychosocial presentation from that of another.

In the social work literature and in anecdotal communications, dysfunction in families is often labeled repulsive, help rejecting, or problematic. This chapter will focus on one type of difficult-to-serve family: the entitled family. A formal definition will be offered, categories of entitled families will be identified, and their etiology will be explored. Case material will be used to present the myriad issues of entitled families, and specific interventions addressing these issues will be proposed, explained, and demonstrated in practical application.

ENTITLEMENT: A DEFINITION FOR CARE MANAGEMENT

To arrive at a definition of entitlement as it pertains to dysfunction in families presenting for care management intervention, melding the current available definitions is necessary. When labeling or defining behaviors, one should be careful to understand that they must all be placed on a continuum from highly functional to totally dysfunctional. Consequently, it is fruitful to begin examining entitlement as a normal coping mechanism.

We constantly engage with others in the social environment around the meeting of a variety of needs. We form spoken and written contracts each time we reach out for help negotiating our physical and social environments, such as buying gasoline, grocery shopping, going to the carwash, taking a cab, or making a doctor's appointment. Because our actions are inextricably bound and driven by our psyches, as we form those contracts we do so with conscious and unconscious beliefs, fantasies, and expectations about the outcomes of these requests, assuming they will be met. Simultaneously, we must balance hope with disappointment rising from some level of awareness that these needs may not be wholly met.

Webster's New World Dictionary defines entitlement as the state or condition of being entitled to rights or benefits specified especially by law or contract. Beginning with our United States Bill of Rights and the Constitution, our entitlement to certain privileges and conditions is clearly outlined. These documents, the basis of our democracy and way of life, enumerate our legal rights as citizens and were motivated by the deeply rooted human need for security. In the legal profession and in business, clients and customers are given written assurances that the products and services requested will be delivered, ensuring that what the customer wants and has asked for will be guaranteed contractually. Federal, state, and local governments have addressed our ingrained need for predictability and expectation by creating entitlement programs, services and resources one can expect as a US wage-earning, tax-paying citizen. Medicare, Medicaid, old age survivors income, veteran's benefits, income maintenance, and aid to dependent children are a few of such benefits or entitlements.

The human sense of entitlement is a construct that helps determine how one approaches life's experiences and defines one's place in the world. A sense of entitlement allows one to set goals, predict outcomes, and feel a sense of control over the environment.

With all other coping mechanisms, the sense of being entitled is functional until it becomes rigidified and produces consistently poor outcomes.[1,2] Without some sense of entitlement, we would be continually anxious, totally disorganized, and prone to crisis.

For geriatric care management practice, the pertinent definition of the entitled family is as follows: the entitled family operates collectively in engaging with others, verbally, nonverbally, and in writing, especially service providers and helping professionals. It expects and demands that specific outcomes, based on preexisting fantasies and magical thinking, be realized. Family members are typically unable to appropriately delay gratification and manage disappointment. Instead, they employ other key defense mechanisms, such as projection, displacement, and reaction formation (see Exhibit 11-1 for a glossary of terms) to assuage their anger and frustration when these outcomes or needs are partially or totally unmet. They engage in the care management relationship without apparent ambivalence, delegating or transferring responsibility for planning and implementing care to a relative or friend, yet simultaneously feel that they must control the relationship, fearing the desired outcome otherwise will elude them.

CATEGORIES OF ENTITLED FAMILIES

Care managers identify their clients as the older or impaired person, but they must also intervene with family members who are directly and indirectly providing care and are thereby dramatically affected by the caregiving relationship. The family pattern of nurturance and care provision is first established by the parent and passed on to the child through repetition in daily life, starting from birth through maturation. Hence, when the adult child comes to the caregiving rela-

Exhibit 11-1 Glossary of Terms[5]

- Borderline personality disorder: This is a commonly diagnosed disorder that is characterized by unpredictable and impulsive behavior as well as sudden changes or shifts in mood. Because of this instability, people with this disorder have a difficult time maintaining relationships and keeping a stable and positive self-image. Some psychologists have suggested that this disorder hugs the line between mood disorders and personality disorders, which may cause some confusion when diagnosing people. The disorder is so commonly diagnosed that as much as 20% of all psychiatric patients are diagnosed with borderline personality disorder. The primary characteristics include (not all of these symptoms have to be present for a person to be diagnosed with the disorder):
  - Unstable and intense interpersonal relationships
  - Chronic fears of abandonment
  - Chronic intense anger and loneliness
  - Self-destructive behavior
  - A range of cognitive problems or distortions such as suspiciousness, unusual feelings of having a sixth sense, and unusual superstitiousness
  - Unstable social relations and repeated failures in job situations
  - Impulsive behavior such as fighting, running away, drug abuse, alcohol abuse, promiscuity, and binge eating
- Countertransference: Countertransference is a situation in which a therapist, during the course of therapy, develops positive or negative feelings toward the patient. These feelings may be the therapist's unconscious feelings that are stirred up during therapy that the therapist directs toward the patient. A therapist might start feeling uneasy about therapy or the patient, unhappy with the way therapy is going, or unhappy with themselves. Just like transference, this is not an uncommon situation in the therapeutic situation. Of course, therapists must not act on any feelings they have.
- Displacement: According to Freudian psychoanalytic theory, displacement is when a person shifts his or her impulses from an unacceptable target to a more acceptable or less threatening target. For example, if you are very angry at your teacher because you did poorly on a test and think the reason for your poor performance is because the teacher asked tricky, unfair questions, you may become anger at your teacher. But, you obviously can't yell at your teacher, hit your teacher, or express your anger in any other hostile way toward the teacher, so you go home and "displace" your anger by punching your little brother instead.
- Narcissistic personality disorder: A pervasive pattern of grandiosity (in fantasy or behavior), need for admiration, and lack of empathy, beginning by early adulthood and present in a variety of contexts. A person with this disorder is preoccupied with fantasies of unlimited success, power, beauty, or ideal love. He or she believes they are special and unique and can only be understood by, or should associate with, other special or high-status people (or institutions). He or she has a sense of entitlement and unreasonable expectations of especially favorable treatment or automatic compliance with his or her expectations and is interpersonally exploitative, envious, and believes that others are envious of him or her. He or she exhibits arrogant, haughty behaviors or attitudes.[4]
- Projection: Projection is one of the defense mechanisms identified by Freud and is still acknowledged today. According to Freud, projection is when someone is threatened by or afraid of their own impulses, so they attribute these impulses to someone else. For example, a person in psychoanalysis may insist to the therapist that he knows the therapist wants to rape some women, when in fact the client has these awful feelings to rape the woman.
- Reaction formation: A defense mechanism where an individual acts in a manner opposite his or her unconscious beliefs. A homosexual who joined a gay hate group would be an example of reaction formation. Freud believed that defense mechanisms helped us cope with the world around us by letting us repress our deepest unconscious fears.
- Transference: Transference is a phenomenon where patients undergoing clinical therapy begin to transfer their feelings of a particular person in their lives to the therapist. For example, the patient may begin to feel the same feelings toward his or her therapist as the patient does for his or her lover. These types of feelings may be positive or negative. The therapist must be aware of this phenomenon and may even be able to use it to help the patient, such as by role playing with the patient.

Source: Winnicott DW. The theory of the patient-infant relationship. 1965.

tionship, he or she reflects back what has been learned from the parent. Essentially the parent or care recipient, in a role reversal relationship with the adult child, is reaping what they themselves had sown. Three basic categories of entitled families result from this dynamic: narcissistic families, rich and famous families, and social welfare model families. Although each category has its own salient features and is used to identify a type of family that care managers encounter, it is possible for entitled families to possess characteristics from one, two, or all three of the categories.

Narcissistic Entitled Families

Entitlement in these families usually develops from a specific kind of "not good enough parenting" in which the parents themselves have struggled with personality disorders, most typically narcissistic or borderline personality disorders that went undiagnosed or were formally diagnosed and untreated.[5] The narcissistic or borderline parent essentially does not experience the child or children as separate and discreet from them and, moreover, uses the children to serve parental needs. Severe boundary issues in which seduction and abandonment are ever-present dynamics and where emotional unpredictability and instability are constant characteristics of this parent–child relationship.[6] The children find themselves in one of two basic relational positions with the parent: (1) the child is elevated to a grandiose, godlike position of perfection in the parent's eyes in order for the parent to fill and fulfill themselves, thereby feeling worthwhile; or (2) the child is devalued in the parent's eyes so that the parent can feel superior and powerful in the world. These children mature into adults who are emotionally impoverished, inflexible, and needy; in the care management

relationship, they present as entitled. Based on their real and intrapsychic experiences, these adult children fear that unless they make inflexible demands, they will receive nothing. An adult child in the first parent–child relational position will present as nasty, aggressive, and devaluing of the service provider. An adult child in the second parent–child relational position will present as essentially needy, insatiable, and will be easily injured by the helping professional. The caregiving adult children of narcissistic entitled families are also often angry and frustrated at having to give care to a parent or parents whom they experienced as ungiving, demanding, intrusive, overpowering, and needy.

Rich and Famous Entitled Families

These families are identified by the parents' socioeconomic, financial, and political prominence. They are families in which all basic needs, services, resources, and creature comforts are obtained via income, assets, abundant discretionary cash flow, or come from political position, station, or power. Once again, the entitlement of the family is passed from the parent to the child, who in turn brings these behaviors and actions to the caregiving milieu and care management relationship. In this category, the entitlement arises out of a family that is accustomed to purchasing everything. They look to pay others to meet their needs (as opposed to families who must themselves find and orchestrate ways to meet basic and complex needs themselves or with the help of the extrafamilial system). Often these families have household staffs: nannies, butlers, drivers, private pilots, cooks, and maids. They may have available to them business and family lawyers and accountants, as well as teams of medical professionals and concierge physicians. Consequently, in almost all situations they are uninvolved in processes, especially those that are difficult, stressful, and time-consuming. Adult children in rich and famous entitled families often were reared by sitters or nannies and do not see their parent as a primary caregiver. Hence, in the role reversal of the caregiving relationship, they do not look to themselves to provide care to the parent, but rather employ others to do so.

Geriatric care managers define themselves as trained healthcare professionals acting as surrogates of the family to address the needs of the elderly or impaired client. Additionally, they ask clients and adult children alike to participate with them toward reaching the goals of the care plan. When these adult children engage care managers to meet their caregiving needs and the needs of their parent, they do so expecting no involvement in processes or outcomes. Further, they hold that paying for services entitles them to positive outcomes, as well as the abject availability, devotion, and attention of the care manager—their employee. A sociological and psychological construct of "I pay you; therefore, I own you" is at play in these relationships. Much of the work of the care manager with a rich and famous entitled family must focus on maintaining control of the process while allowing the perspective of the client and family to *feel* in control.

Social Welfare Model Entitled Families

These families are identified by the parent's life experiences and political, sociocultural, philosophical, unconscious, and conscious beliefs that one's needs and assistance should be subsidized, provided at low cost, or be free of charge. While these families occupy all socioeconomic backgrounds, the parents often were children of the New Deal or hold to left wing, communist, or socialist political viewpoints. As

such, they expect that the government as a part of US citizenship should pay for one's biospsychosocial needs. Thus, they do not easily find value in any service beyond what the federal, local, and state entitlement systems provide. These families regard paying for service as an extravagance and thereby unnecessary, or they find fee-for-service "social services" a direct insult to their socialist political views. In the context of the care management relationship, these families present with the following constructs: "I do not want to pay for a service that I should be getting for free," which is followed by, "I am undeserving to have/purchase/want these 'Cadillac' services," and concluding with "Care managers are 'social servants' who should not charge for these services as it devalues me to pay for something that my beliefs inform me should be free." Consequently, engagement of these elderly or impaired clients is difficult because it is incumbent upon the care manager to help them adjust or bridge a personal, psychological perspective or worldview to get them to consider the need for such a service. Often, it is only the duress of a medical or psychiatric crisis and a resultant hospital stay that promotes any openness toward a care management relationship as other institutional-based professionals have insisted that to regain a previous level of functioning additional support services at home will be necessary. The adult children of these families, often baby boomers, may have adapted and adjusted their politics and worldview as a result of learned behaviors in the post-1960s, a less liberal time during which affluence and personal wealth increased exponentially. These adult children have grown to feel that "creature comforts" are a necessity and therefore outsourcing basic and personal needs is much less of a personal or political affront. Encouraging their parents to bridge their worldview may result in increased guilt feelings in the adult child. These guilt feelings may arise from the idea that they have imposed their changed worldview on their parent(s), thereby distancing themselves from the family and its shared beliefs.

CARE MANAGEMENT WITH THE ENTITLED FAMILY: A STEP-BY-STEP APPROACH

Know Thyself

Work with an entitled family begins well before the family actually engages the care manager for the initial assessment. The initial work really begins with the care manager—with his or her psyche—and an understanding of the focus and parameters of how he or she wants to practice. Before engaging the entitled family, the care manager must want and be ready to work with the difficult-to-serve. He or she must be prepared to withstand the emotional drain of working with families who are demanding, needy, and devaluing. Once that is clear, the practitioner must look at his or her available time and scale back the census of his or her practice in order to accommodate the intensive time commitment that these families require. The care manager must also factor into his or her business plan the high-risk nature of these families as fee-for-service clients. There may likely be an increased need for business support services and more tightly managed business practices to address these clients' overwhelming needs for structure and predictability. With this population, there is a higher rate of termination and accounts receivable issues. If one is prepared for these changes in one's practice, for the inherent increase of the work intruding on one's personal time and the potential for a wide fluctuation in billing, the next step in work-

ing with these families begins with engaging them in an inquiry.

The Inquiry

As in all care management practice, the assessment begins with the inquiry. Although National Association of Professional Geriatric Care Managers (NAPGCM) standards refer to the older person as the client, the call for service is usually made by someone in the family system that perceives the need. It is important from the outset of the call that care managers stay in touch with the feelings that the caller engenders in them. There will be an overriding sense of the caller as demanding, aggressive, and directive with little sense of the care manager as a separate, discreet person with time pressures and a need for involvement, collaboration, and predictability. Moreover, entitled callers place no value on the care manager as a trained professional. Ironically, they do not trust the care manager can understand their unique needs or arrive at the outcomes that they require.

At this point, it is also important for the care manager to begin assessing the degree of this family's entitlement and whether one has the capacity and motivation to work with them. A care manager wanting to engage such families must utilize some key techniques in an attempt to avoid some of the practical pitfalls in the inquiry call. Here are a few such pitfalls:

1. Never allow such inquiries to be taken by untrained or unskilled support staff or junior care managers. Entitled callers want to feel that the expert who, from the outset, has ample time and interest in them and their situation and is attending to them.
2. Do not delay taking the entitled caller's inquiry call, if possible. If the care man-

ager has advance notice about when the call is coming through and will not be available, he or she must make a time when the call can happen at the caller's next convenient hour.

3. Try never to put these callers on hold. Entitled callers often interpret "being on hold" as the care manager having limited time for them. Waiting may cause a narcissistic injury resulting in a rupture in the formation of the initial relationship.

4. Do not try to set limits immediately. Listen to the caller's needs and requests. The reaction to an entitled caller's lack of boundaries and pressing demands is to set limits with them in an effort to protect oneself against feeling enveloped, controlled, overwhelmed, or annihilated.

5. Avoid vagueness. It is imperative to be clear in defining care management and the scope of one's practice, as well as explaining fees and how these are incurred in the care management process.

6. Convey availability for an immediate consultation to discuss the situation further. These clients need to feel as if they are on center stage in the care management relationship.

7. Be action oriented rather than psychoanalytic. Entitled callers want to know what the care manager will do, not what they think or feel or how they assess the caller and situation. Remember that entitled families experience helping professionals as instruments of their needs.

The goal of the inquiry is to provide information on the service to be provided, convey interest in the client's problem and situation, and most importantly, to encourage the caller to decide to engage the care manager for ongoing work. At this juncture, it is important for the care manager to sug-

gest that the adult children, without the older person(s) present, come to the office for a consultation to discuss the situation and need in detail. Depending on the type of entitlement that family members present, their understanding of the need for an initial consultation will vary. For example, narcissistic entitled family members may see the care manager as an extension of themselves, solely involved with their need for gratification; therefore, the care manager should know how to begin without information, further understanding, or a relationship. Rich and famous entitled families may not find value in a consultation because they want no involvement in the process beyond engaging the service and signing service authorizations: "I found you, hired you, and am paying you: *just do it.*" The social welfare model entitled family may not want the consultation unless it is complimentary and find a fee-for-service meeting wounding because it is experienced as an affront to their fantasy of free social service. Nevertheless, the professional must discover a way to engage them for an initial consultation during which the formal assessment will begin and a basic contract for ongoing work will be delineated.

ONGOING WORK WITH THE ENTITLED FAMILY OF EVE ELEGANT

Ongoing work with members of the entitled family is like walking a tightrope. One slip and the care manager can lose control of the situation and be powerless to help anyone. The care manager must track the psychodynamic "pulse" of the explicit, implicit and often conflicting needs and demands of all involved while maintaining a fragile equilibrium in order to realize the primary goal: safety and quality of life for the identified older person. Some of the techniques and challenges are discussed in the case of Eve Elegant and her classic narcissistic entitled family. (See Table 11-1.)

The Clients

Eve Elegant is an 82-year-old white, upper-middle class widow who is "sweet but passive." Her emotionally remote husband died 45 years ago. Eve was a highly intelligent, competent, controlling woman who had managed the home and family finances. After her husband's death she developed his small dress company into a well-known brand in the New York City garment industry, leaving the child rearing of her two daughters, Susan and Joan, to paid nannies. Eve continues to be a medically intact, very attractive woman suffering from early to moderate dementia. Her continued social drinking exacerbates her memory loss, confusion, and bouts of anger and agitation. She has also had some recent nighttime falls.

Susan, a never-married 46-year-old poet, lives in the same city as her mother and is very involved in Eve's day-to-day life. Their relationship has been historically characterized by their mutual inability to gratify each other emotionally. Susan was always met by Eve's disapproval and criticism. Eve's need for her daughter to be a narcissistic reflection of her grandiose sense of self was forever frustrated by Susan's passive, dependent personality.

The younger daughter, Joan, is a married mother of two young children and a very successful attorney. Joan had an equally poor and conflict-laden mother–daughter relationship, but she "gave up" and chose to escape Eve's critical judgment by moving to Dallas years ago. She purports to have resolved issues with her mother by coming to terms with Eve's pathological inability to parent or relate to her daughters and now her

grandchildren. Contact between Eve and Joan's family has been limited to holiday visits and occasional telephone calls until Eve began to decline cognitively. Although Joan expresses concern for her sister's burden, her critical judgment of Susan's ineffective, passive approach is apparent to all. Joan is also ambivalent about allowing the care manager to help Susan to stabilize Eve's situation, because she questions the competence of anyone Susan would select to help her.

The relationship between Joan and Susan has been predictably strained by sibling competition for Eve's unattainable love and recognition. Both daughters employ dysfunctional coping mechanisms—defensive splitting and projection—to manage overwhelming anxieties related to engulfment and abandonment.

Presentation, Problems, Unspoken Requests, Distortions, and Risks

Susan Elegant was referred to the care manager by the homecare agency with whom she had contracted for companion services for her mother. Eve was still going to work several afternoons a week and needed help with getting ready and traveling to the office without getting lost. Susan had been reluctant to discuss Eve's diagnosis of Alzheimer's disease with her mother, and Eve was resistant to having any help in her home. The agency had tried to stabilize the situation, placing a succession of 12 different caregivers over the course of 1 month. The caregivers were either rejected by Eve and Susan or were unwilling to return because of Eve's characteristic abusiveness, made worse by symptoms of sundowning and use of alcohol. Susan had not addressed the alcohol consumption and minimized the behavioral outbursts as being provoked by caregivers who lacked skill and sensitivity.

The family's functional ability to address the presenting problem of securing care for Eve was hampered by both daughters' underlying need to resolve longstanding issues by using the family crisis to gratify unmet emotional needs. (See Table 11-2.) To work successfully, the geriatric care manager had to do the following:

- Engage the client and her daughters, each of whom conveyed qualities or behaviors that were repelling. Eve was verbally abusive and rejecting of homecare workers who were culturally or racial different. Susan was overbearing and intrusive. Joan was cold, rejecting, and devaluing.
- Elicit each member's perception of the presenting problems and expectations.
- Listen to the underlying, unspoken requests of each family member.

- Recognize and reframe the distortions in their perceptions and interpretations of the problems that were barriers to resolution.

Eve's devaluation of the care manager and verbal abusiveness to the homecare workers was understood as an attempt to maintain Eve's sense of esteem and control in the face of her physical and cognitive decline. The care manager's interventions were, therefore, designed to reinforce Eve's sense of security and control over herself and her environment. Susan's intrusiveness and demands for 24-hour contact with the care manager was recognized as a symptom of Susan's difficulty separating from her mother. The care manager had invested time in assuring Susan that she would be a constant support. The care manager was able to interpret Joan's suspiciousness and need to exert excessive control over the care manager's work

Table 11-1 Presentation, Problems, Unspoken Requests, Distortions, and Risks

Family Member	Presentation	Presenting Problems	Unspoken Request
Eve	Initially condescending, hostile, and rejecting of relationship with care manager. Except when in an acutely agitated, paranoid state, Eve was able to engage with care manager around her life accomplishments and her desire to remain functional and active.	Needs help managing her "social calendar" and administrative assistance in the office. Denies inability to manage independent activities of daily living: preparing meals, routine hygiene, selecting clothing, remembering medication, daily money management, and travel.	To maintain her longstanding, but well-protected fragile sense of self by using alcohol to reinforce dysfunctional coping in an attempt to preserve her ego, now fragmenting under the assault of aging and cognitive decline.
Susan	Susan is frantic and dependent, and lacks any insight despite years of psychotherapy.	Mother has always been demanding, critical, and manipulative. The caregivers are unable to tolerate her paranoid outbursts and	To finally realize her mother's love and recognition by being the only one able to "save" Eve.

continues

Table 11-1 Presentation, Problems, Unspoken Request, Distortions and Risks (continued)

Family Member	Presentation	Presenting Problems	Unspoken Request
		behavioral problems. She needs someone who is able to prevent her from ordering from the liquor store.	To gratify her mother's narcissistic needs by purchasing, and thereby identifying with, the "best," om- nipotent care manager and the "all good" homecare worker.
		I am overwhelmed and depleted by caregiving burdens, but the situa- tion requires a "very special" care manager who really "under- stands" this unique sit- uation, and can help me find "the right" caregiver.	To protect the longstand- ing, enmeshed, inter- dependent relationship with her mother by having both the care manager and caregiver fail.
Joan	Joan presents with veiled anger toward her mother and is skeptical and at times cold and dismissive of the care manager's ability to improve an "impossible situation."	Mother has always been demanding, critical, and manipulative; the care manager will never be able to deal with the drinking prob- lem, and caregivers will never be able to tolerate Eve's paranoid outbursts and behav- ioral problems.	To unconsciously obtain her mother's love and approval by merging with Eve's need for control.
		Susan has always been overinvolved in Mother's daily life. This creates more, rather than fewer, problems now. Perhaps a care manager could provide support for Susan and help her cope better.	Joan minimizes the seri- ousness of the alcohol use and sabotages the care manager's ability to form a relationship with Eve by revealing the cost of the care manager service.
		Mother is not able to manage her finances and Susan has been unable to help her pay the bills. I will use my power of attorney to pay her bills and send household cash.	To reinforce her own nar- cissistic need to be the "better sibling," and maintain the rigid boundaries between herself and the other members of her family, Joan implicitly controls her mother's care from a distance. Joan uses her power of attorney and disapproval to ma- nipulate and sabotage the care management process.

Table 11-2 The Care Management Process

Family Member	Distortions	Potential Risk of Mismanagement
Eve	I have no need for help other than for a glamorous companion who functions as a sophisticated servant or a private secretary. I only drink socially and "for business."	If Eve's narcissistic defenses are not penetrated, she will be at risk for liver failure, falls, and other physical injuries, financial exploitation, social isolation, and a precipitous decline in overall wellness and quality of life.
Susan	Mother's behavioral outbursts are caused by a "bad" homecare worker's provocation. Only a very special, "sensitive" caregiver would eliminate the problem. I can't delegate care management responsibility to the care manager because only I "understand" how to assuage my mother's loneliness and "protect" her from the unpleasantness of having a homecare worker in the house. Joan has never been able to cope with mother in the way I have. The care manager should "help Joan understand" what is needed.	Susan compulsively repeats the dysfunctional cycle of seeking and losing approval. As Eve lacks capacity to recognize her deficits, she will reject Susan's efforts to intervene, Susan will avoid confrontation at all costs, and Eve will continue to be at risk, thereby perpetuating Susan's pattern of failure. Susan will compete with the care manager for which one will be successful. She will provoke Joan's disapproval in her unconscious compulsion to repeat patterns established with her mother. This will leave Susan isolated in a merged relationship with Eve. Susan will latch on to a magical "quick fix," but soon will become enraged when interventions do not produce an immediate solution. The care manager and homecare worker will fall from grace and become impotent and worthless.
Joan	The care manager clearly can't engage my mother because she can't get her to stop drinking. Time spent in trying to establish a relationship with Mother is an unnecessary expense. Mother is still able to make decisions and should be told about the cost of having the care manager. It is "unethical" to keep this a secret.	Joan will not confront her mother about her drinking, but will still compete with and undermine the care manager's efforts. Joan will then be pulled into the inevitable crises in her mother's care, exacerbating her fears of engulfment and creating the potential for Eve's neglect and being at risk. Eve is unable to recognize or tolerate the existence of her deficits. Information about the cost of care will be an assault and could fatally rupture the relationship with the care manager.

as a displacement of Joan's characteristic defenses against her mother.

The Care Management Process

The challenge with Eve's family, akin to walking a tightrope over a minefield, was to promote functional behavior that would minimize risk for all in the face of the family's entrenched dysfunctional coping patterns. Family members consciously believed that by resolving their identified problems each would "feel better." Eve demanded an attractive, subservient companion, verbally abusing and ultimately rejecting all candidates that failed to mirror her own narcissism. Joan demanded the care man-

ager "control" the finances but was unwilling to accept the recommendation to cancel Eve's credit cards and was inconsistent in sending payments to the care manager for weekly cash allowance that would have given Eve a sense of control over her affairs. Susan's approach was equally passive–aggressive. She embraced every new suggestion made by the geriatric care manager, but because of her separation issues with her mother, sabotaged the work, often creating a crisis that only she could solve. In response, Joan would become enraged, devaluing the geriatric care manager for not realizing her unrealistic expectation of "freeing Susan of her caregiving burden." Joan further undermined the care management process by

Table 11-3 Goals and Interventions

Family Member	Goals	Interventions
Eve	1. Engage Eve and establish trust. 2. Transfer relationship with care manager to paid caregiver who can help Eve continue to function at the highest level and experience a quality of life, while minimizing risks. 3. Overcome rupture created by being told that she had to pay for care manager's relationship.	1. Convey an interest in Eve, her history, interests, and concerns in order to understand Eve's perception of self; mirror her grandiose self; join Eve in her resistance to any intervention that would undermine her grandiose self. 2. Work with Joan to promote understanding regarding Eve's impaired judgment and the need to invoke Joan's power of attorney to pay for Eve's needed service. 3. Recruit caregivers who physically mirror Eve's sense of self, but don't challenge Eve's grandiosity. 4. After caregivers have been selected (see interventions with Susan) invest in orientation and training beyond traditional homecare curriculum. 5. Introduce caregiver "staff" as "well known" and the "best." 6. Explain that the staff is there to provide "assistance." 7. Provide daily telephone and on-call support to caregivers to provide strategies to manage Eve's behavior.

continues

Family Member	Goals	Interventions
Susan	1. Establish a collaborative relationship with Susan, allowing her to "solve" the problem and maintain her attachment to Eve, thereby minimizing Susan's need to sabotage the care manager's efforts to stabilize the situation.	1. Involve Susan in screening and selecting caregiver candidates. 2. Involve Susan with daily care management work; assign her specific tasks. 3. Don't resolve problems or stabilize Eve's situation without crediting Susan's insight.
Joan	1. Establish a system to provide and account for weekly cash disbursements for use by Eve and the caregivers. 2. Stabilize Eve's day-to-day life to reduce the number of crises that draw Joan in and increase her stress and dysfunction. 3. Contain cost.	1. Provide a detailed written monthly account indicating funds received, cash disbursement with receipt documentation, and a running balance. 2. Provide weekly verbal reports about Eve's behaviors and activities. Report on current or anticipated problems before they erupt. Commiserate with Joan about the issues she has identified. 3. Acknowledge and empathize with Joan's concern about managing the expense of Eve's chronic and probably progressive care needs. Work with Joan about projected long-term care costs, providing alternative ways to pay for service.

sharing information with her mother about the cost of care management services.

The care manager has to establish goals targeted for each member of the family and modify them as the family responds to sequential interventions and each other. In realizing the ultimate goal—promotion of well-being and reduction of risk—the care manager has to be spontaneous, creative, and flexible.

Contracting

Because it sets the initial parameters, expectations, and goals for all further work, contracting is a very important component of working with all clients and families. With the entitled client and family, contracting from the outset is vitally important because these families have complex and complicated fantasies and expectations of the care management process. If these are not presented, explored, and understood, the care manager will fall prey in his or her work to myriad struggles, misunderstandings, impasses, and resultant ruptures throughout the work. These families may not be able to tolerate interruptions of empathic tracking throughout the work, but especially in the beginning phase, so a clear, concise, and detailed contract, preferably in writing, is imperative.[7] The process for contracting should proceed in the following manner:

- Explore the client and family's expectations of service, including their definition of care management and their fantasies and ideas of what the care manager will do for them. Understand that both the older or impaired person and each family member are all "clients." In order not to miss any "request" as to how the service should be delivered, the care manager needs to explore the expectations for each of them—both the explicit expectations (what is directly stated or expressed) and the implicit expectations (the unspoken wish or meaning). Often, that which is not said and therefore unaddressed is the cause for dissatisfaction and termination later. Despite Susan Elegant's explicit request for the care manager to reduce her mother's agitation, supervise the caregivers, and improve her mother's quality of daily life, Susan's implicit wish to maintain the interdependent bond between herself and her mother and to ultimately obtain her mother's approval was demonstrated in Susan's initial actions (overriding orders to caregivers, late-night telephone calls to Eve, and unannounced visits).

- Make sure to acknowledge all of the family members' expectations, even if those requests are unrealistic and cannot be part of the final contract, because all people's anxiety and frustration are assuaged, especially the entitled, by being listened to and understood.

- Begin to identify achievable goals, preparing the family for what will and will not be delivered in the care management process. The care manager consistently advised Susan and Joan that there might be several attempts to find a good care giver "match" for Eve, that a good match, would never be a perfect match, and that even with a good match, the initial process would be rocky and require considerable care management support and intervention. By predicting the possible

obstacles, the care manager helped the family anticipate and ultimately tolerate intermittent disappointment and frustration when expectations were not immediately gratified.

- Listen for the conflicting needs of the adult child and the older or impaired person and help all to feel that what they want will be explored and attempted by the care manager—a construct of "Yes, until it has to be *no*."

- Be specific, clear, and task oriented rather than process oriented, both verbally and in writing, when outlining the goals of the contract. These families should walk away from the consultation with a mutually agreed upon, initial plan of action that they can reflect upon, amend, and discuss—a plan that can be referred to as the work unfolds. Entitled families will be constantly questioning the care manager's motivations and plan; so a written plan is a helpful tool for all in managing ongoing and changing expectations, and it assists in building a positive, working relationship.

- Avoid being pedantic and impersonal as a reaction to the entitled family's need to devalue the care manager and remain in control of the service. Entitled clients and their families often do not see a need for a relationship with the care manager, and so they wish to remain distant, or at the very least parallel, where a constant level of control can be maintained. An expression of empathic acceptance of the client and family's perception of the problem will minimize their need to be defensive.

- Begin to explore responsibility and accountability with regard to the ongoing work. It is the care manager's role to decide with the family what he or she will do and what the family wants to do for itself. Clearly state verbally and in writing, if possible, that the care manager cannot be responsible for outcomes when he or she is not involved in the process or planning. The care manager was able to assess that Joan Elegant was highly ambivalent about her need to feel in control of the finances and her reluctance to get drawn into her mother's life. Initially, Joan had been somewhat unreliable in sending household cash but still held the care manager responsible for her mother's agitation often precipitated when Eve was unable to access her own money. The care manager developed a clear, written plan, which specified the amount of money Joan would deposit in a separate account at the first of every month. The care manager had power of attorney over this account and was able to provide Eve with the limited cash she needed to feel in control.

CARE MANAGEMENT BUSINESS PRACTICES WITH THE ENTITLED FAMILY

Practicing care management with the entitled family is a time-consuming and emotionally taxing venture. It requires the practicing professional to have a high level of experience in the field, as well as a high level of education and psychodynamic understanding. It also requires that the care manager have a carefully designed and staffed practice. Whether it is a solo practice or a group practice, a high level of technical and administrative support is mandatory to sustain work with the entitled family and their persistent and insatiable demands. If one is prepared to provide service to this population, the work with these families begins with business development.

Business Development and Marketing

Generally speaking, entitled families are usually found as a subset of the difficult-to-

serve client and his or her family. These clients are referred for care management services for much the same reasons and from the same sources as the usual and customary client. Examining the anecdotal data from years of care management practice, 70% of care management referrals come from professional sources and, speaking generally, the rest comes from word of mouth. Of those referrals from professional sources, the bulk come from discharge planners and social workers in institutions such as hospitals; nursing homes and their short-term rehabilitation units; primary care physicians; medical specialists such as geriatricians, neurologists, psychiatrists, psychologists, and psychotherapists; community agencies serving the elderly or the chronically ill or impaired; and attorneys and trust officers in financial institutions. Some examples of referral sources are the following:

- Hospital departments of psychiatry: Social workers and discharge planners who are responsible for discharging patients with character disorders. Also target institutions that serve an affluent population, those that have longstanding, stellar reputations, and those that are private pay facilities, meaning private psychiatric units.
- Concierge wings of hospitals: Because of their narcissism and insatiable demands, entitled patients and their families are often found in these specialty services of hospitals.
- The top 10 rehabilitation units: Entitled families want to be in the best situations.
- Top 100 primary care physicians or concierge MD practices: The entitled families are drawn to experts and services that are tailor-made.
- Psychiatrists and neurologists in private practice: Look for professionals who do not take insurance assignments and who have longstanding, high-profile reputations.

- Community agencies: Build referral relationships with the top managers here, such as the CEO or managing directors. Intake, colleagues, and friends of the agency and the board of directors who work with the entitled families presenting for service will call upon these individuals. Entitled families do not feel adequately served unless it is by a director, manager, or person in charge.
- High-profile attorneys: The entitled client or family is often litigious and seeks legal advice to air complaints or ensure that their demands are met.
- Trust departments from top financial and prominent firms: Look for clients in these firms that have a net worth between $1 million and $5 million. The client whose net worth is higher than $5 million may already have a full complement of formal and informal services in place and will have insufficient need to find value in the care management relationship.

Once these referral sources are identified, the sole purpose of the initial business development contact is to let that source know the care manager's interest in the difficult-to-serve population and what, if any, experience he or she has in working with entitled families. It is also important that the care manager have a solid business plan, years of experience in the field, and have generated a word-of-mouth reputation and positive publicity in local newspapers or trade journals. The entitled family usually will not want to work with a new practitioner or one without much public reputation because they will feel this professional's lack of experience will not enable him or her to meet their needs. The care manager's lack of public reputation will be an initial narcissistic injury and make engagement impossible.

Working with Entitled Families and Supervising Care Management Staff

Generally speaking entitled families look to work with prominent and experienced care managers or large, well-staffed care management firms. They fantasize that their needs can only be met by the most experienced or most prominent. Consequently, the solo practitioner must have a solid business with administrative staff and systems in place to provide the care manager with the support needed to face these families' incessant demands and requests. The following conditions must be in place if the care manager and his or her staff are to succeed with these families:

- Anticipate the transferential and countertransferential issues that will arise in the work with these families. Care managers must be clear that they are right for a particular entitled family or must know where and how to refer them to some other practitioner. If the care manager is practicing from within a group practice or firm, he or she must make a clear assessment as to which of the staff are the best for the case. A good initial match between care manager and family is vitally important. Patience, timeliness, empathic listening, and action orientation are mandatory in working with the entitled. Often these families want the "best care manager" and require that a senior staff member or a principle be assigned to them.
- Can the care manager or one of the staff tolerate being devalued in the service of the entitled family's narcissism?
- Ensure that the care manager's caseload is varied, and that he or she has time to devote to each member of these families. If any practitioner has too demanding a caseload or one in which the predominant charac-

teristic is the difficult-to-serve or heavy-care client and family, then he or she will not be able to bear the emotional and time burden of an entitled family.

- Not every care manager will find it exhilarating to "climb Mt. Everest," but the care manager that finds difficult people a challenge may be able to succeed with these families and find great pride in the outcomes of their efforts.
- Consider assigning layers of staff to these families. Multiple relationships can deflect the inherent devaluation and, via the "good cop vs. bad cop" paradigm, allow for strategic interventions to address the demand for accuracy and perfection. If a team approach is used, make sure that consistent and timely collaboration and internal consultation regarding adherence to the care plan is maintained in order to avoid these families' splitting tendencies.
- Be sure to track the family's emotional response to the process and outcomes of the total service provided by the practice—from how calls are handled to what the invoice looks like. Know when to be flexible, and always look to customize the service while staying aware of when limits need to be set.
- Be proactive. Stay ahead of the demands of the entitled client and family by performing an ongoing and continuous assessment of their needs. Do not fall into procrastination as a reaction to their daunting and exhausting demands and unrealistic expectations. With these families know that you can run, but you cannot hide.
- Know when to act and when to listen or react. As Leonie Nowitz, one of the founders of care management practice, says, "Know when to do something, and when to just stand there."
- Last, but not least, make sure to *document*. In working with entitled families, it is im-

portant to be able to accurately report on the progress of the work on a regular basis, as well as to respond quickly when they ask for reporting. Careful and consistent chart documentation will make it possible to meet these families' demands for reporting and allow all staff to be on the same page in the family's eyes, thereby decreasing their dissatisfaction.

Fees and Billing Practices

Because care management is difficult for the entitled family to value and accept, they typically act out their issues about the service via fees and billing practices. Their level of satisfaction and dissatisfaction is reflected in the payment of their bill. As in all work with these families, is it important to balance their need to be in control of the relationship and the services rendered versus their need for these services to be magically delivered in a customized manner devoid of process. To achieve positive outcomes, a structured approach to fees and billing practices is highly recommended.

Setting Fees

- Hourly fees should be commensurate with experience and reputation. If the entitled family needs the "best in the business," then the hourly fee should be on the high side of competitive for the market. This fee structure is best suited and attractive to entitled families of the narcissistic and rich and famous types.
- Consider billing by package (fixed price) or flat rates. For the social welfare model entitled family, flat rates will be much more consistent with their socialist politics and, therefore, more emotionally and psychologically acceptable. Although flat fees desensitize the family to anxiety-provoking detail, they undermine certain

clients' and families' sense of control because there is a lack of detail provided in this billing model. However, flat rates can also engage the narcissistic entitled family by implying the utter availability of the care manager, because hourly time spent is not itemized.

- Taking deposits or retainers protects the care manager and the practice from nonpayment of the bill if the family terminates precipitously. In addition, the family must engage in an exploration of their issues with the care management relationship in the process of asking for a refunded deposit. Often working through their need to terminate will result in a continuation of service.

- Taking prepayments based on anticipated needs outlined in a care plan ensures the family's adherence to the contract and plan and ensures payment for service as it is rendered.

- Taking credit cards for payment ensures that the bill will be paid and continuous accounts receivable calls will be kept at a minimum.

Billing Practices

The Cycle. Entitled families, as well as all families in crisis, respond well to predictability. Hence, billing for care management services should occur on a regular schedule of not less than a monthly cycle. The more frequent the billing cycle, the greater the ability of the practitioner to examine the client's and family's experience of the service.

The Style. The bill and the billing process are concrete representations of the care management product. To these families, an imperfect bill or invoice equals a worthless or nonexistent product. Itemization is mandatory as detailing services and time is important documentation for accountability, but too much detail can become a red flag for certain families, because it encourages their predilection for nit-picking. Because it elaborates how each objective in the care plan was achieved, descriptive invoicing can also help develop the client's sense of pride in ownership of the care management product. Billing by preset time increments is also essential because it documents how much time each objective took to be achieved, and it allows the family to understand the reality of time spent. However, some families will find incremental billing an assault to their narcissism and grandiosity. They may ask, "How can my small problem be so time consuming?" and will extrapolate from this position to, "Anyone with half a brain could solve my problem in two minutes."

Accounts Receivable. Finally, exquisite tracking of fees owed provides a window to the client's experience. Often, entitled families nonverbally indicate their feelings about the care manager and the service by nonpayment or a shift in the timeliness of their payments. For example, a periodic late payment can be a call for the immediate attention of the practitioner. Long-term nonpayment, although usually seen as an indicator of dissatisfaction, in the entitled family could mean that they have stopped paying as they now see the service as so integral in their lives, so given and therefore acceptable, that paying for it would be like paying for the very air that they breathe. Avoiding collection problems with entitled families is crucial. Unaddressed collection problems are tantamount to a breakdown in the empathic tracking of the family. If this occurs, and if a simple refund or courtesy adjustment in their bill will repair the rupture, better to negotiate and make those compromises than to lose the case.

Termination. The long-term success rate with the entitled family is generally poor due to the fact that these families need a level of attention and perfection that most care managers cannot uphold. Usually when these conflicts arise and cannot be resolved or the demands of the family are too great and unceasing, the care manager becomes powerless and thereby worthless in the family's perception. Allowing the entitled family to separate and no longer feel engulfed may actually give the care manager more control. This paradoxical intervention may ameliorate the entitled family's resistance and allow its members to recontract or allow them to continue within the old contract feeling more empowered within the relationship. When the situation and case are unworkable, and all avenues of repair have been exhausted, make certain that the client is offered a referral to a comparable or alternative service. Moreover, make certain to document, in detail, all conversations, e-mails, letters, and face-to-face discussions with all involved to control for positive outcomes and accountability—even when termination is inevitable and unavoidable.

CONCLUSION

Entitled families pose a challenge, creating stress for the professional and taxing the resources of the care management practice. On the other hand, these difficult-to-serve families, if engaged properly, are oddly the model clients and can form the foundation for a thriving geriatric care management business. These are the people who have problems that cannot be solved by traditional agency-based providers. These are the clients who require customization, responsiveness, and creativity. Although the care manager must draw from experience or acquire knowledge that runs the gamut from psychodynamics, family systems, business administration, and human resource management, the investment is worthwhile. Because entitlement is a normal coping mechanism, the geriatric care manager's experience gained from work with these extremely complex families enhances his or her work with all clients.

REFERENCES

1. Freud A. *The Ego and Mechanisms of Defense.* New York, NY: International Universities Press; 1946.
2. Vaillant GE. *Empirical Study of Ego Mechanisms of Defense.* New York, NY: American Psychiatric Press; 1986.
3. *The Psychology Students' Best Friend.* Available at: http://www.AlleyDog.com. Accessed June 3, 2008.
4. American Psychiatric Association. *Quick Reference to the Diagnostic Criteria from DSM–IV.* Washington, DC: American Psychiatric Association; 1994.
5. Winnicott DW. The theory of the parent-infant relationship. In:*The Maturational Processes and the Facilitating Environment.* New York, NY: International Universities Press; 1965.
6. Kernberg O. *Borderline Conditions and Pathological Narcissism.* New York, NY: Jason Aronson; 1975.
7. Bohart AC, Greenberg LS, eds. *Empathy Reconsidered: New Directions in Psychotherapy.* Washington, DC: American Psychological Association; 1997.

CHAPTER 12

Forgiveness with the Aging Family

Cathy Jo Cress and Fred Luskin

Forgiveness appears as spiritual guidance across all religions. In literature from Shakespeare to HBO's ground breaking show *Sopranos*, forgiveness and brutality often rest on the same knife's edge, seeping blood followed by sought-after penance.

In Buddhism followers are asked to forgive themselves. Forgiveness is the central message of Christianity. Believers are taught that Christ died for all of their sins. The Christian model of forgiveness draws from the belief that people should forgive each other like God does—unconditionally.[1] On the day of atonement, the most solemn of Jewish holidays, Jews seek to expiate their sins and achieve a reconciliation with God.[2]

Great literature and a quest for God gives us a body of fables, tales, and stories to scan when trying to map forgiveness in the aging family. At the end of the *Sopranos*, we are left with New Jersey mob boss Tony Soprano struggling to forgive his aging and demented Uncle Junior who shot him in the stomach. The fraught midlife of Tony is plagued with anxiety attacks and childhood scars wreaked, he believes, by his malevolent mother and his Mafioso father. He faces Junior, the only parent figure in his life that appeared to show true love for him, who violated him with a gunshot. Can he forgive this father figure?

In King Lear, a Shakespearean drama about an aging and retiring king, Lear spurns and then casts out his favorite daughter,

Cordelia, whom he expected to care for him in his old age. When Cordelia fails to falsely flatter him as her other two sisters do, as he is about to divide up the kingdom for them, Lear's ego explodes, and what the Greeks called hubris sets him up for the giant fall. He banishes Cordellia and gives her part of his kingdom to his covetous malevolent daughters Regan and Gonerel. When these adult children betray him, Cordelia, now married to a king, comes back with her husband's army to save Lear, forgiving her father for his sins and dying herself in the process.

Before her death with newfound humility Lear begs repentance. "I am a very foolish fond old man," he tells Cordelia and she has "some cause" to hate him. Cordelia's forgiveness ("No cause, no, cause") reconciles the father and daughter, and for a flicker of time, happiness prevails.

Tony Soprano and King Lear along with many midlife family members seek to forgive or be forgiven by other aging family players. This includes parents, relatives, siblings, and the whole feathered train of the aging family. In fact, as the nuclear family breaks down and the boundaries of the family expand to include stepparents, partners, friends, and fictive kin, there are more and more family members who we feel must apologize for hurts.

As has been covered in the other chapters of this book, the aging family—like all families—can generally be divided into two categories: nearly normal and dysfunctional. Both types of aging families are often blocked in their effort to set up adequate parent care and relieve the stress and burden from the family caregivers. The degree of blockage is much more formidable with the dysfunctional family, but the care manager will find his or her best care plan stuck with both aging family groups. Both family groups can benefit from forgiveness techniques, allowing adult children to care for the aging parents.

The nearly normal aging family is a generally nurturing family. This relatively standard group of kin rarely experiences abuse and neglect but does suffer from divorce, which can leave adult children suffering 40 years later, seeking reparation for the hurt they experienced from otherwise nurturing parents (see Chapter 8 on siblings).

To review the hallmarks of the aging functional family: the family nest generally had enough love so the children were not fighting over the limited emotional resources given by the parents. Parent care was by and large nurturing and there was little abuse or neglect. If there were wounds inflicted on the children by parents, siblings, relatives, or anyone in the family, they were not deep enough to still need healing, and there are few thick scars left on the now adult children. This is because, if there were emotional lacerations, they were dealt with right away by the family and healed well with little residual disfigurement.

This aging family successfully transitioned through the developmental stages of their lives: birth, adolescence, marriage, and the first child. All transitions were generally well maneuvered by the entire family. However, the last transition, the need for care of the aging parent or the filial crisis, throws

them off balance, and they do have great difficulty navigating this developmental phase.

Siblings in the nearly normal aging family had standard childhood rivalry and can still be at war over wounds from sisters and brothers. The norms in sibling rivalry, like boys competing with boys (usually spurred on by the parents), occurred and may distance the siblings yet in midlife. The standard of the oldest child taking charge and at times bullying the younger children has occurred. This can spur on sibling rivalry in the midlife present. The youngest child in the aging family, who generally is deemed the favorite by most mothers, still engenders the ire of the other children causing midlife sibling rivalry. There usually is a favorite child, either the youngest, the first born, or a child picked by the parent, and that child in midlife can be harassed and resented still by the midlife adult children. Stepsiblings in the main have many wounds brought on by divorce, and this creates one of the greatest challenges in midlife siblings. All these sibling rivalries can cause parent care issues in the nearly normal family, but generally the nearly normal family can rebalance itself and move forward through midlife. For old parental or siblings issues that block parental care in the nearly normal family, forgiveness techniques can be very valuable to the care manager.

In the dysfunctional aging family there are knife marks left, with deep gouges that never healed. The dysfunctional aging family remains at war with each other; the same bloody roots of dysfunction repeated from one generation to the next. The hallmarks of the dysfunctional aging family, to review from past chapters, are not enough love in the family nest; the children, now at midlife, had to fight for what little nurturance the then young parents could bring to the rickety nest they built. Nurturing is often missing in the dysfunctional aging family because the parents themselves got little nurturing themselves as children and on and on back through the family line. Parental neglect and abuse are frequent in the history of the aging dysfunctional family. The now older parents can suffer now and in the past from serious mental health problems such as schizophrenia or bipolar disorder. Health and addiction problems such as alcoholism are frequent. Family interaction and communication—parental treatment of children, siblings' treatment of each other, stepparent interaction, and interface of everyone in the family—has wrought deep emotional tissue damage that never healed. These families generally negotiated all of life's developmental phases with great difficulty. The role in the family, especially the parental one, was murky with a poor, abusive, or mentally unfit leader of the family. The rules in the family were unfair, ambiguous, or full of double binds. There is deep-seated ambivalence. Finally, the last life transition in the aging family, the care of the declining parent, rocks the family, which had little balance to begin with. They are asked to care for parents who did not care for them, thus wreaking havoc on an already disorganized aging family. In these families care manager forgiveness skills can be crucial in organizing the family enough to render nuturing care to the aging parent.

CASE EXAMPLE: LEN RAMBLER AND VINNIE RAMBLER

Len Rambler is a 63-year-old adult son. His 90-year-old father, Vinnie Rambler, recently had a stroke and is in Better Care Rehabilitation facility for treatment of a severe left-sided stroke and speech therapy. Vinnie hopes to return to his home in Milpitas, California, and have 24-hour care. His only child, Len, lives in New Jersey and has had little to do with his father since his mother died 30 years ago. The father was an engineer, went through AA years ago, and remarried twice. His present wife has early dementia, and it is obvious to the care manager referred by the home health agency hired to provide 24-hour home care that the wife cannot spearhead or manage the care.

At the care manager's request, Len, the adult son, flies in to have a family meeting at the rehab facility. Even though he is the only child and the care manager explains that the stepmother has early dementia and cannot manage the care situation or the family assets, the son balks. He explains that when he was growing up, his father was an alcoholic, and he feels his father never nurtured him. He complains to the care manager that his father never took him to Boy Scouts, never came to school events, and paid little attention to his son's grades or school work. He angrily tells the care manager that he survived this harsh parenting but is reluctant to become involved in either his father's life or his care. Len states that he feels his father ruined his childhood, and even though the father no longer drinks, the adult son wants nothing to do with his father's care.

The care manager suggests that Len seek out a therapist in his local town of Asbury Park, New Jersey, who has aging experience and family therapy training, to work on his anger and hurt. He agrees and she makes a referral. In the meantime the care manager agrees to manage the father's care once Len returns to New Jersey and arranges for a local financial planner and elder law attorney to manage the finances, with Len's approval. Len signs a contract to pay fror the care manager's services. His dad signs a contract with the home health agency for 24-hour care.

Into the mix of pain and strife, a life's end is approaching. This last stage will pass more smoothly for all if forgiveness is invited to play a part. The aging family is unique in the spectrum of families in that death hovers over the cast of characters, threatening to permanently close the play. With this specter of urgency, forgiveness—for whatever it may be—needs to occur before the parent dies if the parent is to be part of forgiveness. Even in the case of aging or midlife siblings, if forgiveness is to be achieved, it needs to be attended to sooner than later because time is ticking more quickly in the aging family. The clock running out elevates the stakes, because if the behavior that caused the wound is not repaired in the family it will probably be passed on to the next generation, and they will wreak the same family misery. There is a cyclic nature of family dysfunction through modeling a parent's or sibling's behavior or interactions. This repeated nature casts a wave over new victims in the future family so that each new generation risks the same fate. Forgiveness can heal some of the wounding and allow people to grow enough not to repeat failed patterns.

Trying to resolve the hurt or wound in the aging family is important because adult children need to achieve filial maturity—the crisis they face with the usually unexpected care of their aging parent. These unforgiven hurts and wounds, most often gouged in childhood, hold adult children back from this filial maturity: seeing their parent for who they are in the here-and-now, an aging family member in need of their care, rather than the haunting, mean parent they experienced 20–40 years ago. Forgiveness in the aging family is critical because these past wounds keep aging siblings living in the haunted past of bullying older brothers and older sisters who had new Macy's prom dresses 30 years ago when the little sister wore hand-me-downs. When aging siblings can't shake themselves out of this past it prevents midlife siblings from working together to care for

their aging parent, and family care for the aging parent is stymied. As a family unit, the midlife siblings often cannot overcome this filial crisis or overcome one of the last developmental phases of the family, the care of an aging parent. Forgiveness is often needed in the aging family to successfully move through this last developmental phase.

This pressure cooker to "make things right," as Sandberg points out,[3] forces professionals who have a background in aging to not only understand the value and the process of forgiveness but to use it as a tool before death stops the clock.

CASE EXAMPLE: HEATHER LOCK AND JANET BUCKSHOT

An adult daughter, Heather Lock, is 57 years old. Her mother, Janet Buckshot, is 75. Heather was born when her mother Janet was 18, and three more siblings were born by the time the mother was 24. Janet was a very young mother, nearly still a child herself, and she did not nurture or hold her first daughter very much as a baby. By the time Heather was 6, she was keeping an eye on the next three children—all toddlers or babies— for her overwhelmed mother. Heather grew up resenting her mother's inept parenting when she was a child, moved out at 16, and has lived at a distance all of her adult life.

Her second oldest sibling, a sister, recently died, and the last two siblings are boys. The mother has been independent and divorced for years. Now she has midstage dementia, which she had hidden from her sons and daughter until she got lost in her car and was taken to the local emergency room by the police who picked her up.

The care manager from the hospital calls Heather and the two boys to the hospital. The two sons always followed the second, now deceased, daughter's lead with the always-difficult mother, but that sister is dead. They are now looking to Heather for guidance because "she is the daughter." But Heather tells the care manager at the hospital, who has called a family meeting in her office, that even though she knows she should take the lead as the daughter, she does not want to. She insists her mother never took care of her as a child, and she was given the hard task of taking care of all her siblings. She is angry that the two brothers who live locally won't step up to the plate with the mother. Heather admits she is mad and stuck. The care manager, who has an excellent background in forgiveness therapy, suggests a second family meeting to be held at her office a few weeks later. In the meantime she gets one of the sons, under her guidance, to accompany Janet Buckshot to the Stanford/VA Alzheimer's Research Center (http://arcc.stanford.edu) at Stanford Hospital to go through a battery of tests for dementia. The care manager also gets the other son to remove Ms. Buckshot's car keys until the results of the test are known. Heather is referred to a professional care manager.

Care managers should count knowledge of forgiveness and an understanding of when and how to use it as a tool as one of the major skills they as professionals should have. Care managers oversee caregiving and attempt to get family members to work together to set up and manage an older person's care needs. The care manager often, with the dysfunctional and nearly normal family, enters a family system because that family is presently "stuck" due to hurts, anger, rage, and resentment of things that happened to the family years ago. These past hurts often bring their unhealed scar tissue into the present and block the care manager's care plan, leaving the older client and their paralyzed midlife family unable to provide care for the older client. The family cannot easily negotiate the filial crisis. When the family caregiver comes to the point of burnout, if forgiveness has not been worked through, it is just one more dif-

ficult burden to lay at the feet of an older person. It can also become just one more very large reason to inappropriately place an older person in a facility.

The care manager needs to help the family let go of these past traumas so that the family can not only get the care the older person needs but also relieve the stress and burden of the family caregiver and other siblings. The care manager also needs to deal with these past traumas that impoverish the family model and move to change that impoverished model before it becomes the program the next family generation uses, thereby passing on the hurt, anger, and unhealed wounds.

If the care manager has a clinical background, she or he can help members resolve the blockage or refer the families to professionals who have the clinical expertise and a background in working with the aging family. In reviewing the literature on forgiveness and the aging family there are several models that the care manager can draw upon. This chapter reviews two that seem particularly useful.

CASE EXAMPLE: MYRNA THREADBARE AND JOHN THREADBARE

Myrna Threadbare is an adult daughter who is 62 years old. She is divorced and has taken back her maiden name. From the time she reached adolescence at 14 to the time she moved out of the house at 18 she was emotionally abused by her father, John Threadbare, every time she went out with a boy. Now Mr. Threadbare is 85 years old. His wife died a year ago, and Mr. Threadbare fell recently and broke his hip. He is evaluated by a geriatrician at the hospital, and he is mentally competent but must have surgery for the broken hip. All his children meet at the emergency room at Stanford Hospital in California. His daughter Myrna was very close to her mother but has kept her distance from her father all her life due to the pain she feels he inflicted on her as a teenager. In fact, she blames him for difficulty she has always had with the men in her life and suspects she has passed this on to her own two daughters who have never married and have a series of aborted relationships with men.

Myrna lives the closest to her father, so it is logical that she takes the lead in his care, according to the care manager the family has just hired to help them with the father's ongoing care. But Myrna is "stuck." She does not want to be the lead family caregiver. The care manager asks the family if they would consider having a family meeting at the hospital to discuss this care. During the meeting Myrna, with the help of the care manager, is able to bring to the surface and experience that pain again, the misery she felt every time she went out with a boy, and her anger at her father. She cannot forgive her father, she tells the care manager and the doctor, who is at the meeting, for ruining her relationship with men. She realizes she is the key sibling to help arrange her father's care, but she is stuck. She is able to see where she is, but the now 60-some woman has prevented herself from being part of her father's care plan. Both the physician and the care manager reframe the problem into the present, around the father's present care needs. Myrna is able to see where she is stuck and unable to be a part of family caregiving. The care manager asks Myna's younger brother if he will oversee the care and he agrees. The care manager suggests a therapist locally where Myrna can work on her feeling of anger and blame toward her father because the care manager uses a "whole family" approach and feels that helping Myrna is integral to helping this family.

Terry Hargrave has developed a model of forgiveness and exoneration for the aging family. Fred Luskin of the Stanford University Forgiveness Project has also developed a model for forgiveness; although not designed specifically for the aging family, it is a hands-on model that can be easily adapted by care managers for aging family members. Both professionals developed their models out of their own experiences of needing to forgive someone after seeing how their own resentments and pain wreaked havoc in their everyday life.

HARGRAVE'S FOUR-STEP MODEL

Hargrave's model involves four steps in which both parties must be involved and the offender cannot be exonerated unless accountability is offered. The aging wrongdoing family member must be willing to tell the wronged family member that this will never occur again. This differs from Luskin's model that asks the wronged person to forgive the offender themselves without requiring the aging wrongdoer to ask for forgiveness. Hargrave's model takes many steps and requires balancing the family ledger. Luskin's model is shorter and releases the wronged person, not necessarily the wrongdoer. Care managers are advised to choose either of these models to help families, or select a professional who can work with the family around forgiveness, helping them move on to the right level of care and relieving the stress of caregivers in the aging family.

Hargrave's model involves four steps that he refers to as stations. All his steps are envisioned in a therapeutic setting, not the client's home where the care manager generally works. If a care manager were to utilize his method with the aging client and the adult child, they should have a clinical background with years of experience and extensive course work in the aging family.

Hargrave's first station is designed to allow the adult child to see what caused the pain in the relationship with their kin years go. It facilitates bringing the damage and pain to the surface or conscience mind. For example, in the previous case Myrna Threadbare, the adult daughter, as a teenager was emotionally abused by her father every time she went out with a boy. Bringing this to the surface and experiencing that pain again can be helpful if it can show the now 62-year-old woman what stops her from being a part of her father's care plan along with other siblings. She will be able, under this step and model, to identify how she is "stuck" and unable to be a part of family caregiving. Hargrave's theory is that being able to bring the pain to the surface and articulate how it occurred can help the adult child guard against this type of injustice in the future. So perhaps Ms. Threadbare will be able to protect herself from future emotionally abusive relationships with men or avoid passing this relationship choice in men on to her own daughters. This step is meant by Hargrave as a protection against future harm. Hargrave states that it is the first step to establishing relational justice. But from the care manager's point of view the adult daughter may be even more unhelpful with parent care after this step. Hargrave states when this pain is brought to the surface, relational distance may occur, meaning the adult child may distance himself or herself further away from the older parent. The purpose of this station is to give the adult insight into harmful behavior that may injure future generations if repeated. Care managers whose goal is to make the care of the parent their first priority may be cautious of this step if, for instance, there is only one child and this child by getting in touch with her childhood hurt may be so alienated that she would not care for her father. Care managers may have to make other arrangements for managing the care as in the case example of Len Rambler and Myra Threadbare. Hargrave states that insight is limited in its ability to heal relationships in that it is primarily meant as protection.

Hargrave's next station is understanding. This second step takes the family member from a conscious reality of what damage was done by the kin (parent or sibling) in the past to a broader idea of how the damage occurred. For example, the adult daughter, Heather Lock, resented her mother's inept parenting when she was a child and has lived at a distance all of her adult life. This daughter, through "understanding" offered by a professional private care manager, may come to the conclusion that the mother was an immature young parent who put way too much responsibility on her oldest child to care for the growing number of younger children in the family. This helps the daughter understand how the damage occurred when she was a child, through giving her the "big picture."

Hargrave's theory is that once the adult child sees the larger picture of what happened to her or his family years ago, she or he might be much more sympathetic to the aging parent as they are now, a frail and vulnerable older person, not in this case the younger immature mother or the internalized parent. This could work to help the adult child move closer to achieving filial maturity by focusing on the past and gaining some understanding of how family history occurred between them and their parent. It could also then help the adult child move toward the present, the here-and-now with their older parent, who may be needing care. They may be able to then choose to be a part of the family care system. But the adult child might have deeper wounds, especially in dysfunctional families, and continue to distance himself or herself from being involved either with the aging parent generally or with the care of the parents. Again the care manager whose goal is to make the care of the parent their first priority may be cautious of this step if, for instance, there is only one child.

Hargrave's theory appears to be that the deeper the hurt in the past the harder it is for the adult child to forgive the wound. So for those who have childhood wounds that are not that deep, the first two steps may be enough to establish exoneration of blame for the injustice and to reestablish a relationship with the aging parent.

For others with deep wounds, Hargrave's first two steps may not be enough to either forgive the family hurt from long ago nor reconnect these adult children with their families.

Hargrave then has a third step called compensation that gives the wrongdoer a chance to compensate for the hurt they caused. Hargrave's third step is meant to reestablish a relationship. Hargrave says that this allows the adult child or wronged person to give the wrongdoer a chance to make amends for the hurt. This can allow the wronged person an opportunity to stop blaming that person. The wronged person must have successfully completed the first two steps and be willing to give up the claim for injustice. Care managers must be aware that in the aging family the older family member must be mentally competent and physically healthy enough to be able to withstand this compensation step. For care managers, establishing this should involve a psychosocial functional assessment and a mental status exam done by the care manager before this step. It could also involve having the older person evaluated by their physician.

For example, adult son Len Rambler had grown up with a father who was an alcoholic and who did a very poor job of nurturing his son; Len survived this harsh parenting but is reluctant to become involved in either his father's life or his care as his father becomes frail and elderly. Len returned to New Jersey and went to a marriage and family therapist who moved Len through Hargrave's first two steps to bring to the surface all these hurts. Len went to the therapist weekly. He then was able to see the larger picture, that the father came from a long line of alcoholics but

himself had done some nurturing such as paying for his son's college, and in spite of his drinking problem he worked hard every day to support his family. By seeing this larger picture now in midlife, Len was more willing to move toward forgiveness and Hargrave's compensation step. During Len's next visit to California a few months later, he met with the care manager at his father's home.

Vinnie, the father, is now home from rehab. His stroke has left him with some left-sided paralysis, but he is able to walk with a cane, speak fairly well, and he is mentally intact. At this point, the care manager, who has been in touch with the marriage and family therapist in New Jersey, works through Hargrave's third step of compensation. She brings the father and son together. The father, with the help of the care manager, speaks to his adult son about his drinking problems and his regret that they led to neglect of his then young son. He asks for the son's forgiveness.

Hargrave's third station is meant to allow the wrongdoer, in this case an aging parent, a chance to make up for the hurt or pain they caused long ago. Hargrave states that this third step is meant to offer compensation for the long ago hurt. This might mean, in a therapeutic setting that includes both the older parent and the midlife adult child, the therapist or highly skilled care manager may help the older person to say they are sorry for the pain they rendered to the then child when they were a young parent. So the alcoholic father, Vinnie Rambler, who is now a 90-year-old frail gentleman, can tell his 60-year-old son, that he realizes he caused his son pain by not being there for him.

What goes along with Hargrave's third step is the requirement that the adult child gives up their claim for injustice, or as Hargrave says, accept a payment plan. This means the adult child must open himself or herself up to the aging parent, which of course risks the possibility of further pain if the now adult parent does not come through as promised. Hargrave' third step can take the form of Len Rambler allowing his teenage sons to see their grandfather for the first time. However, Hargrave points out that this third station runs large risks as well. If it results in more untrustworthy behavior, then what he calls "relational healing" cannot occur. For example, if Len, who was ignored as a child by his alcoholic father, brings his sons to visit the grandfather on several family occasions and Vinnie the grandfather starts to drink again and is not caring or communicative to either his own son or grandchildren, it may only serve to seal the doom of the relationship.

Station four of Hargrave's method underscores the difference between Hargrave's method and Luskin's. Hargrave believes that forgiveness is always what he calls relational, that is, it always involves two people. He conceded that it can occur at times between two people without having to confront or talk to each other, but he says that he strongly feels that it does take two people.[4]

So, Hargrave's fourth station is the act of forgiveness where the wronged person tells the wrongdoer they forgive them and releases the wrongdoer from blame. Hargrave says that at this point the person who was the victim must let the culprit off the hook. The victim must no longer hold the culprit responsible for the pain that was caused. Hargrave says that this makes trustworthiness possible. For example, Vinnie and Len would go through all three steps where the son would bring the childhood neglect to the surface, then through the work of the therapist or the highly skilled care manager, the son might be able to see the larger picture of his father and family and understand the neglect in the context of the larger picture. Thirdly, the fa-

ther might ask for forgiveness in a therapeutic setting, and then the son finally in the fourth step might accept his father's apology and release his father from blame.

LUSKIN'S HEAL METHOD

Luskin believes that forgiveness is for the wronged person not the wrongdoer.[5] This is the major difference in the approaches of Hargrave and Luskin. Luskin also believes that forgiveness can be done without doing it in a therapeutic setting, another difference between the two methods. Luskin's HEAL method involves four steps that can be remembered using the acronym HEAL: Heal, Education, Affirm, and Long term. These steps involve just the person who was wronged, so they can be used on the adult child without involving the older parent. This is a plus for care managers working with adult children with aging parents who are over 85 years of age and too frail or mentally confused to withstand this interaction. It does not require a therapeutic setting and can be initiated by a care manager. The care manager can use Luskin's techniques in the home or conceivably just suggest Luskin's book as an educational resource to the adult child or family member.

Luskin points out that there is a vicious cycle that goes on with a grievance story. Luskin calls a grievance story a story told by a victim that describes the painful things they endured and from which they have not healed. Holding on to and retelling the grievance story does not allow a chance for growth or change. Luskin has a test for a grievance story that includes: Is it being told more than once, sometimes several times a day in your head, with the person who hurt you as the central chapter in the story, and he or she is the villain? Has the story stayed the same for many years, with the story focusing on your pain and what you have lost? These questions come from a list of 12 tests where a positive to answer to the first 11 will qualify the teller as having a grievance story.[6]

Grievance stories, according to Luskin, are based on unenforceable rules. These rules are expectations or demands about people and life that we do not have the power to enforce. For instance, in the case of the adult son, Len Rambler, who was neglected by his alcoholic father, the son did not have the power to make the father treat him well. He was only a child when it happened, and trying to make a parent treat you fairly, a spouse to love you, or a mother nurture you is impossible. When people try to enforce unenforceable rules Luskin says they can become frustrated, bitter, angry, and despondent. Luskin believes that rules warp our judgment because we do not see the damage the rules are causing us in the here-and-now. Luskin compares our grievance to planes in the sky and sees us as air traffic controllers. These grievances or hurts for which we hold people accountable remain as planes flying around in our head, taking up valuable space in our mind with their repetitive paths and endless flying. He suggests that as air traffic controllers we need to make these planes land— let go of our grievances.

Luskin's HEAL method starts out with *H* for *heal*. In this step he asks the wronged person to state what they had hoped would have happened between them and the offender. So, the poorly parented adult daughter, Heather Lock, could say that she had hoped that her mother would have treated her in a loving way when she was a child and had hoped her mother would not have given her so much responsibility to mother her younger siblings when she was only a child herself. In Luskin's version the now adult daughter would state not what had to happen with those unenforceable rules, but what Heather

hoped might have happened. So Luskin is asking the person telling the story to make their story what was hoped for in the past not what had to or should have happened. He also asks that the offended person make this story personal. An example with Heather Lock might be "I had hoped that my Mom would have held me and comforted me when I was a little girl."

Luskin then moves on to the *E* in his heal method—education. In Luskin's model he wants the offended person to acknowledge that they do not always get what they want and accept that reality, no matter how painful it might be. So, the adult child, Heather Lock, might say of her now frail mother, "I understand that my mother did not hold me and comfort me when I was less than 10 years old." The now adult son, Len Rambler, might say, "I understand that my Dad never came to my school events, never became a scout leader when I was a young boy." They can go on to say, "I understand some mothers do not hold and comfort their children" or "I understand that some fathers do not become involved in their children's lives when they are young." The key here with Luskin's method is that sadness should emerge from the offended party but not depression. The adult child has brought their hurt to the surface of their mind. This is like Hargrave's first step where the damage is brought to the surface. What Luskin does is give an intersection that can lead to therapy at this point. If the adult child brings this pain to the surface and experiences not just sadness but depression, Luskin suggests that then the adult child seek a therapeutic intervention or see a physician. We might say that these wrongs are deep tissues scars from the dysfunctional aging family, somewhat like Hargrave's model. This may take the care manager suggesting that the adult child seek a therapist who has a background in aging and depression and be evaluated by their primary physician for depression.

The next step in Luskin's model is *A* for *affirm*. What Luskin wants the person who is offended to do is to focus on the here-and-now, not the negative past. Luskin wants the offended party to move to the present, the here-and-now and out of the past. So, the daughter, Heather Lock, who is now an adult child in her sixties, could say that, instead of focusing on what her mother did not do for her in the past, she will focus on what she can do for her own mother in her eighties and her own adult children.

Therefore, the adult child could reframe her past grievance into what Luskin calls a positive intention. Heather Lock's positive intention could be "I affirm my positive intention to hold my children, even though they are now adults." And even more powerful is to say, "I affirm to hold my aging mother and nurture her in her old age." Or the midlife adult son, Len Rambler, could say to himself, "I affirm to be involved in my aging dad's care." The affirmation shifts the adult child from their obsession with the negative past and moves them to the positive present where they can actually change behavior in the family in the here-and-now. This is especially important to the adult children because they can move to use this affirmation to care for their aging parents. This allows the airplanes flying around in their head to land and space to be cleared for the here-and-now, where the aging family can solve the filial crisis with all siblings on board. It also allows the adult child to let go of the internalized younger parent in their head and see the here-and-now aging parent, which is the crux of filial maturity.

The *L* in the HEAL method is for *long term*. According to Luskin, this station commits the person to long-term practice of his method and the long-term use of it every time the person starts again to dwell on old family hurts.

In aging families, as they regroup and align again around the problems caused by the infirmities of the aging parents, there is much more interaction than perhaps family members have had for decades. Adult children are drawn back into the orbit of the family. By practicing Luskin's HEAL method, the adult child can use his or her positive intention every time the old hurt from his long-ago past surfaces, which is bound to be frequent when adult children start the process of facing the filial crisis of their parent needing care and choosing whether they will be involved in that care. From Luskin's point of view the adult daughter, Heather Lock, who is reenrolled in her mother's care after not seeing her mother regularly for years, can use this method every time her mind reaches back to the past and that painful childhood wound of not being nurtured by her own mother. What Luskin wants her to do each time this hurt surfaces is to tell her story in its new version to herself with its new positive intention: "I affirm my positive intention to hold my children, even though they are now adults." And even more powerfully to say, "I affirm to hold my aging mother and nurture her in her old age."

The last station in the HEAL method is to make a long-term commitment to both use this method, and in addition from Luskin's point of view, to learn new skills that a person needs to succeed. This adult daughter, Heather Lock, may learn from the care manager's assessment to take care better care of herself in order to care for her aging parent and openly nurture her own adult children. The care manager may indeed suggest Heather needs to take care of own level of stress from being involved in her mother's care and having a full-time job and children of her own to nurture. After doing a caregiver assessment the care manager may suggest to Heather that part of the long-term commitment would be to go to a caregiver support group and to take a yoga class. This may help her control the constant stress she is going through to care for so many people in her family, especially a mother who did not care for her. After an assessment, the care manager might advise Heather to go to ongoing therapy to deal with her relationship with her mother. Referring the adult daughter to the caregiver support group dovetails well with Luskin's method because he believes that people who have successfully healed from a similar grievance are good models for others having that similar past pain. Caregiver support groups are valuable, according to Luskin, in that participants can both share their stories and share how they healed or overcame their own pain to reach out and offer care to their parent.

Luskin's theory of blame is that when we are in pain, as many adult children are when they become reengaged with their mother or father over the aging parent's care needs or filial crisis, we blame the current pain on what the person did in the past. This assumes that the offender meant to hurt us and that what happened in the past is the cause of how people feel in the present. By believing this, people use their chronic pain to forestall their healing in their present lives and in their current relationships.

He does not deny that understanding the past is helpful. However, he believes we need to develop life skills in the present to improve our lives and heal those hurts. He states that taking responsibility for one's life creates the opposite of blaming. All these adult children that care managers deal with are people stuck in the past, like Heather Lock or Len Rambler. The care manager can use these methods to get the adult child "unstuck" and move him or her to caring for the aging parent.

The adult daughter, Heather Lock, not nurtured as a little girl and faced with her mother's care, took the care manager's advice and used the HEAL method. By getting involved in a caregiver support group, going to yoga, and having weekly visits to the spa she learned learn to nurture herself and rejoined her siblings in nurturing her mother. She also and reached out to her own now adult children to nurture them in a way that she had not been mothered.

CASE EXAMPLE: BOBBI MEYBERG, RACHEL GITZENBERG, AND ARLENE GITZENBERG

Bobbi Meyberg is a 61-year-old mother of three adult daughters who are all in their late 20s. Two daughters are still in school, one in medical school and the other in dental school. Bobbi, who is a physician, has helped, along with her husband, put all these daughters through school and is still financially supporting her youngest two daughters. Bobbi's husband, Steven, is an attorney. Bobbi's mother, Rachel Gitzenberg, lives alone in New York City, where Bobbi grew up. Ms. Gitzenberg has been a widow for 10 years and is 89 years old. Her other daughter, Arlene, lives in Los Angeles, California. Ms. Gitzenberg has two sons Robin and Mitchell who live outside New York. Mitch sees their mother on holidays and family occasions, and Robin, the youngest, visits his mother twice a week.

Bobbi receives a call one afternoon from her mother's physician. Her mother fainted on the street while shopping and broke her arm. She is in the emergency room of the hospital. Bobbi calls all of her siblings, and only her brother Robin meets her at the emergency room. The medical team decided to set Ms. Gitzenberg's arm and have her spend a few days in the hospital for tests because Rachel's doctor suspects she has early signs of dementia.

This is her second fall in 6 months, and although she has been on a regimen of calcium and medication for osteoporosis for a long time, she has brittle bones and is prone to breaks. Ms. Gitzenberg is forgetful, but at 89 appears to be mentally intact. She is a widow who lived in a loveless marriage for years where she believed that her husband saw other women constantly. They had separate bedrooms for the last 30 years of their marriage. Bobbi has used an agency before when her mother had her last fall, and this agency, Premier Care, has care managers as part of their service. Ms. Gitzenberg has her arm set, recovers in ICU, and then spends several days in the hospital. She is very confused after the surgery. Her daughter, Arlene, flies in from California, and Mitch, Bobbi, Robin, and Arlene meet in the hospital room.

Arlene and Bobbi are on speaking terms, but are very distant. They see each other on family occasions that Arlene has attended sporadically over the years. Arlene moved to California in the 1970s to matriculate at University of Southern California. She met a man and married and dropped out of school. Her husband was in the entertainment industry in the early 70s and subsequently left her for another woman. Arlene raised her daughter alone. That daughter is now in her 20s and single. Arlene has always had a weight problem and has struggled with medical problems related to obesity. She has always felt that Bobbi and her brothers were favored over her. Bobbi excelled in school, where Arlene was a lackluster student. Bobbi has always been high energy, thin, and attractive, and Arlene is overweight. Their mother Rachel depended on Bobbi, then on Mitch and Robin if she had a problem, and rarely called Arlene for help. Arlene believes that Rachel has made remarks over the years that Arlene looks more like a sister-in-law she despised and resembles her ex-husband and his side of the family. But Ms. Gitzenberg has financially helped Arlene for the past 20 years because her daughter's first husband was indicted on stock fraud with his

multimedia company and went to prison. Arlene has never completed her undergraduate degree. She has had occasional jobs as a professional editor for a romance novel writer but none consistently because of her weight-related problems and long history of depression. Bobbi and her sister have been civil to each other but are barely on speaking terms because Arlene has refused to visit her mother since before her mother's first fall, stating she is angry with her mother.

In the hospital room, over their recovering mother, Arlene, Bobbi, Mitch, and Robin discuss their mother's care. Bobbi wants her mother to come home with 24-hour care with the same agency she used after her last fall. Arlene is against this and says her mother needs to move to an assisted living facility where she can get some care when she needs it. Arlene has depended on her mother's financial help over the years and is afraid that the money used for 24-hour care will deplete her mother's resources and thus her own support. Bobbi has power of attorney for health care and tells her siblings that she has decided it is in her mother's best interest to hire 24-hour care and bring her home to her old neighborhood.

Arlene becomes enraged and tells Bobbi that she was always the favorite and is always bossy, and she disagrees with this decision and is going to move from California back to New York and care for her mother. Mitch also has been jealous all his life of his mother's favoritism of Bobbi because he is the oldest boy. He went to medical school but dropped out. He has been a successful real estate agent and broker, yet he was never a doctor, the thing that his parents wanted more than anything, he feels. He sides with Arlene, saying she should be able to try this plan. Bobbi cites the health risks that Arlene faces with her weight. Rachel's physician comes into the room when all four siblings are glowering at each other and tells them he has decided to discharge the mother but only with 24-hour care or to a skilled nursing facility to recover. Bobbi says she has power at attorney and she wants her mother to come home with 24-hour care. Both Arlene and Mitch say she should be released to a skilled nursing facility that is part of an assisted living facility to recover because it will be less expensive.

The physician, seeing the intense family strife, asks the family if a care manager is involved. Bobbi tells him that she has used Premier Services before, and they have a private care manager as part of their services. He writes an order for a Medicare company to follow Ms. Gitzenberg home with PT, OT, tells the family she cannot go home without private 24-hour care, and suggests to all the siblings that they use a care manager. Ms. Gitzenberg is released the next day and the care manager makes a home visit. The care manager suggests a family meeting at the Gitzenberg home and calls all four siblings and asks if they will attend.

Highly skilled care managers who have a clinical background and years of experience can adapt either or both Luskin's and Hargrave's methods. All care managers should know and understand the principles of forgiveness and exoneration in order to make an appropriate referral to a therapist who utilizes forgiveness therapy and has an extensive background in working with aging families. All care managers should know enough about forgiveness to refer family members to Luskin's self-help text, which can be used by just about everyone who is seeking forgiveness information. Hargrave also has a text that is written for laypeople in concert with a therapist. This along with standard self-help from family forgiveness texts should be part of the continuum of care or educational tools and resources a care manager can use to assist aging families.

Siblings disagreeing about the level of care a parent may need is one of the great blockages in implementing a care plan faced by care managers, physicians, and families

themselves. Old wounds between sisters and brothers stop siblings from working together to implement a good parental care plan. Take the case example of Bobbi Meyberg and her mother Rachel and use both Hargrave's and Luskin's methods to try and solve these sibling problems and get Ms. Gitzenberg to the right level of care.

CARE MANAGER USING FORGIVENESS METHODS

When Rachel Gitzenberg gets home and 24-hour care, medical equipment, and client services are in place, the care manager performs a caregiver assessment on Bobbi as the main care provider, and then performs the same assessment on Arlene, who plans to move into her mother's home. Both Mitch and Robin then consent to answer questions for a caregiver assessment as well. The care manager creates a genogram on each sibling, gathering family information, background, and their relationship with the mother. She finds in her assessment that Bobbi Meyberg is always willing to take on her mother's care but is highly stressed by her own medical practice, supporting two adult children through school, and a recent diagnosis of high blood pressure. The care manager finds, in talking with Arlene, that Arlene plans to move back to New York to take care of her mother after she returns to California to settle her affairs. She discovers that Arlene has serious medical problems related to her weight, carries an emotional wound from her childhood, and blames her mother for favoring Bobbi, for not loving her because she looks like her father, who the mother felt was a cheating husband. She also feels that her mother favors Bobbi because she is a physician, is thin, and always did well in school. The care manager also finds that Arlene has been financially dependent on her mother all these years and that the mother has sent her money on a regular basis.

The care manager finds that Mitch has financial worries related to the subprime mortgage crisis and is thinking of switching careers. He resents his older sister Bobbi as well because she became a physician and he dropped out of medical school. He is glad she takes the vast load of family pressure from the mother but still resents Bobbi. He and Arlene have had dinner several times during her visit and he now favors moving Ms. Gitzenberg to an assisted living facility because he wants to preserve his share of his parent's estate for his own retirement, which he sees in a few years. He also has recently been diagnosed with prostate cancer, making him feel like he needs to have as much out of life as he can and looks forward to the money he will inherit from his mother to bolster his retirement.

Rachel owns a brownstone on the Upper East Side of New York that has recently appreciated in value with skyrocketing New York real estate. Robin, the youngest child of Ms. Gitzenberg works for a hedge fund and is financially set for the rest of his life. He has always had a great relationship with his mother because he is the baby. He needs nothing from her estate. He is also glad that big sister Bobbi takes the brunt of the responsibilities for his mother. He wants his mother to be happy and safe. Robin believes his mother is happiest and safest at home.

The care manager asks all the siblings to come to a family meeting at her office in 3 weeks. At the first meeting they discuss their mother's diagnosis first. Her arm is healing well but her osteoporosis continues, and she is at risk for another fall. She also has a confirmed diagnosis of early dementia that accelerated with the recent fall and hospital stay. She is mentally clear now that she has been home for 3 weeks. The care

manager feels that for at least 3 months she will need 24-hour care because of the fall risk. Care needs will be over $12,000 per month. Ms. Gitzenberg has the financial assets to afford this.

The care manager has a background in forgiveness and exoneration. She realizes that Arlene runs large health risks and would be a poor care provider for her mother. She sees that Bobbi has done an excellent job of caring for her mother but needs more support from her siblings because she now has a medical diagnosis. She has spoken with Ms. Gitzenberg on each weekly visit she has made to her home and finds that she wishes to be able to remain in her home of 40 years and has the financial ability to do that for at least 7 years.

In the meetings after reviewing the diagnosis she turns to Robin, who is power of attorney for finances of his mother's estate. He assures everyone that there are adequate finances to keep their mother at home for 7 years. The care manager points out that because Ms. Gitzenberg is 89, she may outlive her estate but that is what she wishes to do. She advises the family to hire an elder law attorney to advise them on Medicaid planning in the event Rachel outlives her assets. She also suggests asking the elder law attorney how the brownstone would be treated by Medicaid.

Bobbi, who is the power of attorney for health care, states that she wishes her mother to remain at home. Arlene speaks up and says that's fine, but she is planning to move back to New York and care for her mother during the day. She expects to be paid for her services. Mitch speaks up and says he backs Arlene's plan. Bobbi becomes angry and accuses Arlene of wanting to use her mother's money for herself. She also accuses Mitch of backing Arlene because he himself is having financial difficulties. Robin is largely silent. The care manager has several choices.

Scenario 1

The care manager refers the family to a family therapist with experience in working with aging families and who has a background in facilitating forgiveness among family members. The family therapist works with the siblings through four meetings. The therapist takes the family through Hargrave's four steps. Hargrave's first station is designed to allow the adult child to see what caused the pain in the relationship with their kin years go. It facilitates bringing the damage and pain to the surface or conscious mind. It is meant to give insight into what caused the family pain years ago and bring the pain into the present. With the therapist's prompting, she is able to get Mitch and Arlene to tell Bobbi their story and to have Bobbi hear their pain.

Arlene is able to verbalize her anger at her mother for favoring Bobbi and her jealousy of Bobbi for always being more successful and more attractive than Arlene. She says that she herself looks like her father and that is why her mother does not favor or love her. The therapist gets Mitch to express his anger and jealousy at Bobbi for finishing medical school when he never did and for being his parents' favorite when he indeed was the oldest boy and deserved that love.

Bobbi is at first shocked by her sister's and brother's anger and becomes defensive. But with the help of the therapist she starts to have insight into how her siblings would experience this anger and hurt. The therapist helps her to understand that it is not her fault that she was the oldest and became a high achiever and a physician, but the therapist helps her to understand how this could wound her sister and brother. On the other hand, the therapist helps both Mitch and Arlene see that birth order or drive were not Bobbi's fault, and to see how her role as oldest, which she had no control over, led to jeal-

ousy and hurt of the middle two children. They are also all able to see with the insight of the therapist that Bobbi was a young child when their parents had a happy marriage. Bobbi spent 5 years with no competition for love in her family nest. The middle two children came along 5 and 7 years later when their parents' marriage was beginning to fail, and the father was away from home much more. They had to compete with Bobbi for attention when Rachel had two babies in diapers. So, all began to see that Bobbi just got happier parenting and more of it, something none of these children had control over.

Hargrave's third station is meant to allow the wrongdoer, in this case the sister, a chance to make up for the hurt or pain she caused long ago. Hargrave states that this third step is meant to offer compensation for the long ago hurt. This might mean the therapist or highly skilled care manager may help the older person to say they are sorry for the pain they rendered to the then child when they were a young parent. With the therapist's prompting, Bobbi is able tell Arlene and Mitch that she is sorry that they had a much harder perhaps less parentally loved childhood. She also says she understands how they felt angry with her for getting more love and attention from their parents. Bobbi says she understands how they feel. She also says that she loves them both very much and siblings mean so much to her as they are all getting older.

At this point Arlene, who has been living with her mother for 3 weeks and is exhausted from what small amount of care she was able to give, tells Bobbi that she appreciates Bobbi caring enough for her sister to say she hears her pain. With the prompting of the therapist, Arlene says she wants to set aside her blaming of Bobbi all these years and work out a new relationship with her sister. Bobbi is also able with the therapist's help to explain that she herself has new health problems from all the pressure she is under and that she needs their help and support as well. The therapist then brings up the next hurdle: the family has to make decisions about the mother's care. The therapist has spoken to the doctor and the care manager with a HIPAA-compliant release. She knows both the care manager and the physician think that the best place for Ms. Gitzenberg is her own home of 40 years, with 24-hour care.

With this Arlene becomes agitated again and turns to her sister and younger brother and says they have plenty of money, and they don't have to worry about finances, but that Mom has always helped her, and if all the money goes for Mom's care, what is she going to do?

Hargrave's fourth station is the act of forgiveness where the wronged person tells the wrongdoers they forgive them and releases them from blame. Hargrave says that at this point the person who was the victim must let the culprit off the hook. The victim must no longer hold the culprit responsible for the pain that was caused. Hargrave says that this makes trustworthiness possible.

The care manager has spoken with Robin about his sister Arlene's financial difficulties. Robin has consulted with his mother's attorney, a new elder law attorney, his mother's financial planner, and with his own attorney. Robin has agreed to send Arlene the same amount of money his mother has been sending her for as long as Rachel remains at home. He is asking that he be reimbursed out of the proceeds of the sale of the mother's home when she moves out or dies. Bobbi speaks up and says that when her youngest daughter is through medical school in 2 years, she will have some extra funds and can also help Arlene. Arlene is overwhelmed by the love her siblings have shown to her at that moment and breaks down and cries. She agrees to the plan of keeping the mother at home and absolves her sister of all of the blame she has heaped on her for all these years.

Rachel is well enough to attend the last family meeting. Arlene is preparing to go back to California, has a referral to a new physician in LA, and a therapist. She and Bobbi just planned and helped celebrate Rachel's 90th birthday. At the meetings, with the therapist's help, Arlene is able to say to Rachel that she had always hoped that she would hold and care for her more when she was little but she understands that Rachel had three children, two in diapers at the time. Rachel who loves to reminisce, tells them all the story of what it was like to wash diapers with a wringer washer and no dryer so that the diapers froze on the line. Arlene also says that she had always hoped that she would love her even if she looked like Aunt Fran. Rachel laughs and says, "No, you look like my sister Esther. You're pretty, like my side of the family."

Scenario 2

Examine this scenario a second way. We will have a care manager with clinical skills and years of experience in care management and aging using Luskin's method in a family meeting in her office with all the siblings present. Luskin's HEAL method starts out with *H* for *heal*. In this step he asks the wronged person to state what they had hoped would have happened between them and the offender. So, the care manager prompts Arlene to say that she hoped that her mother would have treated her in a loving way when she was a child. In Luskin's version the now adult daughter would say in a positive way what she hoped would have happened, instead of what did not occur. Luskin is asking the person telling the story to make their story what was hoped for in the past, not what had to or should have happened. He also asks that the offended person make this story personal. An example with Arlene might be, "I had hoped that my Mom would have praised me more when I was a little girl," which Arlene is able to say to her siblings.

The care manager then moves on to the *E* in Luskin's HEAL method—*education*. In Luskin's method he wants the offended person to acknowledge that they do not always get what they want and accept that reality, no matter how painful it might be. So, the care manager helps Arlene say, "I understand that my mother was unable to hold and love me as much as I wished when I was a little girl. I accept that things do not always go my way." And Mitch can say, "I understand that my Dad did not encourage me when I was a little boy and my Mom did not spend a lot of time being loving to me." They can go on to say, "Many mothers do not love and encourage their children to their children's satisfaction," or "I understand that many fathers do not become involved in their children's lives when they are young." The key here with Luskin's method is that sadness should emerge from the offended party but not depression. If depression emerges, then the client should see a physician and or therapist. Another way of saying it is the adult child now needs to grieve the loss that was first experienced in childhood. The adult child has brought the hurt to the surface of their mind. This is like Hargrave's first step where the damage is brought to the surface.

In this case Arlene is able to talk about her bouts of depression during her life and how depressed she is right now. The care manager is able to suggest that she see a local physician for an evaluation of her depression and her weight problem, which might be related. Mitch is able to say he is just sad about what has been revealed.

A second family meeting is held a few weeks later with the care manager moderating the meeting. The next step in Luskin's model is *A* for *affirm*. What Luskin wants the person who is offended to do is to focus on the here-and-now, not the negative past. Luskin wants the offended party to move to the present, the here-and-now and out of the past.

Instead of focusing on what her mother did not do for her in the past, Arlene is prompted to focus on what she could do for her own life, which includes her mother. She is able to talk about how she thought she could move in with her mother and participate in her care, but after 3 weeks she realizes she is exhausted and concerned about her own health. So, she agrees to her sister Bobbi's plan but states she is still very worried about the money because she needs the financial support that the mother has been sending to her.

But she is able to see that her sister Bobbi has been a huge help to her mother and to her by taking all the responsibility for her mother all these years. She says that she wants to thank her sister for this and help her in whatever small way she can for the care. This is discussed and the care manager suggests that, as Arlene has spent many of her working years as a private editor of fiction, Arlene start an e-newsletter about their mother with information she will receive weekly from the care manager, Bobbi, Mitch, and Robin. By Arlene focusing on what she can do in the present for the situation she is able to say she will do a family newsletter.

The adult child could reframe the past grievance into what Luskin calls a positive intention. The adult daughter's positive intention could be "I affirm my positive intention to help my sister even though there are only small ways to offer that assistance." But even more poignantly Arlene is able to say, "I affirm to support my aging mother and my desire to nurture her in her old age." So, the affirmation shifts the adult child from their obsession with the negative past and moves them to the positive present where they can actually change behavior in the family in the here-and-now if they choose to. This is especially important to the aging family because they can move to use this affirmation to care for their aging parents. This allows the airplanes flying around in their heads to land and space to be cleared for their actual lives instead of blame from things that happened generations ago, all of which helps to solve the filial crisis with all siblings on board.

The *L* in Luskin's HEAL method is for *long term*. According to Luskin, this station commits the person to the long-term practice of these useful methods and the commitment to practice each time the person starts again to dwell on old family hurts.

In the Gitzenberg family, when they reorganized again around their mother's fall and diagnosis of early dementia, there was more interaction than the family members had had for many years. Adult children are drawn back to the center of the family, the parent. By practicing the *L* in Luskin's HEAL method, the adult child can use his or her positive intention every time the old hurt from the long-ago past surfaces, which happens more intensely around the filial crisis of their parent needing care, and choose whether they will be involved in care. From Luskin's point of view this is imperative for Arlene who is drawn into in her mother's care and reasserts her wound from her mother not loving her enough as a child and her subsequent habit of blaming her older sister Bobbi. Arlene can use this method every time her mind reaches back to the past and that painful childhood wound of not being nurtured enough by her own mother when she as a child needed care. What Luskin wants her to do is, each time this hurt surfaces, have Arlene tell her story in its new version to herself with its new positive intention, which would be "I affirm to support my aging mother and nurture her in her old age," which she will prove by writing the family newsletter about Ms. Gitzenberg's care from California.

The *L* in the HEAL method means to make a long-term commitment to both use this method and to learn new skills a person needs to manifest that positive intention. For Arlene to nurture her mother and be a part of the circle of sibling care to help her family nurture Ms. Gitzenberg, she must also care for herself. Because she is morbidly overweight, she has agreed with the care manager's suggestion of going to a physician in New York who can assess both her weight problems and her chronic depression. She also agrees to get a referral to a physician in Los Angeles and a therapist in LA who specializes in depression. Arlene also expresses an interest in biofeedback tools suggested by the care manager and says she will look into hypnosis for her depression and weight problems when she returns to LA. She also agrees to explore education resources suggested by the care manager, including forgiveness literature. All four siblings agree to take advantage of technological resources for caregivers and to participate in conference calls every week for 3 months after the last family meeting in New York with the care manager. They will use Care Pages (www .carepages.com) for the conference calling. All four siblings agree to get their mother a Jitterbug (www.jitterbugdirect.com), an easy-to-use cell phone, so they can all call her on a regular basis, and a Presto printer (www.presto.com) so that Arlene can send her the newsletter and they can all send digital pictures of the grandchildren to Ms. Gitzenberg.

Bobbi Meyberg, the oldest daughter, who is the main care provider in the family and has borne the brunt of the family's caring for Ms. Gitzenberg, has a recent diagnosis of high blood pressure, perhaps brought on by stress. The care manager gets Bobbi's agreement to take long-term care of herself, fulfilling the *L* in Luskin's HEAL theory. She agrees to take advantage of emotional support tools suggested by the care manager including joining a support group for family caregivers. She also acknowledged a need for self-care, considering all the stress she is under with her mother, her two daughters in graduate school, and her own medical practice. She agrees to get a weekly massage, join a yoga class, and renew her membership in her gym, where she likes spinning. Bobbi agrees to take advantage of educational tools suggested by the care manager and buys a number of self-help books including Luskin's *Forgive for Good* and Hargrave's *The Aging Family*. She also is interested in online resources in New York State and agrees to research online through the New York State aging site (http://aging.state.ny.us/links/index.htm).

Mitch acknowledges he is sad in discovering his parents had lesser time to care for him because he was born close to Arlene and because at that time his parents' marriage was beginning to unravel. He feels no need for counseling like Arlene but decides that he will also join a support group to bolster Bobbi, the main care provider and learn more himself. They decide to go together to a meeting that is held near where they both live. He agrees to pursue educational resources by buying Luskin's self-help book *Forgive for Good*, visit his mother once every two weeks, and call her weekly. He agrees to send digital pictures of his family through Presto because he really enjoys digital photography.

Robin agrees to make a long-term commitment, the *L* in Luskin's HEAL, in the following way: As the most wealthy child he agrees to work with his attorney and Arlene's attorney and his mother's New York elder law attorney to draw up an agreement to lend Arlene the amount her mother has given her each year so that his mother's income can be used for her 24-hour care. This money will be debited against Arlene's share of their mother's brownstone in New

York, which has greatly appreciated in value in the past few years. They all agree that Arlene may still have money coming to her after that. Robin, who has an excellent relationship with his mother since he is the last born and a favorite, will visit his mother twice a week, as he has for years. He agrees to call her three times a week on her new Jitterbug. Robin agrees to take over paying his mother's bills from Bobbi, with his mother's financial planner and attorney doing oversight. He agrees to e-mail Arlene once a week with a financial report of his mother's bills and with the help of the financial planner do a monthly balance sheet to go in the newsletter.

Filial maturity—solving the filial crisis of parents needing care—has been achieved in all of these families by the addition of forgiveness and exoneration techniques. In the case of Len Rambler, whose alcoholic father neglected him as a child in the 1950s, he went to a marriage and family therapist in New Jersey who used Hargrave's four forgiveness stations. The therapist worked with the California care manager long distance, with Len's and Vinnie's agreement. By seeing this larger picture, this now midlife son was more willing to move toward forgiveness, and with the guidance of the care manager in California, Hargrave's compensation step occurred, when Vinnie asked his forgiveness and Len exonerated his father from further blame. Len affirmed to treat his own children in a more positive way, having insight into his own compulsive workaholic behavior, where he neglected his own sons much like his father neglected him. Len also affirmed to treat his father in a more positive way by visiting him in California on a regular basis and allowing his teenage sons to see their grandfather for the first time. Len also agreed to continue counseling with the therapist to explore his own compulsive behavior so he did not pass this on to his sons, affirming his commitment to treating himself and his own sons in a positive way and take care of himself and his family. Len was able to let his airplanes land.

Heather Lock is 57 years old was born when her mother Janet was 18 followed by three more siblings by the time the mother Janet was 24. sHer aging mother Janet now has midstage dementia which she hid from her sons and daughter until she got lost in her car and was taken to the local emergency room by the police who picked her up. This prompts Heather's filial crisis: Can she help her other siblings care for her mother, who she feels never cared for her?The care manager from the hospital calls Heather and her siblings to the hospital for a family meeting and suggested a second family meeting to be held at her office. The care manager, knowing Luskin's techniques, worked with Heather Heather, with the help of the care manager trained in forgiveness, and Luskin's techniques was able to forgive her mother, let the airplanes in her head land, and make a long-term commitment to nurture her now aging mother before her mother died. With the care manager's guidance, Heather connected with another care manager at Avenidas in Palo Alto. That care manager helped enroll Janet in their adult day program and arrange senior transportation to get there. Heather was then able to allow herself to attend Christmas with the family for the first time in 25 years. Heather and her brothers were able to solve their filial crisis, take care of their mother's growing dependency and safety risk, and Heather, by being able to work through forgiveness, was able to move from the past to the present and affirm her need to care for herself, her children, and her mother in the here and now.

Forgiveness is a major tool that can be used by a care manager. If the care manager has very sophisticated clinical skills and years of experience in the field of care management, the care manager can use any one of the forgiveness models to help aging families themselves. If they do not have this level of experience and training they can select a therapist who has training in aging and a background in forgiveness to work with the family. Investigate your community and your continuum of care to find out which marriage and family therapists specialize in aging, then call them and ask about their training in forgiveness models. No matter what the care manager's clinical background, education is a major tool a care manager should use. Referring families to forgiveness literature such as Luskin's book and Hargrave's multiple books is an important choice for care managers in working with aging families.

SUMMARY

Change is one of the hardest things we face as human beings, and families are no different. Yet, as Darwin told us, "It is not the strongest of the species that will survive, nor the most intelligent, but those who are adaptive to change." Forgiveness is the path to change. It allows the aging family to regroup, use its power as the workhorse of our society, and mobilize members to care for aging family members.

Forgiveness brings siblings together. It can move adult children, violated in the past, towards flawed aging parents who need them. Forgiveness is a time traveler that moves aging family members, frozen in the past, into the present. It helps us see siblings and parents in the here and now and provides opportunities to work together caring for the parent. Forgiveness makes aging family members healthier both emotionally and physically. It is a wonderful tool for the change agent—the care manager—a critical tool in her or his toolbox.

REFERENCES

1. Krause N, Ingersol-Dayton B. Religion and the process of forgiveness in later life. *Review of Religious Research*. 2001;42(3):253.
2. The Holy Bible: King James Version. 2000 Leviticus 23
3. Sandberg JG. It isn't fair: Helping older families balance their ledgers before the note comes due. *Family Relations*;48(2):177.
4. Hargrave TD, Anderson WT. *Finishing Well*. New York, NY: Brunner Mazel:157.
5. Luskin F. *Forgive for Good, A Proven Prescription for Health and Happiness*. San Francisco, CA: Harper; 2002. Pg 37
6. Luskin F. *Forgive for Good, A Proven Prescription for Health and Happiness*. San Francisco, CA: Harper; 2002: Introdroduction v11.

RESOURCES FOR PROFESSIONALS WHO OFFER THERAPY INVOLVING FORGIVENESS MODELS

Individual Counseling

American Association of Marriage, Family Therapists—www.aamft.org

National Association of Social Workers—www.nasw.org

American Psychological Association—www.apa.org

Psychiatric Interventions

American Association of Geriatric Psychiatrists—www.aagpgpa.org

Training and CEUs in forgiveness techniques—www.learningtoforgive.com

Terry Hargrave's Web site—www.terry hargrave.com

Literature

Hargrave T. *Forgiving the Devil, Coming to Terms With Damaged Relationships*. Phoenix, AZ: Zeigm, Tucker & Theisen; 2001.

Hargrave T. *Families and Forgiveness*. New York, NY: Brunner Mazel; 1994.

Hargrave T, Anderson WT. *Finishing Well*. New York, NY: Brunner Mazel; 1992.

Luskin F. *Forgive for Love, The Missing Ingredients for Healthy and Lasting Relationships*. San Francisco, CA: Harper; 2008.

Luskin F. *Forgive For Good, A Proven Prescription for Health and Happiness*. San Francisco, CA: Harper; 2002.

Index